T0362212

Current Topics in Critical Care for the Anesthesiologist

Editors

ATHANASIOS CHALKIAS
MARY L. JARZEBOWSKI
KATHRYN ROSENBLATT

ANESTHESIOLOGY CLINICS

www.anesthesiology.theclinics.com

Consulting Editor
LEE A. FLEISHER

March 2023 • Volume 41 • Number 1

ELSEVIER

1600 John F. Kennedy Boulevard • Suite 1800 • Philadelphia, Pennsylvania, 19103-2899

http://www.theclinics.com

ANESTHESIOLOGY CLINICS Volume 41, Number 1
March 2023 ISSN 1932-2275, ISBN-13: 978-0-323-96193-6

Editor: Joanna Collett
Developmental Editor: Arlene Campos

Anesthesiology Clinics (ISSN 1932-2275) is published quarterly by Elsevier Inc., 360 Park Avenue South, New York, NY 10010-1710. Months of issue are March, June, September, and December. Periodicals postage paid at New York, NY and at additional mailing offices. Subscription prices are $100.00 per year (US student/resident), $386.00 per year (US individuals), $478.00 per year (Canadian individuals), $740.00 per year (US institutions), $936.00 per year (Canadian institutions), $100.00 per year (Canadian student/resident), $513.00 per year (foreign student/resident), $498.00 per year (foreign individuals), and $936.00 per year (foreign institutions). To receive student and resident rate, orders must be accompanied by name of affiliated institution, date of term, and the *signature* of program/residency coordinator on institutions letterhead. Orders will be billed at individual rate until proof of status is received. Foreign air speed delivery is included in all *Clinics'* subscription prices. All prices are subject to change without notice. POSTMASTER: Send address changes to *Anesthesiology Clinics,* Elsevier Health Sciences Division, Subscription Customer Service, 3251 Riverport Lane, Maryland Heights, MO 63043. Customer Service (orders, claims, online, change of address): Elsevier Health Sciences Division, Subscription Customer Service, 3251 Riverport Lane, Maryland Heights, MO 63043. **Tel:1-800-654-2452 (U.S. and Canada); 314-447-8871 (outside U.S. and Canada). Fax: 314-447-8029. E-mail: journalscustomerservice-usa@elsevier.com (for print support); journalsonlinesupport-usa@elsevier.com (for online support).**

Reprints. For copies of 100 or more of articles in this publication, please contact the Commercial Reprints Department, Elsevier Inc., 360 Park Avenue South, New York, NY 10010-1710. Tel.: 212-633-3874; Fax: 212-633-3820; E-mail: reprints@elsevier.com.

Anesthesiology Clinics, is also published in Spanish by McGraw-Hill Inter-americana Editores S. A., P.O. Box 5-237, 06500 Mexico D. F., Mexico.

Anesthesiology Clinics, is covered in *MEDLINE/PubMed (Index Medicus), Current Contents/Clinical Medicine, Excerpta Medica, ISI/BIOMED,* and *Chemical Abstracts*.

Contributors

CONSULTING EDITOR

LEE A. FLEISHER, MD, FACC, FAHA
Robert D. Dripps Professor and Chair of Anesthesiology and Critical Care, Professor of Medicine, Perelman School of Medicine, University of Pennsylvania, Philadelphia, Pennsylvania, USA

EDITORS

ATHANASIOS CHALKIAS, MD, MSc, PhD, FESC, FAcadTM, FCP, FESAIC
Assistant Professor, Department of Anesthesiology, Faculty of Medicine, University of Thessaly, Larisa, Greece; Outcomes Research Consortium, Cleveland, Ohio, USA

MARY L. JARZEBOWSKI, MD
Clinical Assistant Professor, Department of Anesthesiology, University of Michigan, Department of Veterans Affairs Ann Arbor Healthcare System, Ann Arbor, Michigan, USA

KATHRYN ROSENBLATT, MD, MHS
Assistant Professor of Anesthesiology and Critical Care Medicine, Departments of Anesthesiology and Critical Care Medicine, and Neurology, Johns Hopkins School of Medicine, Baltimore, Maryland, USA

AUTHORS

PROMISE ARIYO, MD, MPH
Assistant Professor, Johns Hopkins University, Baltimore, Maryland, USA

TALIA K. BEN-JACOB, MD, MSc
Associate Professor, Department of Anesthesiology, Division of Critical Care, Cooper Medical School of Rowan University, Camden, New Jersey, USA

SUZANNE BENNETT, MD, FCCM
Associate Professor, Department of Anesthesiology, University of Cincinnati College of Medicine, Cincinnati, Ohio, USA

ALISHA BHATIA, MD
Assistant Professor, Department of Anesthesiology, Rush University Medical Center, Chicago, Illinois, USA

EDWARD BITTNER, MD, PhD, MSEd, FCCM
Associate Professor of Anesthesia, Harvard Medical School

JASON C. BRAINARD, MD, FCCM
Associate Professor, Department of Anesthesiology, University of Colorado Hospital, Aurora, Colorado, USA

JERRAD BUSINGER, MD
Associate Professor of Anesthesiology and Critical Care, Chief, Division of Anesthesia Critical Care, Fellowship Director, Anesthesia Critical Care, University of Louisville Hospital, Louisville, Kentucky, USA

ATHANASIOS CHALKIAS, MD, MSc, PhD, FESC, FAcadTM, FCP, FESAIC
Assistant Professor, Department of Anesthesiology, Faculty of Medicine, University of Thessaly, Larisa, Greece; Outcomes Research Consortium, Cleveland, Ohio, USA

PINXIA CHEN, MD
Department of Anesthesiology and Critical Care Medicine, St. Luke's University Health Network, Bethlehem, Pennsylvania, USA

CHRISTOPHER CHOI, MD
Assistant Professor, Department of Anesthesiology and Pain Management, The University of Texas Southwestern Medical Center, Dallas, Texas, USA

JARVA CHOW, MD, MS, MPH
Assistant Professor, Department of Anesthesia and Critical Care, University of Chicago, Chicago, Illinois, USA

ELIZABETH K. COTTER, MD, MPH
Assistant Professor, Department of Anesthesiology, Pain and Perioperative Medicine, University of Kansas Medical Center, Kansas City, Kansas, USA

MONICA DA SILVA, MD
Department of Anesthesiology and Perioperative Medicine, University of Alabama at Birmingham, Birmingham, Alabama, USA

ALLISON DALTON, MD
Associate Professor, Department of Anesthesia and Critical Care, Section of Critical Care Medicine, University of Chicago, Chicago, Illinois, USA

KRASSIMIR DENCHEV, MD
Clinical Assistant Professor, Department of Anesthesiology, Wayne State University, Pontiac, Michigan, USA

RANJIT DESHPANDE, MD, FCCM, MBBS
Assistant Professor, Department of Anesthesiology, Yale School of Medicine, New Haven, Connecticut, USA

SUHAS DEVANGAM, MD
Department of Anesthesiology, Division of Critical Care, University of Michigan Medical School, Ann Arbor, Michigan, USA

MURTAZA DIWAN, MD
Assistant Professor, Department of Anesthesiology, University of Michigan, Ann Arbor, Michigan, USA

DAVID J. DOUIN, MD
Department of Anesthesiology, University of Colorado School of Medicine, Aurora, Colorado, USA

JENNIFER ELIA, MD
Assistant Professor, Department of Anesthesiology, University of California, Irvine School of Medicine, Orange, California, USA

BABAR FIZA, MD
Department of Anesthesiology, Division of Critical Care Medicine, Emory School of Medicine, Atlanta, Georgia, USA

CARTER M. GALBRAITH, MD
Division of Critical Care Medicine, Department of Anesthesiology and Perioperative Medicine, The University of Alabama at Birmingham, Birmingham, Alabama, USA

LEE GOEDDEL, MD, MPH
Department of Anesthesiology and Critical Care Medicine, Johns Hopkins School of Medicine, Baltimore, Maryland, USA

JONATHAN GOMEZ, MD, MS
Clinical Fellow, Department of Anesthesiology and Critical Care Medicine, Johns Hopkins School of Medicine, Baltimore, Maryland, USA

RACHEL HAMMER, DO
Assistant Professor, Department of Anesthesiology, Emory University, Atlanta, Georgia, USA

CHRISTINA J. HAYHURST, MD
Division of Anesthesiology Critical Care Medicine, Department of Anesthesiology, Vanderbilt University Medical Center, Nashville, Tennessee, USA

MADA F. HELOU, MD
Program Director for Anesthesiology, Associate Professor of Anesthesiology, Critical Care Intensivist, Department of Anesthesiology and Perioperative Medicine, Case Western Reserve University School of Medicine, University Hospitals Cleveland Medical Center, Cleveland, Ohio, USA

ERIN HENNESSEY, MD, MEHP
Clinical Associate Professor, Stanford University

MEGAN HENLEY HICKS, MD
Assistant Professor, Department of Anesthesiology, Wake Forest University School of Medicine, Atrium Health Wake Forest Baptist Medical Center, Winston-Salem, North Carolina, USA

JOSE HUMANEZ, MD
Assistant Professor, Department of Anesthesiology, University of Florida College of Medicine–Jacksonville, Jacksonville, Florida, USA

MARY L. JARZEBOWSKI, MD
Clinical Assistant Professor, Department of Anesthesiology, University of Michigan, Department of Veterans Affairs Ann Arbor Healthcare System, Ann Arbor, Michigan, USA

AALOK K. KACHA, MD, PhD
Associate Professor, Department of Anesthesia and Critical Care, Section of Critical Care Medicine, Department of Surgery, Section of Transplant Surgery, University of Chicago, Chicago, Illinois, USA

KUNAL KARAMCHANDANI, MD, FCCP, FCCM
Associate Professor, Department of Anesthesiology and Pain Management, The University of Texas Southwestern Medical Center, Dallas, Texas, USA

ASHISH K. KHANNA, MD, MS, FCCP, FCCM, FASA
Associate Professor and Vice-Chair for Research, Department of Anesthesiology, Wake Forest University School of Medicine, Atrium Health Wake Forest Baptist, Director Perioperative Outcomes and Informatics Collaborative (POIC), Winston-Salem, North Carolina, USA; Outcomes Research Consortium, Cleveland, Ohio, USA

SARAH KHORSAND, MD, FASA
Assistant Professor, Department of Anesthesiology and Pain Management, The University of Texas Southwestern Medical Center, Dallas Texas, USA

BRENT KIDD, MD
Assistant Professor, Department of Anesthesiology, University of Kansas Medical Center, Kansas City, Kansas, USA

MICHAEL E. KIYATKIN, MD
Assistant Professor, Department of Anesthesiology, Albert Einstein College of Medicine, Montefiore Medical Center, Bronx, New York, USA

JOHN C. KLICK, MD, FCCP, FASE, FCCM
Associate Professor, Department of Anesthesiology, University of Vermont Medical Center, University of Vermont Larner College of Medicine, Burlington, Vermont, USA

RAFAL KOPANCZYK, DO
Assistant Professor, Department of Anesthesiology, The Ohio State University Wexner Medical Center, Columbus, Ohio, USA

ALAN KOVAR, MD
Assistant Professor, Oregon Health Sciences University

SHREYAJIT R. KUMAR, MD
Assistant Professor of Clinical Anesthesiology, Department of Anesthesiology, Weill Cornell Medicine, Department of Anesthesiology, NewYork-Presbyterian Hospital, New York, New York, USA

HOWARD LEE, MD
Department of Anesthesiology, Northwestern University Feinberg School of Medicine, Northwestern Memorial Hospital, Chicago, Illinois, USA

GRETCHEN LEMMINK, MD
Assistant Professor, Department of Anesthesiology, University of Cincinnati College of Medicine, Cincinnati, Ohio, USA

RON LEONG, MD
Clinical Assistant Professor of Anesthesiology, Thomas Jefferson University Hospital, Sidney Kimmel Medial College, Philadelphia, Pennsylvania, USA

CHRISTOPHER MAHROUS, MD
Department of Anesthesiology, Cooper Medical School of Rowan University, Camden, New Jersey, USA

LUCAS MEUCHEL, MD
Fellow, Oregon Health Sciences University

HALEY MIRANDA, MD
Assistant Professor, Department of Anesthesiology, Pain and Perioperative Medicine, University of Kansas Medical Center, Kansas City, Kansas, USA

DOMAGOJ MLADINOV, MD, PhD
Assistant Professor, Department of Anesthesiology, Perioperative and Pain Medicine, Brigham and Women's Hospital, Boston, Massachusetts, USA

FRANK M. O'CONNELL, MD, FACP, FCCP, FCCM
Anesthesiology, Atlanticare Regional Medical Center, Pomona, New Jersey, USA

LOUISA J. PALMER, MBBS
Department of Anesthesiology, Division of Critical Care, Brigham and Women's Hospital, Boston, Maryland, USA

KIMBERLY F. RENGEL, MD
Division of Anesthesiology Critical Care Medicine, Department of Anesthesiology, Vanderbilt University Medical Center, Nashville, Tennessee, USA

KATHRYN ROSENBLATT, MD, MHS
Assistant Professor of Anesthesiology and Critical Care Medicine, Departments of Anesthesiology and Critical Care Medicine, and Neurology, Johns Hopkins School of Medicine, Baltimore, Maryland, USA

VEENA SATYAPRIYA, MD
Assistant Professor, Department of Anesthesiology, The Ohio State University Wexner Medical Center, Columbus, Ohio, USA

MARA A. SERBANESCU, MD
Department of Anesthesiology, Duke University Hospital, Durham, North Carolina, USA

ARCHIT SHARMA, MD, MBA, FASE
Division of Cardiothoracic Anesthesia, Solid Organ Transplant, and Critical Care, Department of Anesthesia, University of Iowa Carver College of Medicine, Iowa City, Iowa, USA

LIANG SHEN, MD, MPH
Assistant Professor of Clinical Anesthesiology, Department of Anesthesiology, Weill Cornell Medical College, New York, New York, USA

SHAHLA SIDDIQUI, MD, MSc, FCCM
Department of Anesthesia, Critical Care and Pain Medicine, Beth Israel Deaconess Medical Center, Harvard Medical School, Boston, Massachusetts, USA

MATTHEW SIGAKIS, MD
Department of Anesthesiology, Division of Critical Care, University of Michigan Medical School, Ann Arbor, Michigan, USA

JORDAN SISCEL, MD
Assistant Professor, Department of Anesthesiology, University of Kansas Medical Center, Kansas City, Kansas, USA

LAUREN SUTHERLAND, MD
Assistant Professor, Columbia University Irving Medical Center, New York, New York, USA

MADIHA SYED, MD
Assistant Professor of Anesthesiology, Department of Intensive Care and Resuscitation, Anesthesiology Institute, Cleveland Clinic Foundation, Cleveland, Ohio, USA

CHRISTOPHER W. TAM, MD
Assistant Professor of Clinical Anesthesiology, Department of Anesthesiology, Montefiore Medical Center, Bronx, New York, USA

BRANT M. WAGENER, MD, PhD
Divisions of Critical Care Medicine, and Molecular and Translational Biomedicine, Department of Anesthesiology and Perioperative Medicine, The University of Alabama at Birmingham, Birmingham, Alabama, USA

LINDSAY A. WAHL, MD
Department of Anesthesiology, Northwestern University Feinberg School of Medicine, Northwestern Memorial Hospital, Chicago, Illinois, USA

WILLIAM JOHN WALLISCH, MD
Assistant Professor, Department of Anesthesiology, University of Kansas Medical Center, Kansas City, Kansas, USA

MATTHEW A. WARNER, MD
Assistant Professor, Department of Anesthesiology and Perioperative Medicine, Mayo Clinic, Rochester, Minnesota, USA

PEGGY WHITE, MD
Associate Professor, University of Florida

AHMED ZAKY, MD, MSc, MPH, MBA, FASA
Department of Anesthesiology and Perioperative Medicine, University of Alabama at Birmingham, Birmingham, Alabama, USA

Contents

> Shock in the critically ill patient is common and associated with poor outcomes. Categories include distributive, hypovolemic, obstructive, and cardiogenic, of which distributive (and usually septic distributive) shock is by far the most common. Clinical history, physical examination, and hemodynamic assessments & monitoring help differentiate these states. Specific management necessitates interventions to correct the triggering etiology as well as ongoing resuscitation to maintain physiologic milieu. One shock state may convert to another and may have an undifferentiated presentation; therefore, continual re-assessment is essential. This review provides guidance for intensivists for management of all shock states based on available scientific evidence.

> Acute ischemic stroke is a neurologic emergency that requires precise care due to high likelihood of morbidity and mortality. Current guidelines recommend thrombolytic therapy with alteplase within the first 3 to 4.5 hours of initial stroke symptoms and endovascular mechanical thrombectomy within the first 16 to 24 hours. Anesthesiologists may be involved in the care of these patients perioperatively and in the intensive care unit. Although the optimal anesthetic for these procedures remains under investigation, this article will review how to best optimize and treat these patients to achieve the best outcomes.

> Traumatic brain injury is a devastating event associated with substantial morbidity. Pathophysiology involves the initial trauma, subsequent inflammatory response, and secondary insults, which worsen brain injury severity. Management entails cardiopulmonary stabilization and diagnostic imaging with targeted interventions, such as decompressive hemicraniectomy,

intracranial monitors or drains, and pharmacological agents to reduce intracranial pressure. Anesthesia and intensive care requires control of multiple physiologic variables and evidence-based practices to reduce secondary brain injury. Advances in biomedical engineering have enhanced assessments of cerebral oxygenation, pressure, metabolism, blood flow, and autoregulation. Many centers employ multimodality neuromonitoring for targeted therapies with the hope to improve recovery.

Mechanical circulatory support (MCS) devices provide temporary or intermediate- to long-term support for acute cardiopulmonary support. In the last 20 to 30 years, tremendous growth in MCS device usage has been seen. These devices offer support for isolated respiratory failure, isolated cardiac failure, or both. Initiation of MCS devices requires the input from multidisciplinary teams using patient factors and institutional resources to guide decision making, along with a planned "exit strategy" for bridge to decision, bridge to transplant, bridge to recovery, or as destination therapy. Important considerations for MCS use include patient selection, cannulation/insertion strategies, and complications of each device.

Perioperative arrests are both uncommon and heterogeneous and have not been described or studied to the same extent as cardiac arrest in the community. These crises are usually witnessed, frequently anticipated, and involve a rescuer physician with knowledge of the patient's comorbidities and coexisting anesthetic or surgically related pathophysiology ultimately leading to better outcomes. This article reviews the most probable causes of intraoperative arrest and their management.

Strategies for the intraoperative ventilator management of the critically ill patient focus on parameters used for lung protective ventilation with acute respiratory distress syndrome, preventing or limiting the deleterious effects of mechanical ventilation, and optimizing anesthetic and surgical conditions to limit postoperative pulmonary complications for patients at risk. Patient conditions such as obesity, sepsis, the need for laparoscopic surgery, or one-lung ventilation may benefit from intraoperative lung protective ventilation strategies. Anesthesiologists can use risk evaluation and prediction tools, monitor advanced physiologic targets, and incorporate new innovative monitoring techniques to develop an individualized approach for patients.

Postoperative respiratory failure has a multifactorial etiology, of which atelectasis is the most common mechanism. Its injurious effects are magnified by surgical inflammation, high driving pressures, and postoperative pain. Chest physiotherapy and noninvasive ventilation are good options to prevent progression of respiratory failure. Acute respiratory disease syndrome is a late and severe finding, which is associated with high morbidity and mortality. If present, proning is a safe, effective, and underutilized therapy. Extracorporeal membrane oxygenation is an option only when traditional supportive measures have failed.

Patient blood management (PBM) is a systematic, evidence-based approach to improve patient outcomes by managing and preserving a patient's own blood and minimizing allogenic transfusion need and risk. According to the PBM approach, the goals of perioperative anemia management include early diagnosis, targeted treatment, blood conservation, restrictive transfusion except in cases of acute and massive hemorrhage, and ongoing quality assurance and research efforts to advance overall blood health.

Delirium, an acute, fluctuating impairment in cognition and awareness, is one of the most common causes of postoperative brain dysfunction. It is associated with increased hospital length of stay, health care costs, and mortality. There is no FDA-approved treatment of delirium, and management relies on symptomatic control. Several preventative techniques have been proposed, including the choice of anesthetic agent, preoperative testing, and intraoperative monitoring. Frailty, a state of increased vulnerability to adverse events, is an independent and potentially modifiable risk factor for the development of delirium. Diligent preoperative screening techniques and implementation of prevention strategies could help improve outcomes in high-risk patients.

Fluid therapy is an integral component of perioperative care and helps maintain or restore effective circulating blood volume. The principal goal of fluid management is to optimize cardiac preload, maximize stroke volume, and maintain adequate organ perfusion. Accurate assessment of volume status and volume responsiveness is necessary for appropriate and judicious utilization of fluid therapy. To accomplish this, static and dynamic indicators of fluid responsiveness have been widely studied. This review discusses the overarching goals of perioperative fluid management, reviews the physiology and parameters used to assess fluid responsiveness, and provides evidence-based recommendations on intraoperative fluid management.

microbial dysbiosis as a key driver of clinical outcomes. Finally, the authors address the intersection of nutrition and the microbiome, exploring the use of supplemental pre-, pro-, and synbiotics to influence microbial composition and improve outcomes in critically ill and postsurgical patients.

Massive trauma remains the leading cause of mortality among people aged younger than 45 years. In this review, we discuss the initial care and diagnosis of trauma patients followed by a comparison of resuscitation strategies. We discuss various strategies including use of whole blood and component therapy, examine viscoelastic techniques for management of coagulopathy, and consider the benefits and limitations of the resuscitation strategies and consider a series of questions that will be important for researchers to answer to provide the best and most cost-effective therapy for severely injured patients.

A second epidemic of burnout, fatigue, anxiety, and moral distress has emerged concurrently with the coronavirus disease 2019 (COVID-19) pandemic, and critical care physicians are especially affected. This article reviews the history of burnout in health care workers, presents the signs and symptoms, discusses the specific impact of the COVID-19 pandemic on intensive care unit caregivers, and attempts to identify potential strategies to combat the Great Resignation disproportionately affecting health care workers. The article also focuses on how the specialty can amplify the voices and highlight the leadership potential of underrepresented minorities, physicians with disabilities, and the aging physician population.

ANESTHESIOLOGY CLINICS

FORTHCOMING ISSUES

June 2023
Pain/Palliative Care
Ronald Gary Pearl and Sean Mackey,
Editors

September 2023
Geriatric Anesthesia
Shamsuddin Akhtar, *Editor*

December 2023
Perioperative Safety Culture
Matthew D. McEvoy and James
Abernathy, *Editors*

RECENT ISSUES

December 2022
Vascular Anesthesia
Megan P. Kostibas, and
Heather K. Hayanga, *Editors*

September 2022
Orthopedic Anesthesiology
Philipp Lirk and Kamen Vlassakov, *Editors*

June 2022
Total Well-being
Alison J. Brainard and Lyndsay M. Hoy,
Editors

SERIES OF RELATED INTEREST

Critical Care Clinics

THE CLINICS ARE AVAILABLE ONLINE!
Access your subscription at:
www.theclinics.com

Foreword

Critical Care: Key Information for Providing High-Quality Perioperative Care

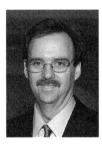

Lee A. Fleisher, MD, FACC, FAHA
Consulting Editor

The COVID-19 pandemic has taught us that understanding critical care is essential for all providers of anesthesia. At the beginning of the pandemic, many anesthesiologists worldwide were pulled from empty operating rooms to help take care of critically ill patients on ventilators in both the intensive care unit (ICU) and sometimes the operating room itself. The last several years have also led to patients with increasing complexity and severity of disease presenting to the operating room. In this issue of *Anesthesiology Clinics of North America*, a group of outstanding contributors wrote a series of articles on both intraoperative and postoperative care of complex patients and problems. Importantly, the authors also discuss the health and well-being of ICU physicians, which is critical in light of the previous couple of years. These articles bring important issues of interest to all practicing anesthesiologists.

In order to commission an issue on critical care, I engaged three amazing critical care anesthesiologists from diverse institutions who together chair the Scientific Writing Subcommittee of the Society of Critical Care Anesthesiologists. Athanasios Chalkias, MD, MSc, PhD is an Assistant Professor of Anesthesiology at the Faculty of Medicine of the University of Thessaly, Greece. As Dr Chalkias is a physician-scientist, his clinical activity and research are dedicated to anesthesiology, intensive care medicine, cardiovascular dynamics, resuscitation, translational intensive care medicine and anesthesiology, and translational physiology. He is a member of the Guidelines Committee and the Trauma and Resuscitation Scientific Forum of the European Society of Anaesthesiology and Intensive Care. Mary Jarzebowski, MD is a Clinical Assistant Professor at the University of Michigan and the VA Ann Arbor Healthcare System, where she practices critical care medicine and anesthesiology. She completed her anesthesiology residency at Rush University Medical Center in

Anesthesiology Clin 41 (2023) xv–xvi
https://doi.org/10.1016/j.anclin.2022.12.001
1932-2275/23/© 2022 Published by Elsevier Inc.

Chicago and a fellowship in critical care medicine at Northwestern University. Her research interests involve emergency airway management as well as mechanisms and clinical outcomes associated with sedation and analgesia in critically ill patients. Kathryn Rosenblatt, MD, MHS is Assistant Professor of Anesthesiology and Critical Care Medicine and Neurology at the Johns Hopkins University School of Medicine and serves as co-director of the neurosurgical anesthesia fellowship. She completed a residency in anesthesiology at SUNY Upstate Medical University and fellowships in both neuroanesthesia and neurocritical care at Johns Hopkins. She also completed a research fellowship, earning an MHS in Clinical Investigation at the Johns Hopkins Bloomberg School of Public Health. Dr Rosenblatt's research interests include cerebral autoregulation monitoring to improve outcomes from sepsis and sepsis-associated encephalopathy.

Lee A. Fleisher, MD, FACC, FAHA
3400 Spruce Street, Dulles 680
Philadelphia, PA 19104, USA

E-mail address:
Lee.Fleisher@pennmedicine.upenn.edu

Preface

Current Topics in Critical Care for the Anesthesiologist

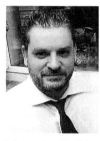
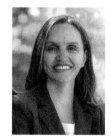
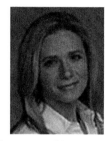

Athanasios Chalkias, MD, MSc, PhD, FESC, FAcadTM, FC, FESAIC
Mary L. Jarzebowski, MD
Kathryn Rosenblatt, MD, MHS

Editors

Anesthesiologists are leaders in perioperative medicine who are responsible for overseeing the care of patients undergoing surgical procedures. With a deep understanding of physiology and pharmacology, coupled with expert resuscitation and procedural skills, anesthesiologists are also particularly well-suited to practicing critical care medicine in medical, surgical, transplant, cardiothoracic, and neurological intensive care units (ICUs). Critical care anesthesiologists continue to expand in number and breadth of practice internationally.

The specialties of anesthesiology and critical care medicine have evolved significantly over recent decades and are integral parts of the patient care continuum. The committed involvement of critical care anesthesiologists in the COVID-19 pandemic further increased public awareness of the role and importance of this specialty in high-acuity patient care, as well as in research, education, policy and implementation, and leadership.

The scope of anesthesiology expertise throughout the world is broad. While the bulk of anesthesiologists in the United States practice as intraoperative care specialists, anesthesia care encompasses all aspects of perioperative medicine and has done so for decades. Modern ICUs began as respiratory care units to provide ventilatory support during large-scale poliomyelitis epidemics around the world. It was a small group of anesthesiologists who started the first United States–based respiratory care unit in the 1950s. Nearly seventy years later, anesthesiologists continue to move between the operating room and the ICU, and lately in great volume, to meet the health care demands of the COVID-19 pandemic.

The same pattern exists for the growing number of critically ill patients moving between the ICU and the operating room. With improvements in short-term survival

Anesthesiology Clin 41 (2023) xvii–xviii
https://doi.org/10.1016/j.anclin.2022.10.001
1932-2275/23/© 2022 Published by Elsevier Inc.
anesthesiology.theclinics.com

from acute and critical illness, as well as advances in surgical technology that allow intervention on more complex patients, anesthesiologists frequently encounter critically ill patients requiring surgical interventions. The perioperative management of these patients necessitates unmatched vigilance due to diminished physiologic reserve, high comorbidity burden, the systemic response to surgery, administration of anesthetics, and/or the available resources. Anesthesiologists of all subspecialties continue to care for critically ill patients during surgery, a trend that is likely to continue given the rising comorbidity burden of today's population.

Anesthesiology Clinics is pleased to introduce a special issue dedicated to critical care medicine for the anesthesiologist. This issue utilizes the breadth of expertise that is represented in our unique specialty, represented here by comprehensive review articles from members of the Society of Critical Care Anesthesiologists. It is our hope that this content helps anesthesiologists navigate the complexities of our patient population as we strive to improve outcomes for the highest acuity patients.

Athanasios Chalkias, MD, MSc, PhD, FESC, FAcadTM, FC, FESAIC
Department of Anesthesiology
Faculty of Medicine
University of Thessaly
Biopolis, 41500
Larisa, Greece

Mary L. Jarzebowski, MD
Department of Anesthesiology
VA Ann Arbor Healthcare System
2215 Fuller Road
Ann Arbor, MI 48105, USA

Kathryn Rosenblatt, MD, MHS
Department of Anesthesiology
Critical Care Medicine, and Neurology
School of Medicine
Johns Hopkins University
Baltimore, MD 21287, USA

*All authors contributed equally to this article

E-mail addresses:
thanoschalkias@yahoo.gr (A. Chalkias)
mjarzebo@med.umich.edu (M.L. Jarzebowski)
krosenb3@jhmi.edu (K. Rosenblatt)

Not all Shock States Are Created Equal

A Review of the Diagnosis and Management of Septic, Hypovolemic, Cardiogenic, Obstructive, and Distributive Shock

Sarah Khorsand, MD[a], Mada F. Helou, MD[b],
Veena Satyapriya, MD[c], Rafal Kopanczyk, DO[c],
Ashish K. Khanna, MD, MS, FCCP, FCCM, FASA[d,e,f],*

KEYWORDS

- Shock • Diagnosis • Management • Intervention • Types

KEY POINTS

- Shock is a common entity present in up to a third of all critical care patients.
- Clinical history and physical examination may help differentiate the type of shock. Assessment of relevant hemodynamic variables, such as blood pressure, heart rate, cardiac output, filling pressures, systemic vascular resistance, measures of flow or perfusion, and oxygen extraction further assist in diagnosis and management. Point-of-care ultrasound is routinely used in the early assessment of shock.
- Specific management of shock states involves correction of the triggering etiology and goal-directed resuscitation.
- One shock state may convert to another or may have an undifferentiated presentation; therefore, frequent re-assessment is necessary.

[a] Department of Anesthesiology and Pain Management, University of Texas at Southwestern Medical Center, 3605 Vancouver Drive, TX 75229, USA; [b] Department of Anesthesiology and Perioperative Medicine, Case Western Reserve University School of Medicine, University Hospitals Cleveland Medical Center, Cleveland Medical Center, 11100 Euclid Avenue, Cleveland, OH 44106, USA; [c] Department of Anesthesiology, The Ohio State University Wexner Medical Center, N437 Doan Hall, 410 W. 10th Avenue, Columbus, OH 43210, USA; [d] Department of Anesthesiology, Section on Critical Care Medicine, Wake Forest Baptist Medical Center, 1 Medical Center Boulevard, 9th Floor Janeway Tower, Winston-Salem, NC 27157, USA; [e] Perioperative Outcomes and Informatics Collaborative (POIC), 1 Medical Center Boulevard, Winston-Salem, NC, 27157, USA; [f] Outcomes Research Consortium, 9500 Euclid Avenue, Cleveland, OH 44195, USA
* Corresponding author. Department of Anesthesiology, Section on Critical Care Medicine, Wake Forest Baptist Medical Center, 1 Medical Center Boulevard, 9th Floor Janeway Tower, Winston-Salem, NC 27157.
E-mail address: akhanna@wakehealth.edu

Anesthesiology Clin 41 (2023) 1–25
https://doi.org/10.1016/j.anclin.2022.11.002
anesthesiology.theclinics.com
1932-2275/23/© 2022 Elsevier Inc. All rights reserved.

INTRODUCTION

The characteristic definition of circulatory shock is the combination of hypotension and hypoperfusion that amounts to progressive failure of oxygen utilization at the cellular level and organ system failure. Shock remains one of the most common causes of emergent intensive care admission across the world.[1] Typical pathophysiological variants of shock are most commonly distributive or vasodilatory followed by cardiogenic, hypovolemic, and obstructive (**Fig. 1**, **Table 1**). Mixed shock, specifically

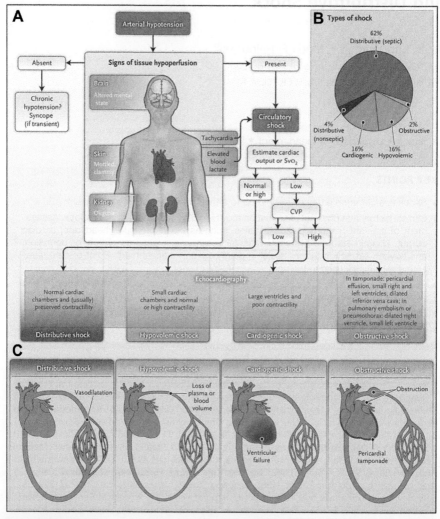

Fig. 1. Pathophysiology and diagnosis of shock states. Clinical assessment of various shock states begins with understanding that mean arterial pressure is the product of cardiac output and systemic vascular resistance. Signs of hypotension manifest as tissue hypoperfusion leading to a combination of delayed capillary refill time, clammy and mottled extremities, elevated blood lactate and organ system changes such oliguria, altered mental status, and tachycardia.2 Categorization of the specific shock syndrome requires an assessment of volume status or cardiac filling pressures and cardiac output or surrogates such as mixed venous oxygenation2. (Used with permission from Vincent JL, DeBacker D; NEJM 2013.)

Table 1
Basic diagnostic and management elements of shock states

Shock State	SVR	HR	CO	CVP/Preload	ScvO₂	Examination/Findings[b]	Treatment
Distributive	↓	↑	Varies[a]	↓	↑	Septic: Febrile, leukocytosis, possible focal infection. Anaphylaxis: rapid onset, urticaria, hives, febrile, swelling, bronchospasm. Neurogenic shock: spinal cord injury, loss of sensation and motor tone, altered reflexes	Septic: Empiric antibiotic, fluids, vasoconstrictors, source control. Anaphylaxis: stop culprit, epinephrine, steroids, fluids. Neurogenic shock: surgical stabilization, BP augmentation
Cardiogenic	↑	↑	↓	↑	↓	Cold extremities, rales, elevated JVD, slow capillary refill	Inotropic support; pacing if bradycardic; treat arrythmia; mechanical support if indicated
Obstructive	↑	↑	↓	↓	↓	Elevated JVD, tachycardic, distant heart sounds, pulsus paradoxus, electrical alternans	Decompress tension pneumothorax; pericardiocentesis; pulmonary thrombectomy
Hypovolemic	↑	↑	↓	↓	↓	Hemorrhage, possible insensible losses, low JVD, dry mucus membranes	Hemorrhage control if applicable; fluid resuscitation

Abbreviations: BP, blood pressure; CO, cardiac output; CVP, central venous pressure; HR, heart rate; JVD, jugular venous distension; ScvO₂, central venous oxygen saturation; SVR, systemic vascular resistance.

[a] *Early septic shock,* usually increased; *late septic shock* with low preload, may be decreased despite hyperdynamic state; *septic cardiomyopathy,* will be decreased; *anaphylactic shock:* usually increased hyperdynamic unless stress-induced cardiac dysfunction; *neurogenic shock:* depends on level of injury and whether sympathetic cardiac accelerators involved.

[b] All shock states will have overlap of: low urine output, altered mental status.

sepsis or septic vasodilatory shock in the setting of preexistent cardiogenic shock is associated with worse outcomes.[2,3] Whatever the etiology, both short-term and long-term organ dysfunction secondary to shock comes with high mortality for the patient and a substantial economic burden to any health care system.[4] This review evaluates types of shock divided into the traditional pathophysiological categories and provides evidence-based guidance for the treatment and management of each.

Evolution of Shock Management

The last decade has witnessed an exponential growth in available literature specific to resuscitation targets and hemodynamic thresholds of shock. An investigation of nearly 9,000 critically ill patients across several intensive care unit (ICU) systems in the United States identified the earliest increased risk of myocardial injury, acute kidney injury, and mortality at a mean arterial pressure (MAP) of 85 mm Hg.[5] Another investigation of several thousand postoperative intensive care patients identified a nonlinear increase in myocardial injury and mortality at pressures higher than the traditional norm of 65 mm Hg.[6] A multicenter, randomized trial of 424 with septic shock determined that a resuscitation strategy targeting normalization of capillary refill time, compared with a strategy targeting serum lactate levels, did not reduce all-cause 28-day mortality.[7]

The role of continuous noninvasive and minimally invasive monitoring for shock is in a state of rapid evolution. New, well-validated measurement techniques are able to complement traditional measures such as the pulmonary artery catheter (PAC).[8] In addition, the use of mechanical circulatory support devices and extracorporeal systems to manage various degrees of cardiogenic shock has rapidly increased worldwide.[2] Further, new vasopressors and increased data for adjuvant therapy and other innovative treatments are available. for shock patients such as steroids and other innovative therapy to help support organ systems is now available for these patients.[9–11] For example, angiotensin II as an agent to effectively support blood pressure may allow for a reduction in other vasopressors and have a substantial survival benefit in the high-renin phenotype of shock.[12,13] Delay in the initiation of vasopressin has been associated with a significant increase in mortality thereby ushering in an era of early and appropriate multimodal use of vasopressors and adjuvants.[14–17] Traditional measures of perfusion such as lactate have been consistently questioned and serum renin has emerged within the limitation of a nonpoint-of-care assay as a superior measure of organ perfusion and prognosis in critically ill patients with shock.[18–21]

Distributive Shock

Vasodilatory or distributive shock is characterized by tissue hypoxemia and low systemic vascular resistance and concomitant high cardiac output (CO) and high heart rate.[22] More than 90% of distributive shock is septic shock and usually manifests as a high output state.[23] However, other causes of nonseptic vasodilatory shock, including post-cardiopulmonary bypass vasoplegia, anaphylaxis, neurogenic shock, and pancreatitis are important clinically relevant examples. Treatment of distributive shock varies by cause, but usually requires vasoconstrictors, fluids, and in some cases may necessitate inotropes as well.

Septic Shock

Epidemiology and pathophysiology

The Third International Consensus Definitions for Sepsis and Septic Shock (Sepsis-3) defined septic shock as a lactate greater than 2 mmol/L and hypotension requiring vasoconstrictors to maintain MAP > 65 mm Hg despite adequate volume resuscitation.

Stated otherwise, septic shock is characterized by a life-threatening organ dysfunction caused by the dysregulated host response to sepsis resulting in regional hypoxia and mitochondrial dysfunction.[24] The Sepsis-3 taskforce found wide variability in mortality associated with septic shock, from 20% up to 80%, with an average mortality of 40%.[25] Early sepsis may have a subtle presentation, as CO is generally preserved and may be hyperdynamic. Extremities are warm and skin is flushed. Septic shock presents with hypotension, temperature > 38.3° C or < 36° C, tachycardia, and tachypnea. CO progressively drops as the disease course evolves, with myocardial depression and a low flow state, whereby skin may be mottled with the decreased capillary refill. This is more common in patients on prolonged high-dose vasopressors, where catecholamine-induced myocardial injury and microcirculatory flow impairment is common.[26] Exposure to increasing amounts of catecholamines upwards of 0.8 to 1.0 mcg/kg/min of norepinephrine equivalents may be associated with a 50% to 80% 30-day mortality.[26–29] Laboratory workup shows elevated lactate, and central venous oxygen saturation due to reduced tissue extraction. Where there is clinical equipoise, an elevated procalcitonin may help confirm the presence of sepsis.[30] In nonintensive care settings, a quick-SOFA (qSOFA) score of 2 or more in the presence of altered mental status, respiratory rate > 22/min, or systolic blood pressure (SBP) < 100 mm Hg, portends a poor outcome in the setting of infection.[31]

End-organ dysfunction resulting from septic shock yields myriad conflicting management goals for the intensivist, and these overlap with other shock states. Briefly, acute kidney injury, cardiac demand ischemia, altered mental status, and gut hypoperfusion result from hypoperfusion. Lactic acidosis impairs vascular tone via intracellular signaling and increased the expression of nitric oxide synthase. It also causes a decreased responsiveness to endogenous and exogenous catecholamines.[32] Uremia worsens altered mental status and airway protection. Shock liver can make lactate interpretation difficult, as both increased production and decreased clearance will elevate lactate. Septic cardiomyopathy (SCM) is a spectrum of disease, ranging from right and/or left ventricular (LV) dilation and dysfunction to myocardial injury and cardiogenic shock, independent of cardiac ischemia. Pathophysiology is likely multifactorial, and preexisting reduced ejection fraction (EF) and coronary artery disease increase the risk of developing SCM during sepsis.[33] Inotropic support for SCM has not been shown to be beneficial, though has not been well-studied in overt sepsis-induced cardiogenic shock. The mixed-shock state this can produce may be better elucidated with the use of a PAC, and the use of temporary mechanical support may be considered.[34]

Diagnosis and Management

Serial tests of end-organ perfusion, such as lactate and central venous oxygenation, assist in diagnosis of septic shock. In addition to standard ICU monitors, patients with rapid decompensation or those who require vasoactive medications benefit from an arterial line.[35] Important clinical endpoints include renal clearance and urine output, mentation, and capillary refill. Monitoring response to a fluid challenge is important to avoid complications of fluid overload. This can be done with continuous monitoring of endpoints such as stroke volume variation (SVV) and pulse pressure variation (PPV).[36] Any change in shock symptomatology should necessitate re-evaluation for a mixed shock state, with a transthoracic echocardiogram and cardiac biomarkers including troponins, B-type natriuretic peptide (BNP), and N-terminal pro-B-type natriuretic peptide (NT-proBNP).[33]

The management of vasodilatory shock is a step-wise approach (**Fig. 2**). Early initiation of antibiotics and source control is the cornerstone of care for sepsis.[37]

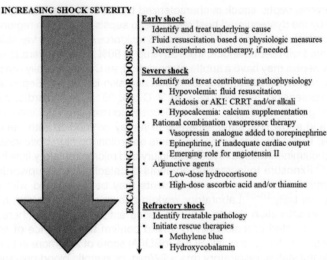

INCREASING SHOCK SEVERITY

ESCALATING VASOPRESSOR DOSES

Early shock
- Identify and treat underlying cause
- Fluid resuscitation based on physiologic measures
- Norepinephrine monotherapy, if needed

Severe shock
- Identify and treat contributing pathophysiology
  - Hypovolemia: fluid resuscitation
  - Acidosis or AKI: CRRT and/or alkali
  - Hypocalcemia: calcium supplementation
- Rational combination vasopressor therapy
  - Vasopressin analogue added to norepinephrine
  - Epinephrine, if inadequate cardiac output
  - Emerging role for angiotensin II
- Adjunctive agents
  - Low-dose hydrocortisone
  - High-dose ascorbic acid and/or thiamine

Refractory shock
- Identify treatable pathology
- Initiate rescue therapies
  - Methylene blue
  - Hydroxycobalamin

Fig. 2. A simplified approach to management of refractory vasodilatory shock. (Used with permission from: Jentzer JC et al., Chest 2018.)

Antibiotics should target the suspected infection and address patient risk factors, including prior susceptibilities and resistance and risk of health care-acquired pathogens. Source control, medically, surgically or via percutaneous intervention where possible, is vitally important.[38]

Goal-directed therapy should be followed with lactate and central venous oxygen saturation as endpoints of perfusion, as well as improvement in capillary refill time. The importance of continual re-evaluation of volume status and further boluses as needed cannot be over-emphasized. The "ROSE" model of fluid resuscitation in septic shock offered by Malbrain and colleagues[39] emphasizes a four-phase sequence for therapy. The four phases *R*esuscitation, *O*ptimization, *S*tabilization, and *E*vacuation are to be balanced appropriately while considering the benefits and risks of overdoing any one of these. Although and/or once euvolemia is achieved, the use of vasoconstrictors starting with norepinephrine is recommended to maintain adequate end-organ perfusion with an MAP goal of greater than 65 mm Hg.[40] Vasopressin may be added as a second agent over escalating doses of norepinephrine. Norepinephrine has stood the test of time as the primary vasopressor for septic shock, though trials comparing this agent with vasopressin as a first-line therapy have not shown a difference in outcomes[41] and may suggest that vasopressin preserves renal function better.[42] Recent evidence has pointed to the detrimental effects of a delay in initiation of vasopressin, being associated with a near 20% increase in mortality for every 10 mcg/min of norepinephrine usage.[15] Understanding the evolution of early multimodal vasopressor therapy is relevant as we move to a more precision medicine-based approach to the management of septic shock.[16,17]

Angiotensin II has been seen to improve hemodynamics and decrease background vasopressor use in a phase III trial published in 2017.[13] Since then significant new evidence using real-world and post hoc data has supported survival benefit in a cohort of patients with septic acute kidney injury (AKI),[43] appropriately resuscitated patients already on vasopressin,[44] those with serum renin greater than population median,[12] and also for responders to very low dose Angiotensin-II.[45] Although the phase III trial reported no difference in serious adverse events attributable to vascular thromboses, the authors did report an overall difference in all vascular events that did not favor

Angiotensin II.[13,46] This has not been seen in real-world utilization studies reported so far.[47]

Lastly, the use of stress dose corticosteroids is recommended in patients who require ongoing vasopressor infusion to maintain MAP greater than 65 mm Hg. Hydrocortisone 200 mg/d dosed 50 mg every 6 hours is a typical regimen and has been shown to increase vasopressor-free days.[48]

Anaphylactic Shock

Epidemiology and pathophysiology

Anaphylaxis and anaphylactoid reactions produce rapid multisystem organ failure through mast cell activation. Fatal anaphylaxis is quite rare with less than one death in 1 million reports in the United States; however, the overall incidence is around 5%.[49] Symptoms relate to mast cell degranulation and the release of histamine, tryptase, heparin, tumor necrosis factor, and other inflammatory mediators. Clinical signs include rash, bronchorrhea, bronchospasm, status asthmaticus, swelling, low venous tone and massive fluid extravasation resulting in low preload, tachycardia and depressed myocardial function.[50] A diagnosis of anaphylaxis is made when the following criteria are met: a rapid and sudden progression of symptoms involving skin and/or mucosa, as well as life-threatening airway, breathing, or circulation problems.[51] An elevated blood serum tryptase greater than 1.2x baseline sent within the first hour of exposure is considered confirmatory though use of this laboratory result is imperfect. The need for improved biomarkers of anaphylaxis exists.[52] Symptoms typically peak quickly, but may present with a biphasic pattern hours or days after exposure to the offending agent, and vary rarely symptoms may linger for days or weeks. The degree of resultant shock may be profound and its course difficult to predict. Tissue hypoxemia and ischemia may result in end-organ damage despite maximal pharmacologic support. Stress-induced cardiomyopathy has been described in several case reports as has coronary vasospasm.[53,54]

Monitoring

Rapid recognition and treatment require cessation of the offending agent and first and foremost intramuscular epinephrine (by injection into the mid-lateral thigh, 0.01 mg/kg of a 1:1000 (1 mg/mL) solution to a maximum of 0.5 mg in adults and 0.3 mg in children), as delay in epinephrine administration can increase risk of mortality. A second dose of epinephrine may be administered to adults and children with severe anaphylaxis whose symptoms are not relieved by an initial dose. Intravenous epinephrine may be dosed instead of intramuscular as 50 μg at a time for adults and 1 μg/kg for children.[55] High-volume fluid administration may be required. Oxygen should be administered, and the airway should be secured as quickly as possible if needed. Steroids and antihistamines address mast cell degranulation but are not first-line therapy. Bronchodilators may be used to treat bronchospasm. In severe reactions, epinephrine infusion as well as vasoconstrictors should be added for continued support of CO and perfusion pressure. In rare cases, the use of mechanical circulatory support to optimize tissue perfusion is needed using intra-aortic balloon pump, veno-venous extracoporeal membrane oxygenator (VV-ECMO), and veno-arterial extracoporeal membrane oxygenator (VA-ECMO).[56]

Neurogenic Shock

Epidemiology and pathophysiology

Neurogenic shock, the subset of physiologic effects resulting from spinal shock, usually results from traumatic spinal cord injury. It can present within minutes and last for weeks after spinal cord injury. Neurogenic shock carries an incidence of approximately 30% in cervical spinal cord injury. This entity is characterized by hypotension due to loss of spinal cord reflexes below the level of the injury and a loss of sympathetic tone.[57] It is caused by loss of descending sympathetic pathways resulting in predominant parasympathetic tone, leading to reduced venous return, bradycardia, and decreased vascular resistance.[58]

Monitoring

Patients with neurogenic shock should be monitored in an ICU with continuous blood pressure measurements, telemetry and pulse oximetry. These patients have a high incidence of respiratory failure, particularly in mid-thoracic SCI and above.[59] Patients with thoracic SCI and above have a higher incidence of severe bradycardia and bradyarrhythmia.[22]

Management

Early surgical stabilization is key to treating and stabilizing spinal cord injury and resultant neurogenic shock. Despite a paucity of evidence, maintaining MAP of 80 to 90/ mm Hg with the use of vasoconstrictors is recommended to augment spinal cord perfusion pressure.[60] The use of the appropriate agent here may be determined by factors such as high spinal injury where preference would be for additional inotropy via norepinephrine, whereas in other situations phenylephrine with unopposed alpha agonism may be appropriate. However, functional outcomes suggest that if a spinal cord injury and resultant neurogenic shock are profound enough, the use of vasoconstrictors does not confer improved functional status despite increasing spinal cord perfusion pressure.[61] High-dose methylprednisolone has been used for the treatment of neurogenic shock but the evidence in favor is scarce and the infectious complications profound.[62] Overall, supportive care is recommended to maintain end-organ perfusion and an appropriate heart rate.

Cardiogenic Shock

Epidemiology and pathophysiology

Cardiogenic shock is a low output state due to primary cardiac dysfunction leading to systemic decompensation, end-organ dysfunction, and secondary myocardial injury. Known cardiac dysfunction with SBP < 80 to 90 mm Hg, a cardiac index < 1.8 L/min/ m^2 without support and < 2.2 L/min/m^2 with support, and signs of tissue hypoperfusion are hallmarks of cardiogenic shock.[63–67] Despite advances in care, mortality remains high and to the tune of 40% to 67%.[68] The Society of Cardiovascular Angiography and Interventions (SCAI) has developed a tiered classification system to standardize the definition and severity of cardiogenic shock to allow for more timely risk stratification and interventions and ultimately improved outcomes (**Table 2**)[69]

The most common cause of cardiogenic shock is acute coronary syndrome (ACS) and resultant LV dysfunction, which accounts for up to 81% of cardiogenic shock patients, followed by acute decompensated heart failure. (**Box 1**)[67,70] Hemodynamic phenotypes reflect the effects of cardiogenic shock on cardiac function and systemic vascular resistance (SVR) and end-organ perfusion. "Cold and wet" is the classically described presentation of cardiogenic shock and denotes the presence of cool extremities and pulmonary congestion due to LV failure and compensatory peripheral vasoconstriction, often poorly tolerated by a struggling pump.[66] "Cold and dry" CS, as the term suggests, correlates with poor systemic perfusion in the absence of pulmonary congestion and is often responsive to diuretic therapy. The systemic inflammatory response that occurs in cardiogenic shock is often underappreciated and is

Table 2
Society of Cardiovascular Angiography and Interventions classification of cardiogenic shock

CS Stage	Physical Examination	Biochemical Markers	Hemodynamics	
A. At risk	Normal CVP, no rales, warm, good peripheral pulses, normal mentation	Normal labs, lactate and renal function	SBP > 100 or normal for patient. If done: CI ≥ 2.5, CVP < 10, S_vO_2 ≥ 65%	At risk for CS: large acute MI or prior infarct, worsening heart failure symptoms
B. Beginning CS	Increased CVP, good peripheral pulses, normal mentation	Minimal renal functional impairment, elevated BNP	SBP < 90 or MAP < 60 or > 30 decrease, HR ≥ 100. If done: CI ≥ 2.2, S_vO_2 ≥ 65%	Clinical evidence of hypotension or tachycardia without hypoperfusion
C. Classic CS	May include any: Looks unwell, panicked, ashen, volume overload, rales, Killip class 3 to 4, cold/clammy, altered MS, decreased UO	May include any: Lactate > 2, doubling creatinine or 50% drop in GFR, increased LFT's or elevated BNP	May include any: SBP > 90, MAP <60 or >30 decrease, and drugs/device used to maintain BP above target, CI < 2.2, P_{pao} ≥ 15, CVP/P_{pao} ≥ 0.8, PAPI < 1.85, CPO ≤ 0.6	Clinical signs of hypoperfusion that requires intervention pharmacologically or with temporary MCS, typically with hypotension
D. Deteriorating/doom	Any of Stage C and deteriorating	Any of Stage C with progressive worsening	Any of Stage C and require multiple pressors and/or mechanical circulatory support to maintain flow	Not responding to initial interventions in Stage C
E. Extremis	No SBP without resuscitation or maximal support to sustain ROSC, PEA or refractory VT/VT	"Trying to die," pH ≤ 7.2, lactate ≥ 5	SBP without resuscitation, pulseless electrical activity, refractory VT/VF, hypotension despite maximal support	Near pulselessness and/or cardiac collapse or CPR, with or without initiation of ECMO, mechanical ventilation, pacing, etc.

Abbreviations: BNP, brain natriuretic peptide; CI, cardiac index; CPO, cardiac power output; CS, cardiogenic shock; CVP, central venous pressure; ECMO, extracorporeal membrane oxygenation; GFR, glomerular filtration rate; LFTs, liver function tests; MAP, mean arterial pressure; MCS, mechanical circulatory support; MI, myocardial infarction; MS, mental status; PAPI, pulmonary artery pulsatility index; P_{pao}, pulmonary artery occlusion pressure; SBP, systolic blood pressure; SCAI, society for cardiovascular angiography and intervention; S_vO_2, mixed venous O_2 saturation; UO urine output, VT/VF, ventricular tachycardia/fibrillation.
Modified from Baran, et al.[69,128]

Box 1
Etiologies of cardiogenic shock

I. Ischemic:
  a. Acute myocardial infarction secondary to LV or RV infarct
  b. Mechanical complication of ischemic infarct

II. Nonischemic
  a. Acute on chronic decompensated heart failure
  b. Acute decompensated heart failure
    i. Chronic ischemia
    ii. Dilated cardiomyopathy
    iii. Myocarditis
    iv. Stress induced cardiomyopathy (Takutsubo)
    v. Pregnancy associated heart disease
      1. Peripartum cardiomyopathy
      2. Coronary artery disease
  c. Post cardiotomy cardiogenic shock
  d. Post cardiac arrest myocardial stunning
  e. Septic cardiomyopathy
  f. Myocardial Contusion
  g. Dynamic LVOT obstruction
    i. Hypertrophic obstructive cardiomyopathy
    ii. Hypertensive cardiomyopathy
    iii. Takutsubo

Abbreviations: LV, left ventricular; LVOT, left ventricular outflow tract; RV, right ventricular.

Adapted from Van Diepen et al.[67]

---

described as "wet and warm," where peripheral vasodilation predominates. Cor pulmonale, isolated right ventricular (RV) failure, is beyond the scope of this review, but the presence and degree of RV and LV failure also affects the clinical presentation of CS. These are important to identify early on, as these parameters determine management strategies (eg, type of inotropic support, afterload reduction, diuretic use, etc.).

Diagnosis

Serial troponins and electrocardiogram (ECG) are essential investigations in cardiogenic shock to identify acute coronary syndrome (ACS) and myocardial necrosis.[67] If evidence of ST elevation Myocardial Infarction (STEMI) or other changes concerning ACS are noted, emergent coronary angiography and determinations of revascularization needs are warranted. Conversely, ST and non-ST abnormalities can also signify myocarditis, decompensated heart failure, or other structural disorders that cause CS.[66,71] Elevations in cardiac biomarkers BNP and NT-proBNP are seen in patients with LV and RV dysfunction but it is important to note that elevations are seen in all shock states and are linked to worse outcomes, regardless of the type of shock. As such, it is not recommended to use BNP or pro-BNP to assess treatment response in cardiogenic shock.[72] Lactate elevations are independently associated with increased mortality in cardiogenic shock and frequent monitoring to assess response to therapies is recommended.[67] Reuda and colleagues[73] analyzed identified 4 key proteins (liver-type fatty acid-binding protein, beta-2-microglobulin, fructose-bisphosphate aldolase B, and SerpinG1) that combined (CSP4) had significant predictive value for short-term mortality in cardiogenic shock when used in conjunction with contemporary risk scoring tools. This may guide shock teams in targeted care for patients with cardiogenic shock and warrants further study.

In addition to standard ICU monitoring and arterial pressure monitoring, PAC should be strongly considered as clinical presentations often correlate and drive decision-making in the management of cardiogenic shock. Thermodilution CO is readily obtained and values measured assist in the calculation of cardiac power output, cardiac power index (CPI) and pulmonary artery pulsatility index (PAPI). Mixed oxygen saturation (SvO_2) is reduced in cardiogenic shock but can also reflect anemia, hypoxemia, or increased oxygen consumption.

Echocardiography will provide EF and degree of biventricular dysfunction and will detect structural and valvular issues contributing to cardiogenic shock and to confirm the placement of mechanical circulatory support (MCS) devices.[67] In addition to rapid detection of gross functional abnormalities, point of care ultrasound (POCUS) can be useful in ruling out common alternative diagnoses, for example, cardiac tamponade or pneumothorax. The presence of three or more B-lines in at least 2 regions of the lung bilaterally on POCUS in the presence of lung sliding points toward pulmonary congestion due to cardiogenic acute pulmonary edema.[74]

Management

The goals of management are to restore perfusion to the myocardium and end organs while treating the underlying cause of failure. If ACS is present based on data available early invasive treatment and reperfusion is the mainstay of treatment. Importantly, emergent revascularization compared with medical therapy in patients with cardiogenic shock has shown mortality benefits across multiple racial and ethnic subgroups.[67,75]

In general, best practices propose that cardiac index should be kept above 2.2 L/min/m^2 and MAP goals > 65 mm Hg. However, further studies are needed to determine ideal goals in CS. Although the use of right atrial pressures and pulmonary artery wedge pressures are poor predictors of fluid response, overall trends along with correlation with echocardiographic findings, physical examination, and biochemical markers may be useful.

Although catecholamines may transiently improve hemodynamics, they are associated with worse long-term outcomes in patients with heart failure with reduced ejection fraction (HFrEF),[76] potentially due to their arrhythmogenicity and increased myocardial oxygen consumption. A recent randomized control trial looking at the use of dobutamine versus milrinone in cardiogenic shock found no difference in outcomes.[77] Thus, benefits of a catecholamine-sparing agent in this setting should be weighed against the need for rapid titration and possibility of concomitant renal failure in shock. Although sinus tachycardia is often a compensatory mechanism seen in cardiogenic shock due to HFrEF, new-onset tachyarrhythmias (eg, atrial fibrillation) may require urgent cardioversion. Lastly, negative inotropes (eg, beta-blockers) should be avoided in cardiogenic shock and consideration of chemical or electrical pacing is warranted if bradyarrhythmias are contributing to hypoperfusion.

If indicated, judicious challenges of 250 to 500 mL are recommended to avoid overstressing the failing pump. Conversely, fluid removal with furosemide and/or the addition of a thiazide diuretic should be considered if increased congestion and overall total body volume is elevated.

Respiratory failure occurs when cardiogenic pulmonary edema impairs gas exchange and worsens shunt. Because venous return is reduced both to the left and right ventricles with positive pressure ventilation (PPV), the overall effect on CO is variable and dependent on other factors which include preload, afterload, severity of left and RV dysfunction and degree of interventricular interdependence. Positive pressure ventilation can improve oxygenation and thereby decrease RV afterload by decreasing hypoxic pulmonary vasoconstriction as well as LV afterload. Noninvasive PPV is often used initially when respiratory insufficiency presents in cardiogenic shock and may decrease likelihood of endotracheal intubation. However, intubation is often unavoidable, especially if it is compounded by the presence of chronic respiratory comorbidities and other acute issues such as aspiration, altered mental status risk, facial trauma or deformities, severe hemodynamic instability or recent GI or upper airway surgery where noninvasive positive pressure ventilation is contraindicated.[78] Moderate to high PEEP (5 to 15 cm H20) may improve overall CO and end-organ perfusion in afterload dependent LV failure.[79] Low tidal volume (4 to 6 mL/kg) is lung protective, and daily assessments to minimize sedation and increase mobility are important in this setting.[78]

Although beyond the scope of this review, if hemodynamic support is inadequate despite maximal medical management, temporary MCS should be considered. Cannulation strategies, physiologic effects, and amount of support vary based on the type of MCS initiated. Early initiation of MCS may confer survival benefit.[80] Given the high mortality in cardiogenic shock and the risks and substantial costs associated initiation of temporary MCS, shock algorithms and multidisciplinary expertise at regional hubs are particularly useful as they allow for early involvement of clinical experts and time-sensitive, patient-centered decision-making on appropriate treatment and support strategies.[59] If no recovery is observed on MCS, temporary MCS can serve as a bridge to advanced therapies with transplantation or durable support devices or bridge to decision as further workup is obtained. Neurologic uncertainty or multisystem organ failure prohibits advanced therapies candidacy, goals of care discussions should occur, and consideration of withdrawal of support should be initiated if there is poor chance of recovery without an exit strategy on MCS.

Obstructive Shock

Epidemiology and pathophysiology

Obstructive shock is caused by a physical impediment of blood flow in the cardiovascular system.[81] It is the least common type of shock, constituting about 2% of all shock states.[82] Tension pneumothorax (TP), cardiac tamponade, and pulmonary embolism (PE) comprise the majority of obstructive shock cases, but any obstruction that restricts venous return, prevents diastolic filling, or severely elevates afterload can result in obstructive shock.[82–84] Grouping based on location, mechanism, or cardiac consequences has been used[81,85–87] with categorization centered around effects on ventricular preload and afterload being most intuitive for an anesthesiologist (**Boxes 2 and 3**).

Diagnosis and Management

Patient presentation varies depending on etiology, acuity, and severity.[81,85–87] Initially, symptoms may be nonspecific, such as shortness of breath or chest pain. In addition, initial physiologic perturbations may be limited to compensatory responses like tachycardia and tachypnea. Physical examination frequently reveals jugular venous distention, abnormal auscultatory findings, and cool extremities.[81,85–87] As the obstruction progresses, hemodynamic indices resemble low-output states, with laboratory values consistent with oxygen supply and demand mismatch. Intravascular volume and cardiac contractility are usually preserved; however, CO, stroke volume (SV), and MAP are decreased.[81,85–87] Finally, systemic vascular resistance and central venous pressure (CVP) are usually increased, whereas wedge pressure varies based on etiology. For patients in extremis, diagnosis is clinical in nature, and treatment should not be delayed for diagnostics. Therapies most often consist of pharmacotherapy followed in quick succession with percutaneous or surgical relief of the obstruction.[81,85–87]

Box 2
Etiologies of obstructive shock

Impaired Preload/Diastolic Filling
  Mediastinal Tumors[129]
  SVC Syndrome[130]
  Tension Pneumo/hemothorax
  Right Sided Cardiac Herniation—vascular torsion[131]
  Left Sided Cardiac Herniation—LV compression/compromise[131]
  Cardiac Tamponade
  Constrictive Pericarditis[81]
  Cardiac Tumors[132]
  Severe Pulmonary Hypertension—effect on the LV[81]
  Massive PE—effect on the LV
  High Grade Abdominal Compartment Syndrome—effect on venous return[133]
  Auto-PEEP/Excessive Intrathoracic Pressure[85]
  Giant Hiatal Hernia[83]

Elevated Afterload
  Massive PE—effect on the RV
  Severe Pulmonary Hypertension—effect on the RV
  Aortic Occlusion[84]
  Coarctation of the Aorta[134]
  High Grade Abdominal Compartment Syndrome—effect on the LV[133]

Abbreviations: LV, left ventricle; PE, pulmonary embolism; PEEP, positive end-expiratory pressure; RV, right ventricle.

Box 3
Etiologies of hypovolemic shock

Extracellular Fluid Loss
  External Losses—Insensible Losses
    Open abdominal procedures
    Hyperthermia
    Respiratory System
  Internal Losses—Gastrointestinal or Renal
    Prolonged NPO times
    Persistent vomiting
    Persistent diarrhea
    Diabetes Insipidus
    Polyuric phase of acute tubular necrosis recovery

Loss of Whole Blood
  Hemorrhagic Shock—Perioperative, Gastrointestinal, Maternal or Vascular Rupture
    Postoperative bleeding
    Esophageal Varices
    Gastrointestinal Ulcers
    Uterine atony
    Placental abruption
    Aneurysmal rupture
  Traumatic Hemorrhagic Shock
    Includes the presence of soft tissue injury in addition to active hemorrhage, for example, motor vehicle collision

Tension Pneumothorax

Epidemiology and pathophysiology

Development of tension pneumothorax is uncommon with poorly quantified incidence.[88,89] Most commonly, it is observed in trauma, ARDS, and mechanically ventilated populations, but a simple pneumothorax can convert to tension physiology if one-way valve communication exists between the alveolus and pleura. Tension pneumothorax occurs when trapped air accumulates in the pleural space, increasing intrapleural pressure above the atmospheric pressure, leading to ipsilateral lung collapse and mediastinal compression with contralateral shift.[88]

Diagnosis and Management

Cyanosis, tracheal deviation, decreased breath sounds, percussion hyperresonance, and subcutaneous emphysema point toward the diagnosis of TP.[88] As TP evolves, compensatory mechanisms are frequently successful in maintaining stability in spontaneously breathing patients.[6,90] Conversely, pneumothorax developed during mechanical ventilation progresses to hemodynamic instability up to 70% of cases.[88-90] Elevated peak and plateau airway pressures, with decreasing lung compliance may be observed. Utilization point-of-care ultrasonography (POCUS) may facilitate faster diagnosis of a pneumothorax, with higher sensitivity than a chest radiography (79% vs 40%) and similar specificity (98% vs 99%).[91] POCUS findings suggestive of pneumothorax include lack of lung sliding and lung pulse, presence of lung point, and barcode sign on motion mode (M-mode).[92] Nonetheless, TP is a clinical diagnosis and treatment should not be delayed to obtain imaging. Therapy consists of emergent placement of large-bore needle into the anterior second intercostal space in the midclavicular line, followed by a percutaneous, small-bore thoracostomy catheter.[93,94]

Cardiac Tamponade

Epidemiology and pathophysiology

Cardiac tamponade is a feared consequence of any pericardial content accumulation, including blood, clot, pus, chyle, and gas.[95-98] It is characterized by restriction of cardiac filling due to elevation of intrapericardial pressure. Initial compensatory responses include elevation of systemic and pulmonary venous pressures, and tachycardia. As left and RV diastolic, right atrial, and wedge pressures equalize, early diastolic filling (Y-descent) fades and ventricular filling (X-descent) becomes predominant. With progression, pulsus paradoxus results due to ventricular interdependence.[95,97]

Diagnosis and Management

Diagnosis of cardiac tamponade is also clinical in nature, but echocardiography is used in most instances.[95,97] Classically, physical examination may reveal muffled heart tones, jugular venous distention, and systolic inspiratory variation of greater than 10 mm Hg, but these may be difficult to appreciate in a perioperative setting.[95,97] Microvoltage and electrical alternans may be seen on ECG with large effusions.[95,97] Pulsus paradoxus maybe still be observed on an arterial line tracing by monitoring inspiratory and expiratory area under the curve. High value occurring on inspiration and low on expiration in mechanically ventilated patients has been previously coined as reversed pulsus paradoxus but is nothing different than what is commonly described by anesthesiologists as PPV.[99,100] Echocardiographic imaging shows diastolic collapse of the right ventricle (highly specific), systolic collapse of the right atrium (early sign), plethoric inferior vena cava (IVC) with hepatic flow reversal, and respiratory variation of mitral and/or tricuspid valve inflow velocities have been classically associated with tamponade physiology.[101]

Recognizing cardiac tamponade after cardiac surgery is especially problematic and requires a high degree of suspicion.[102] Because the pericardial sac is often left open and in communication with pleural spaces preventing large fluid collections, it is usually a localized pocket of clot pressing on one cardiac chamber that causes cardiac tamponade. In effect, an insidious presentation ensues. Gradually worsening hypotension, low CO, increasing filling pressures, and increasing inotropic and pressor support are encountered. Worsening lactic acidosis is also observed, but classic equalization of pressures usually does not occur.[102] To aid in diagnosis, transesophageal echocardiography (TEE) is frequently used with success, but its limitations should be understood, as it may be insufficient to find regional clots, appreciate tissue edema, or illustrate chamber collapse when contaminant cardiac pathology is present.[102]

Treatment requires evacuation of the pressurized pericardial content. This can be achieved with percutaneous or surgical techniques.[95,97] Although awaiting definitive treatment, patients should be temporized with the enhancement of venous return with volume administration or leg elevation, promotion of chronotropy/inotropy and systemic venous pressure with epinephrine boluses, and reduction of intrathoracic pressure by limiting tidal volume and positive end-expiratory pressure (PEEP).[102]

Pulmonary Embolism

Epidemiology and pathophysiology
PE may result in obstructive shock when two or more lobar arteries and at least 50% to 60% of vascular bed are affected, elevating pulmonary vascular resistance.[81] Resultant acute elevation of RV afterload leads to chamber enlargement and myocardial failure. In effect, a decrease in early diastolic filling and preload of the LV leads to a reduction in SV and CO.[81,85]

Diagnosis and Management
Patient presentation varies with severity. Patients with altered mental status, hypotension, elevated cardiac troponins, and BNP are at increased risk of mortality and adverse outcomes.[103,104] Use of tools like Pulmonary Embolism Severity Index (PESI), or simplified PESI (sPESI) is encouraged as they can aid in risk stratification and therapy selection.[104]

Although computed tomography pulmonary angiography is a diagnostic gold standard, POCUS may be used as a bedside tool to rule-in a diagnosis of a PE. POCUS has a high specificity and low sensitivity for the diagnosis, and relies on indirect evidence like RV failure or deep venous thrombosis.[105] RV dysfunction on POCUS can be recognized by evaluating tricuspid annular plane systolic excursion (TAPSE), lateral tricuspid annular systolic velocity (S'), or short pulmonary flow acceleration and low tricuspid regurgitant pressure gradient (60/60 sign).[106] Pressure overload of the RV can be recognized by septal flattening in systole. The size of the RV can be qualitatively estimated by comparison to the neighboring LV.[105] Free wall akinesis with apical sparing (McConnell's sign) is frequently associated with a diagnosis of a PE, but its specificity lies in recognition of acute right heart strain, regardless of the cause.[106,107] Rarely, thrombus-in-transit may be observed and is the only pathognomonic ultrasonographic finding indicative of an acute PE in a symptomatic patient.[108]

PE with hypotension (massive PE) is the most severe type, where hypotension is defined as SBP less than 90 mm Hg for > 15 minutes.[109] Patients with hypotension, shock, myocardial dysfunction, and low risk of bleeding should undergo systemic thrombolytic therapy.[109] Catheter-based thrombus removal may be an option in patients with high risk for bleeding or failed systemic thrombolysis.[109] Surgical embolectomy may also be of benefit.[110] Given that therapies frequently depend on local expertise, standardization of in-hospital care is now recommended. Development of Pulmonary Embolism Response Teams (PERT) helps to improve quality, efficiency, and multidisciplinary communication, resulting in improved outcomes.[111,112]

Hypovolemic Shock

Hypovolemic shock is from a loss of intravascular volume, either directly from the loss of whole blood or indirectly from extracellular volume loss, that leads to inadequate organ perfusion[8,86,113] Ultimately, all types of hypovolemic shock decrease preload, which leads to a deficit in perfusion pressure and consequently, macrocirculation and microcirculation suffer. The resulting poor circulation results in decreased tissue perfusion and triggering of an inflammatory cascade.[86] External fluid losses include insensible losses (eg, open surgical abdominal procedures or hyperthermia). Internal fluid losses include gastrointestinal causes (eg, prolonged *nil per os* [NPO] times, persistent vomiting, or diarrhea) and renal causes (eg, diabetes insipidus [DI], polyuric phase of acute tubular necrosis recovery).[86] Hypovolemic shock that is due to the loss of whole blood is termed hemorrhagic shock, and when associated with soft tissue injury is termed traumatic hemorrhagic shock. Traumatic hemorrhagic shock is more common than nontraumatic causes of blood loss.[86,113] Hemorrhagic shock includes perioperative hemorrhage (eg, postoperative bleeding), gastrointestinal hemorrhage (eg, varices, ulcers), maternal hemorrhage (eg, uterine atony, placental abruption), and vascular rupture (eg, aneurysm).[86,114] Traumatic hemorrhagic shock includes soft tissue injury in addition to active hemorrhage. This distinction is important because the presence of soft tissue injury has additional implications on the effects of shock.[115] For instance, available evidence shows that soft tissue injury increases the likelihood of disruption of the blood-endothelium interactions, and may accelerate coagulopathy through mechanisms that exacerbate tissue hypoxia.[115]

Epidemiology and Pathophysiology

The pathophysiology of hypovolemic shock that is due to the loss of extracellular fluid varies according to the underlying cause. However, in all these cases daily fluid loss exceeds daily intake. The primary method of water intake is through the consumption of fluids and food, and the primary method of water loss is through urine, sweat, and stool. Fluid loss that is easily quantified is termed sensible loss, such as urine output. Fluid loss that is not easily measured is termed insensible loss, and is estimated to reach up to 800 mL/d. Insensible fluid loss largely occurs through water excretion in the stool, skin, and respiratory system.[116] Prolonged NPO times contribute to hypovolemia by decreasing intake in the context of continued sensible and insensible fluid loss.

Profound sensible losses can also lead to hypovolemic shock, as is seen with DI. DI is a condition where there is either a defect in the production or utilization of antidiuretic hormone (ADH), the key posterior pituitary polypeptide that is responsible for the conservation of fluid at the distal convoluted tubule. In central DI, there is a deficiency of ADH. In nephrogenic DI, ADH levels are normal; however, the kidney is unable to respond to the hormone. In both types of DI, patients release large volumes of dilute urine. If untreated, these patients are at risk for hypovolemic shock.[117]

Hemorrhagic Shock and Traumatic Hemorrhagic Shock

The pathophysiology of hemorrhagic and traumatic hemorrhagic shock has been under study for many years, and the effects are far-reaching on the tissue level, vascular level, and cellular level. On the tissue level, hemorrhage leads to hypovolemia, which in turn leads to reflex vasoconstriction. This vasoconstriction leads to decreased blood flow to vital organs and consequent multisystem organ failure in severe cases.[114] Hemorrhage also affects the vascular endothelium in both a local and generalized fashion.[115] Locally, thrombus formation is promoted through platelet activation, and the consequent formation of a platelet thrombin plug and the site of injury.[118] However systemically, the glycocalyx is shed due to the increased catecholamines and oxygen debt.[119] Glycocalyx shedding can lead to increased fibrinolytic activity and auto-heparinization, which lead to coagulopathy.[115] Of note, glycocalyx shedding combined with leukocyte-endothelial interactions also results in capillary leak syndrome.[86] Coagulopathy is compounded by decreased platelet numbers as well as decreased platelet activity.[114] The soft tissue injury in traumatic hemorrhagic shock contributes to and likely accelerates coagulopathy, possibly through mechanisms that worsen tissue hypoxia.[115] The hypothermia and acidosis found in trauma patients also exacerbate active bleeding.[86]

Effects are also complex at the cellular level. In both hemorrhagic and traumatic hemorrhagic shock, the acute reduction of red blood cell quantity causes inadequate oxygen delivery to cells, thereby forcing transition to anaerobic metabolism.[115,120] Byproducts and wastes including lactic acid, inorganic phosphates, and oxygen radicals begin to accumulate leading to acidosis. As cellular metabolism begins to fail, dying cells release damage-associated molecular patterns (DAMPs, alarmins, and other intracellular molecules) that activate the innate immune system thereby triggering a systemic inflammatory response.[121]

Diagnosis and Management

Elevated lactate and base deficit are a characteristic finding in hemorrhagic shock. However, acid-base balance ultimately depends on the underlying cause of the hypovolemic shock. For example, gastrointestinal losses can result in metabolic alkalosis, such as in the case of persistent vomiting. In hemorrhagic shock hemoglobin and hematocrit are usually severely decreased. However, if hemoconcentration is present, these values will be increased.[115]

PPV in appropriately ventilated patients in sinus rhythm is regarded as a useful measure of volume responsiveness. PPV reliability can be compromised by elevated respiratory rates, RV failure, and decreased chest wall compliance. Trends in CVP monitoring over time are also frequently used to assess intravascular volume status. CVP values should be interpreted in the context of ventilator settings and can be compromised by patient chest wall compliance and RV function as well. With the current ubiquity of ultrasound, measurement of the inferior vena cava throughout the respiratory cycle has also become another indicator for intravascular volume status.[115]

Laboratory studies frequently reveal evidence of pre-renal kidney injury: elevated blood urea nitrogen, serum creatinine, and urine osmolality; reduced urine sodium with fractional excretion of sodium less than 1%; and high or low serum sodium and potassium depending on the underlying cause.[115] In hemorrhagic shock, platelet counts can be decreased mainly due to dilutional effects and hemoglobin and hematocrit will be low unless hemoconcentration is present. International normalized ratio (INR), Prothrombin time (PT), and activated partial thromboplastin time (aPTT) can be elevated and fibrinogen levels can be decreased.[122] Thromboelastography is an excellent tool for the monitoring of clot formation and can help guide transfusion decision-making.

The "Stop the Bleed" concept of successful treatment of hypovolemic shock ultimately depends on the definitive correction of the underlying cause, and on the ability to temporize the patient with balanced resuscitation and vasopressors in the interim. To help temporize initial bleeding, the American College of Surgeons began the STOP THE BLEED campaign. The purpose of the initiative is to educate the public on hemorrhage control tactics following manmade or natural disasters.[123] The program improved the confidence and willingness of laypersons to render aid, and showed increased tourniquet use following program rollout.[124]

En route to the hospital, it is preferable to avoid aggressive resuscitation with crystalloid solutions to avoid clotting factor dilution, hemodilution and the consequent exacerbation of hypoxia.[114] If fluid administration alone is insufficient to restore adequate perfusion (SBP <80 mm Hg), it may be necessary to temporize blood pressure with vasopressors. Although there remains controversy regarding the optimal time to initiate vasopressors as well as choice of agent, norepinephrine has been suggested as first line.[125] This due to its sympathomimetic properties as well the potential benefit of splanchnic venoconstriction and movement of blood volume to the central circulation thereby increasing venous return and CO. Importantly phenylephrine, often used in clinical practice may have opposing effects on the splanchnic pre-portal and hepatic veins, thereby decreasing venous return and consequent downstream effects. In the hospital, definitive bleeding control is priority as well as adequate restoration of euvolemia via balanced resuscitation. Blood products are transfused in ratios that resemble whole blood, usually at a 1:1:1 ratio of packed red blood cells, fresh frozen plasma, and platelets. Massive transfusion protocols initiated at this rate improve morbidity and mortality of trauma patients in hemorrhagic shock.[126]

SUMMARY

Shock is a common and often life-threatening problem in the critically ill. Early diagnosis and intervention are a cornerstone for all flavors of this pathophysiological state. Multimodal therapeutics, new diagnostic tools, and consistent evidence-based protocolized practices have been shown to improve outcomes. A single patient may transition from one shock state to another; therefore, a vigilant approach that involves close and repeated re-evaluation is always a necessity. Future work is needed to fill current gaps in available guidelines for the management of shock, such as clear recommendations for nonseptic vasodilatory shock, timing of initiation of vasopressors in relationship to fluids and adjuvants, and management of shock in patients with RV failure or those on mechanical circulatory support.[14,38] Appropriate resuscitation goals continue to evolve as we explore the interplay between microcirculatory and macrocirculatory dysfunction and the role of optimal blood pressure, flow dynamics, and peripheral perfusion as therapeutic targets.[127]

CLINICS CARE POINTS

- Shock classically presents in one of the four categories of distributive (high output), hypovolemic, obstructive or cardiogenic, each of which can be diagnosed with clinical presentation, hemodynamic monitoring, point of care ultrasound and clinical laboratory parameters including biomarkers.

- Shock states can often evolve from one form to the other with minimal direct and obvious signs or symptoms. This necessiatates continual monitoring and re-evaluation of therapy including flexibility with diagnostics.

- Several new therapeutics have come to the forefront for management of all types of shock, and there is benefit to tailor therapy to type of insult while we await further higher level of evidence and robust trials.

DISCLOSURE

Supported by internal funds only. Dr A.K. Khanna is a consultant for Edwards Life-sciences, Caretaker Medical, Retia Medical, Philips Research North America, GE Healthcare, Baxter, and Medtronic. He is supported by an NIH, United States/NCATS KL2 award for a pilot trial of continuous hemodynamic and oxygenation monitoring on hospital wards and a Wake Forest Center for Hypertension and Vascular Research grant for evaluation of the renin angiotensin system in septic shock. The Department of Anesthesiology at Wake Forest School of Medicine is funded by Edwards Lifesciences, United States, Masimo, United States and Medtronic. Other authors do not have relevant personal financial interests. All authors contributed to drafting and reviewing the article, and all concur with the submitted version.

REFERENCES

1. Mayr FB, Talisa VB, Balakumar V, et al. Proportion and cost of unplanned 30-day readmissions after sepsis compared with other medical conditions. JAMA 2017; 317(5):530–1.
2. Berg DD, Bohula EA, van Diepen S, et al. Epidemiology of shock in contemporary cardiac intensive care units. Circ Cardiovasc Qual Outcomes 2019;12(3): e005618.
3. Jentzer JC, Bhat AG, Patlolla SH, et al. Concomitant sepsis diagnoses in acute myocardial infarction-cardiogenic shock: 15-year national temporal trends, management, and outcomes. Crit Care Explor 2022;4(2):e0637.
4. Gershengorn HB, Garland A, Gong MN. Patterns of daily costs differ for medical and surgical intensive care unit patients. Ann Am Thorac Soc 2015;12(12): 1831–6.
5. Maheshwari K, Nathanson BH, Munson SH, et al. The relationship between ICU hypotension and in-hospital mortality and morbidity in septic patients. Intensive Care Med 2018;44(6):857–67.
6. Khanna AK, Maheshwari K, Mao G, et al. Association Between Mean Arterial Pressure and Acute Kidney Injury and a Composite of Myocardial Injury and Mortality in Postoperative Critically Ill Patients: A Retrospective Cohort Analysis. Crit Care Med 2019;47(7):910–7.
7. Hernandez G, Ospina-Tascon GA, Damiani LP, et al. Effect of a resuscitation strategy targeting peripheral perfusion status vs serum lactate levels on 28-day mortality among patients with septic shock: the ANDROMEDA-SHOCK randomized clinical trial. JAMA 2019;321(7):654–64.
8. Saugel B, Thiele RH, Hapfelmeier A, et al. Technological assessment and objective evaluation of minimally invasive and noninvasive cardiac output monitoring systems. Anesthesiology 2020;133(4):921–8.
9. Annane D, Renault A, Brun-Buisson C, et al. Hydrocortisone plus fludrocortisone for adults with septic shock. N Engl J Med 2018;378(9):809–18.
10. Marik PE, Khangoora V, Rivera R, et al. Hydrocortisone, vitamin C, and thiamine for the treatment of severe sepsis and septic shock: a retrospective before-after study. Chest 2017;151(6):1229–38.
11. Venkatesh B, Finfer S, Cohen J, et al. Adjunctive Glucocorticoid Therapy in Patients with Septic Shock. N Engl J Med 2018;378(9):797–808.
12. Bellomo R, Forni LG, Busse LW, et al. Renin and survival in patients given angiotensin II for catecholamine-resistant vasodilatory shock. a clinical trial. Am J Respir Crit Care Med 2020;202(9):1253–61.

13. Khanna A, English SW, Wang XS, et al. Angiotensin II for the treatment of vaso-dilatory shock. N Engl J Med 2017;377(5):419–30.
14. Ammar MA, Ammar AA, Wieruszewski PM, et al. Timing of vasoactive agents and corticosteroid initiation in septic shock. Ann Intensive Care 2022;12(1):47.
15. Sacha GL, Lam SW, Wang L, et al. Association of catecholamine dose, lactate, and shock duration at vasopressin initiation with mortality in patients with septic shock. Crit Care Med 2022;50(4):614–23.
16. Wieruszewski PM, Khanna AK. Early multimodal vasopressors-are we ready for it? Crit Care Med 2022;50(4):705–8.
17. Wieruszewski PM, Khanna AK. Vasopressor choice and timing in vasodilatory shock. Crit Care 2022;26(1):76.
18. Gleeson PJ, Crippa IA, Mongkolpun W, et al. Renin as a marker of tissue-perfusion and prognosis in critically Ill patients. Crit Care Med 2019;47(2):152–8.
19. Jeyaraju M, McCurdy MT, Levine AR, et al. Renin kinetics are superior to lactate kinetics for predicting in-hospital mortality in hypotensive critically Ill patients. Crit Care Med 2022;50(1):50–60.
20. Khanna AK. Tissue perfusion and prognosis in the critically Ill-is renin the new lactate? Crit Care Med 2019;47(2):288–90.
21. Khanna AK. Renin Kinetics and Mortality-Same, Same But Different? Crit Care Med 2022;50(1):153–7.
22. Ince C. The microcirculation is the motor of sepsis. Crit Care 2005;9(Suppl 4):S13–9.
23. Vincent JL, De Backer D. Circulatory shock. N Engl J Med 2014;370(6):583.
24. Singer M, Deutschman CS, Seymour CW, et al. The third international consensus definitions for sepsis and septic shock (Sepsis-3). JAMA 2016;315(8):801–10.
25. Shankar-Hari M, Phillips GS, Levy ML, et al. Developing a New Definition and Assessing New Clinical Criteria for Septic Shock: For the Third International Consensus Definitions for Sepsis and Septic Shock (Sepsis-3). JAMA 2016;315(8):775–87.
26. Singh T, Khan H, Gamble DT, et al. Takotsubo Syndrome: Pathophysiology, Emerging Concepts, and Clinical Implications. Circulation 2022;145(13):1002–19.
27. Brown SM, Lanspa MJ, Jones JP, et al. Survival after shock requiring high-dose vasopressor therapy. Chest 2013;143(3):664–71.
28. Jenkins CR, Gomersall CD, Leung P, et al. Outcome of patients receiving high dose vasopressor therapy: a retrospective cohort study. Anaesth Intensive Care 2009;37(2):286–9.
29. Auchet T, Regnier MA, Girerd N, et al. Outcome of patients with septic shock and high-dose vasopressor therapy. Ann Intensive Care 2017;7(1):43.
30. Gregoriano C, Heilmann E, Molitor A, et al. Role of procalcitonin use in the man-agement of sepsis. J Thorac Dis 2020;12(Suppl 1):S5–15.
31. Seymour CW, Liu VX, Iwashyna TJ, et al. Assessment of clinical criteria for sepsis: for the third international consensus definitions for sepsis and septic shock (Sepsis-3). JAMA 2016;315(8):762–74.
32. Kimmoun A, Novy E, Auchet T, et al. Hemodynamic consequences of severe lactic acidosis in shock states: from bench to bedside. Crit Care 2015;19:175.
33. Beesley SJ, Weber G, Sarge T, et al. Septic Cardiomyopathy. Crit Care Med 2018;46(4):625–34.

34. George P, Srivastava MC, Ludmir J, et al. Augmenting Function for Infarction from Infection: Impella 2.5 for Ischemic Cardiogenic Shock Complicating Sepsis. Case Rep Cardiol 2017;2017:8407530.

35. Cecconi M, De Backer D, Antonelli M, et al. Consensus on circulatory shock and hemodynamic monitoring. Task force of the European Society of Intensive Care Medicine. Intensive Care Med 2014;40(12):1795–815.

36. Cecconi M, Parsons AK, Rhodes A. What is a fluid challenge? Curr Opin Crit Care 2011;17(3):290–5.

37. Seymour CW, Gesten F, Prescott HC, et al. Time to Treatment and Mortality during Mandated Emergency Care for Sepsis. N Engl J Med 2017;376(23): 2235–44.

38. Evans L, Rhodes A, Alhazzani W, et al. Surviving Sepsis Campaign: International Guidelines for Management of Sepsis and Septic Shock 2021. Crit Care Med 2021;49(11):e1063–143.

39. Malbrain M, Van Regenmortel N, Saugel B, et al. Principles of fluid management and stewardship in septic shock: it is time to consider the four D's and the four phases of fluid therapy. Ann Intensive Care 2018;8(1):66.

40. Hamzaoui O, Scheeren TWL, Teboul JL. Norepinephrine in septic shock: when and how much? Curr Opin Crit Care 2017;23(4):342–7.

41. Russell JA, Wellman H, Walley KR. Vasopressin versus norepinephrine in septic shock: a propensity score matched efficiency retrospective cohort study in the VASST coordinating center hospital. J Intensive Care 2018;6:73.

42. Gordon AC, Mason AJ, Thirunavukkarasu N, et al. Effect of Early Vasopressin vs Norepinephrine on Kidney Failure in Patients With Septic Shock: The VANISH Randomized Clinical Trial. JAMA 2016;316(5):509–18.

43. Tumlin JA, Murugan R, Deane AM, et al. Outcomes in Patients with Vasodilatory Shock and Renal Replacement Therapy Treated with Intravenous Angiotensin II. Crit Care Med 2018;46(6):949–57.

44. Wieruszewski PM, Wittwer ED, Kashani KB, et al. Angiotensin II Infusion for Shock: A Multicenter Study of Postmarketing Use. Chest 2021;159(2):596–605.

45. Ham KR, Boldt DW, McCurdy MT, et al. Sensitivity to angiotensin II dose in patients with vasodilatory shock: a prespecified analysis of the ATHOS-3 trial. Ann Intensive Care 2019;9(1):63.

46. Senatore F, Jagadeesh G, Rose M, et al. FDA Approval of Angiotensin II for the treatment of hypotension in adults with distributive shock. Am J Cardiovasc Drugs 2019;19(1):11–20.

47. Chow JH, Wittwer ED, Wieruszewski PM, et al. Evaluating the evidence for angiotensin II for the treatment of vasoplegia in critically ill cardiothoracic surgery patients. J Thorac Cardiovasc Surg 2022;163(4):1407–14.

48. Evans L, Rhodes A, Alhazzani W, et al. Surviving sepsis campaign: international guidelines for management of sepsis and septic shock 2021. Intensive Care Med 2021;47(11):1181–247.

49. Mikhail I, Stukus DR, Prince BT. Fatal anaphylaxis: epidemiology and risk factors. Curr Allergy Asthma Rep 2021;21(4):28.

50. Brown SG. The pathophysiology of shock in anaphylaxis. Immunol Allergy Clin N Am 2007;27(2):165–75.

51. Wyckoff MH, Singletary EM, Soar J, et al. 2021 International consensus on cardiopulmonary resuscitation and emergency cardiovascular care science with treatment recommendations: summary from the basic life support; advanced life support; neonatal life support; education, implementation, and teams; first

aid task forces; and the COVID-19 working group. Resuscitation 2021;169: 229–311.

52. Passia E, Jandus P. Using baseline and peak serum tryptase levels to diagnose anaphylaxis: a review. Clin Rev Allergy Immunol 2020;58(3):366–76.

53. Cha YS, Kim H, Bang MH, et al. Evaluation of myocardial injury through serum troponin I and echocardiography in anaphylaxis. Am J Emerg Med 2016;34(2): 140–4.

54. Wei J, Zhang L, Ruan X, et al. Case report: takotsubo syndrome induced by severe anaphylactic reaction during anesthesia induction and subsequent high-dose epinephrine resuscitation. Front Cardiovasc Med 2022;9:842440.

55. Soar J, Pumphrey R, Cant A, et al. Emergency treatment of anaphylactic reactions–guidelines for health care providers. Resuscitation 2008;77(2):157–69.

56. Chan-Dominy AC, Anders M, Millar J, et al. Extracorporeal membrane modality conversions. Perfusion 2015;30(4):291–4.

57. Ruiz IA, Squair JW, Phillips AA, et al. Incidence and natural progression of neurogenic shock after traumatic spinal cord injury. J Neurotrauma 2018; 35(3):461–6.

58. Furlan JC, Fehlings MG, Shannon P, et al. Descending vasomotor pathways in humans: correlation between axonal preservation and cardiovascular dysfunction after spinal cord injury. J Neurotrauma 2003;20(12):1351–63.

59. Casha S, Christie S. A systematic review of intensive cardiopulmonary management after spinal cord injury. J Neurotrauma 2011;28(8):1479–95.

60. Hadley MN, Walters BC, Grabb PA, et al. Blood pressure management after acute spinal cord injury. Neurosurgery 2002;50(3 Suppl):S58–62.

61. Martin ND, Kepler C, Zubair M, et al. Increased mean arterial pressure goals after spinal cord injury and functional outcome. J Emerg Trauma Shock 2015; 8(2):94–8.

62. Hurlbert RJ, Hadley MN, Walters BC, et al. Pharmacological therapy for acute spinal cord injury. Neurosurgery 2015;76(Suppl 1):S71–83.

63. Hochman JS, Sleeper LA, Webb JG, et al. Early revascularization in acute myocardial infarction complicated by cardiogenic shock. SHOCK Investigators. Should We Emergently Revascularize Occluded Coronaries for Cardiogenic Shock. N Engl J Med 1999;341(9):625–34.

64. Ponikowski P, Voors AA, Anker SD, et al. 2016 ESC Guidelines for the diagnosis and treatment of acute and chronic heart failure: The Task Force for the diagnosis and treatment of acute and chronic heart failure of the European Society of Cardiology (ESC)Developed with the special contribution of the Heart Failure Association (HFA) of the ESC. Eur Heart J 2016;37(27):2129–200.

65. Thiele H, Zeymer U, Neumann FJ, et al. Intraaortic balloon support for myocardial infarction with cardiogenic shock. N Engl J Med 2012;367(14):1287–96.

66. Vahdatpour C, Collins D, Goldberg S. Cardiogenic shock. J Am Heart Assoc 2019;8(8):e011991.

67. van Diepen S, Katz JN, Albert NM, et al. Contemporary management of cardiogenic shock: a scientific statement from the american heart association. Circulation 2017;136(16):e232–68.

68. Jentzer JC, van Diepen S, Barsness GW, et al. Cardiogenic shock classification to predict mortality in the cardiac intensive care unit. J Am Coll Cardiol 2019; 74(17):2117–28.

69. Baran DA, Grines CL, Bailey S, et al. SCAI clinical expert consensus statement on the classification of cardiogenic shock: This document was endorsed by the American College of Cardiology (ACC), the American Heart Association (AHA),

the Society of Critical Care Medicine (SCCM), and the Society of Thoracic Surgeons (STS) in April 2019. Catheter Cardiovasc Interv 2019;94(1):29–37.

70. Harjola VP, Lassus J, Sionis A, et al. Clinical picture and risk prediction of short-term mortality in cardiogenic shock. Eur J Heart Fail 2015;17(5):501–9.

71. Javanainen T, Tolppanen H, Lassus J, et al. Predictive value of the baseline electrocardiogram ST-segment pattern in cardiogenic shock: Results from the Card-Shock Study. Ann Noninvasive Electrocardiol 2018;23(5):e12561.

72. Mueller C, McDonald K, de Boer RA, et al. Heart failure association of the european society of cardiology practical guidance on the use of natriuretic peptide concentrations. Eur J Heart Fail 2019;21(6):715–31.

73. Rueda F, Borras E, Garcia-Garcia C, et al. Protein-based cardiogenic shock patient classifier. Eur Heart J 2019;40(32):2684–94.

74. Picano E, Scali MC, Ciampi Q, et al. Lung ultrasound for the cardiologist. JACC Cardiovasc Imaging 2018;11(11):1692–705.

75. Palmeri ST, Lowe AM, Sleeper LA, et al. Racial and ethnic differences in the treatment and outcome of cardiogenic shock following acute myocardial infarction. Am J Cardiol 2005;96(8):1042–9.

76. Dooley DJ, Lam PH, Ahmed A, et al. The role of positive inotropic drugs in the treatment of older adults with heart failure and reduced ejection fraction. Heart Fail Clin 2017;13(3):527–34.

77. Mathew R, Di Santo P, Jung RG, et al. Milrinone as compared with dobutamine in the treatment of cardiogenic shock. N Engl J Med 2021;385(6):516–25.

78. Masip J, Peacock WF, Price S, et al. Indications and practical approach to non-invasive ventilation in acute heart failure. Eur Heart J 2018;39(1):17–25.

79. Alviar CL, Miller PE, McAreavey D, et al. Positive pressure ventilation in the cardiac intensive care unit. J Am Coll Cardiol 2018;72(13):1532–53.

80. Basir MB, Schreiber TL, Grines CL, et al. Effect of early initiation of mechanical circulatory support on survival in cardiogenic shock. Am J Cardiol 2017;119(6):845–51.

81. Parrillo JD,RP. Critical care medicine: principles of diagnosis and management in the adult. 5th edition. Philadelphia: Elsevier; 2019.

82. De Backer D, Biston P, Devriendt J, et al. Comparison of dopamine and norepinephrine in the treatment of shock. N Engl J Med 2010;362(9):779–89.

83. Baig M, Nada K, Aboueisha A, et al. An atypical cause of obstructive shock. Am J Respir Crit Care Med 2021;203(4):e7–8.

84. Grip O, Wanhainen A, Bjorck M. Acute Aortic Occlusion. Circulation 2019;139(2):292–4.

85. Gropper MA, Miller RD, Eriksson LI, et al. Miller's anesthesia. 9th ed. edition. Philadelphia: Elsevier; 2019.

86. Standl T, Annecke T, Cascorbi I, et al. The Nomenclature, Definition and Distinction of Types of Shock. Dtsch Arztebl Int 2018;115(45):757–68.

87. Haseer Koya H, Paul M. Shock. In: StatPearls. Treasure Island: FL; 2022.

88. Vincent J-L, Abraham E, Kochanek P, et al. Textbook of critical care. 6th edition. Philadelphia: Elsevier; 2011.

89. Roberts DJ, Leigh-Smith S, Faris PD, et al. Clinical Presentation of Patients With Tension Pneumothorax: A Systematic Review. Ann Surg 2015;261(6):1068–78.

90. Leigh-Smith S, Harris T. Tension pneumothorax–time for a re-think? Emerg Med J 2005;22(1):8–16.

91. Alrajab S, Youssef AM, Akkus NI, et al. Pleural ultrasonography versus chest radiography for the diagnosis of pneumothorax: review of the literature and meta-analysis. Crit Care 2013;17(5):R208.

92. Ka FHL, Hagopian L, Wayman D, et al. Sonographic diagnosis of pneumo-thorax. J emergencies, Trauma Shock 2012;5(1).
93. Kulvatunyou N, Erickson L, Vijayasekaran A, et al. Randomized clinical trial of pigtail catheter versus chest tube in injured patients with uncomplicated trau-matic pneumothorax. Br J Surg 2014;101(2):17–22.
94. Chang SH, Kang YN, Chiu HY, et al. A Systematic Review and Meta-Analysis Comparing Pigtail Catheter and Chest Tube as the Initial Treatment for Pneumo-thorax. Chest 2018;153(5):1201–12.
95. Little WC, Freeman GL. Pericardial disease. Circulation 2006;113(12):1622–32.
96. Fink RJ. Pneumopericardium causing pericardial tamponade. Clin Case Rep 2020;8(12):3571–2.
97. Shabetai R. Pericardial effusion: haemodynamic spectrum. Heart 2004;90(3): 255–6.
98. Adekile A, Adegoroye A, Tedla F, et al. Chylothorax and chylopericardial tampo-nade in a hemodialysis patient with catheter-induced superior vena cava steno-sis. Semin Dial 2009;22(5):576–9.
99. Teboul J-L, Monnet X, Chemla D, et al. Arterial pulse pressure variation with me-chanical ventilation 2018.
100. Malahfji M, Arain S. Reversed Pulsus Paradoxus in Right Ventricular Failure. Methodist Debakey Cardiovasc J 2018;14(4):298–300.
101. Alerhand S, Carter JM. What echocardiographic findings suggest a pericardial effusion is causing tamponade? Am J Emerg Med 2019;37(2):321–6.
102. Kaplan JA, Cronin B, Maus T. Kaplan's essentials of cardiac anesthesia for car-diac surgery. Second edition. Philadelphia, PA: Elsevier; 2018.
103. Coutance G, Cauderlier E, Ehtisham J, et al. The prognostic value of markers of right ventricular dysfunction in pulmonary embolism: a meta-analysis. Crit Care 2011;15(2):R103.
104. Natanzon SS, Fardman A, Chernomordik F, et al. PESI score for predicting clin-ical outcomes in PE patients with right ventricular involvement. Heart Vessels 2022;37(3):489–95.
105. Fields JM, Davis J, Girson L, et al. Transthoracic Echocardiography for Diag-nosing Pulmonary Embolism: A Systematic Review and Meta-Analysis. J Am Soc Echocardiogr 2017;30(7):714–723 e714.
106. Patel VI, Miles M, Shahangian S, et al. McConnell's sign: Echocardiography in the management of acute pulmonary embolism. Clin Case Rep 2021;9(10): e04994.
107. Walsh BM, Moore CL. McConnell's Sign Is Not Specific for Pulmonary Embolism: Case Report and Review of the Literature. J Emerg Med 2015;49(3):301–4.
108. Squizzato A, Galli L, Gerdes VE. Point-of-care ultrasound in the diagnosis of pul-monary embolism. Crit Ultrasound J 2015;7:7.
109. Kearon C, Akl EA, Ornelas J, et al. Antithrombotic therapy for VTE disease: chest guideline and expert panel report. Chest 2016;149(2):315–52.
110. Neely RC, Byrne JG, Gosev I, et al. Surgical embolectomy for acute massive and submassive pulmonary embolism in a series of 115 patients. Ann Thorac Surg 2015;100(4):1245–51 ; discussion 1251-1242.
111. Wright C, Goldenberg I, Schleede S, et al. Effect of a multidisciplinary pulmo-nary embolism response team on patient mortality. Am J Cardiol 2021;161: 102–7.
112. Witkin AS, Harshbarger S, Kabrhel C. Pulmonary embolism response teams. Semin Thromb Hemost 2016;42(8):857–64.
113. Taghavi S, Askari R. Hypovolemic Shock. In: StatPearls. Treasure Island: FL; 2022.

114. Cannon JW. Hemorrhagic Shock. N Engl J Med 2018;378(4):370–9.
115. White NJ, Ward KR, Pati S, et al. Hemorrhagic blood failure: Oxygen debt, coagulopathy, and endothelial damage. J Trauma Acute Care Surg 2017;82(6S Suppl 1):S41–9.
116. McNeil-Masuka J, Boyer TJ. Insensible Fluid Loss. In: StatPearls. Treasure Island: FL; 2022.
117. Hui C, Khan M, Radbel JM. Diabetes Insipidus. In: StatPearls. Treasure Island: FL; 2022.
118. Hoffman M, Cichon LJ. Practical coagulation for the blood banker. Transfusion 2013;53(7):1594–602.
119. Johansson PI, Henriksen HH, Stensballe J, et al. Traumatic Endotheliopathy: A Prospective Observational Study of 424 Severely Injured Patients. Ann Surg 2017;265(3):597–603.
120. Barbee RW, Reynolds PS, Ward KR. Assessing shock resuscitation strategies by oxygen debt repayment. Shock 2010;33(2):113–22.
121. Zhang Q, Raoof M, Chen Y, et al. Circulating mitochondrial DAMPs cause inflammatory responses to injury. Nature 2010;464(7285):104–7.
122. Ishikura H, Kitamura T. Trauma-induced coagulopathy and critical bleeding: the role of plasma and platelet transfusion. J Intensive Care 2017;5(1):2.
123. Surgeons ACo. Stop the bleed. American College of Surgeons. Available at: https://www.stopthebleed.org/about-us/. Accessed June 27, 2022.
124. Nichols R, Horstman J. Recommendations for Improving Stop the Bleed: A Systematic Review. Mil Med 2022;187(11–12):e1338–45.
125. Spahn DR, Bouillon B, Cerny V, et al. The European guideline on management of major bleeding and coagulopathy following trauma: fifth edition. Crit Care 2019; 23(1):98.
126. Cantle PM, Cotton BA. Balanced resuscitation in trauma management. Surg Clin North Am 2017;97(5):999–1014.
127. Khanna AK, Karamchandani K. Macrocirculation and Microcirculation: the "batman and superman" story of critical care resuscitation. Anesth Analg 2021;132(1):280–3.
128. Baran DA, Grines CL, Bailey S, et al. SCAI clinical expert consensus statement on the classification of cardiogenic shock: this document was endorsed by the American College of Cardiology (ACC), the American Heart Association (AHA), the Society of Critical Care Medicine (SCCM), and the Society of Thoracic Surgeons (STS) in April 2019. Catheter Cardiovasc Interv 2019;94(1):29–37.
129. Bourcier S, Villie P, Nguyen S, et al. Venoarterial extracorporeal membrane oxygenation support rescue of obstructive shock caused by bulky compressive mediastinal cancer. Am J Respir Crit Care Med 2020;202(8):1181–4.
130. Adi O, Ahmad AH, Fong CP, et al. Shock due to superior vena cava obstruction detected with point of care ultrasound. Am J Emerg Med 2021;48:374 e371–3.
131. Mehanna MJ, Israel GM, Katigbak M, et al. Cardiac herniation after right pneumonectomy: case report and review of the literature. J Thorac Imaging 2007; 22(3):280–2.
132. Parlow S, Cheung M, Verreault-Julien L, et al. An unusual case of obstructive shock. JACC Case Rep 2021;3(18):1913–7.
133. Pereira BM. Abdominal compartment syndrome and intra-abdominal hypertension. Curr Opin Crit Care 2019;25(6):688–96.
134. Mendelson J. Emergency department management of pediatric shock. Emerg Med Clin North Am 2018;36(2):427–40.

Perioperative Management of the Acute Stroke Patient

From Door to Needle to NeuroICU

Alisha Bhatia, MD[a],*, Jerrad Businger, MD[b]

KEYWORDS

- Ischemic stroke • Mechanical thrombectomy • Anesthesia • Perioperative
- Critical care • Outcome

KEY POINTS

- Initial assessment, stabilization, and resuscitation are essential to optimize perfusion to affected areas of the brain.
- Treatment of acute ischemic stroke with intravenous tissue-type plasminogen activator is beneficial for select patients up to 4.5 hours after onset of symptoms, while, beyond this window, mechanical thrombectomy in selected patients may improve disability outcomes.
- Anesthesia technique should be tailored to the individual but general anesthesia can be implemented without concerns if strict adherence to intraprocedural blood pressure management with systolic blood pressure goals greater than 140 mm Hg is maintained.
- Postoperative optimization of physiology is crucial and hypotension, hypovolemia, hypoxemia hyperthermia, and hyperglycemia should be treated aggressively.

INTRODUCTION

Stroke is a leading cause of death and disability in the United States. Approximately 795,000 individuals suffer from a new or recurrent stroke in the United States each year.[1] Although early recognition of symptoms is essential for seeking timely care, knowledge of these symptoms as well as risk factors for developing stroke is lacking among the general population. Initial neurologic assessment for acute ischemic stroke (AIS), stabilization, and resuscitation are essential to optimize perfusion to affected areas of the brain.[2] According to the American Heart Association/American Stroke Association, these initial assessments and treatments are best performed through

[a] Department of Anesthesiology, Rush University Medical Center, 1645 West Congress Parkway, Jelke 736, Chicago, IL 60612, USA; [b] Division of Anesthesia Critical Care, Anesthesia Critical Care, University of Louisville Hospital, 530 S. Jackson Street/ RM. C2A01, Louisville, KY 40202, USA
* Corresponding author.
E-mail address: Alisha_bhatia@rush.edu

Anesthesiology Clin 41 (2023) 27–38
https://doi.org/10.1016/j.anclin.2022.11.001
1932-2275/23/© 2022 Elsevier Inc. All rights reserved.

multidisciplinary collaboration. On arrival to the hospital, emergency medicine, neurology, neurointerventional, and anesthesia teams play essential roles in the evaluation of patients with acute ischemic stroke (AIS) and treatment with intravenous (IV) and intra-arterial therapies.

PREOPERATIVE CONSIDERATIONS

Treatment of AIS with IV tissue-type plasminogen activator has proven to be beneficial for select patients up to 4.5 hours after onset of symptoms.[3] The greatest benefits, including reduced in-hospital mortality, reduced symptomatic intracerebral hemorrhage, and increased independent ambulation at discharge occur when the drug is administered early after stroke onset and decline with time. The DAWN (DWI or CTP Assessment with Clinical Mismatch in the Triage of Wake-Up and Late Presenting Strokes Undergoing Neurointervention with Trevo) trial demonstrated that mechanical thrombectomy beyond this initial window, within 6 to 24 hours of last known well, in patients with clinical deficits that are disproportionately severe relative to the infarct volume, also had improved disability outcomes at 90 days.[4]

Initial assessment of an AIS patient should include a complete history and physical, if possible, with prompt attention to any airway and circulatory needs, and completion of the National Institutes of Health Stroke Scale (NIHSS), as shown in **Table 1**.[5] All patients should undergo imaging to evaluate for intracranial hemorrhage before initiation of IV thrombolysis. Due to the time-sensitive nature of these interventions, noncontrast head computerized tomography (CT) is effective.[6] MRI can be useful in instances in which the onset of symptoms is unclear, for example, in "wake up" strokes or if the time at which the individual was last known to be well is unknown. However, immediate care should not be delayed for this form of imaging.[7] Noninvasive vessel imaging is recommended for patients who meet criteria for mechanical thrombectomy. CT angiogram has been shown to be more accurate than magnetic resonance angiogram, so it is reasonable to pursue this study before obtaining laboratory studies in patients who do not have a history of renal failure.[8] The Alberta Stroke Program Early CT Score (ASPECTS) measures the early extent of ischemic changes on imaging. When applied to noncontract head CTs, it correlates with the extent of final infarct on follow-up imaging in patients with large vessel occlusion (LVO).[9] A normal brain has an ASPECTS of 10, and the score falls as more areas are affected by infarct. A complete middle cerebral artery (MCA) infarct would have a score of 0. An increase in dependence for activities of daily living is seen with an ASPECTS of 7 or less. Multiple studies have demonstrated that with an ASPECTS of 6 or greater, no additional perfusion studies are needed before thrombectomy.[10,11] Additional workup, including blood glucose, troponin, and electrocardiogram, can also be obtained for patients with AIS but should not preclude the initiation of thrombolytics.

During assessment for thrombolytics, patients should also be assessed for all resuscitative needs, including respiratory and hemodynamic support. Blood glucose should be checked to ensure that neurologic symptoms are not due to hypoglycemia or hyperglycemia. Supplemental oxygen should be provided as needed but only to treat hypoxia. Intubation should not be delayed in patients with potential airway compromise. Hypotension and hypovolemia should be avoided in all patients with AIS.[12] In patients receiving thrombolytics, systolic blood pressure (SBP) should be lowered to less than 185 mm Hg and diastolic blood pressure (DBP) should be lowered to less than 110 mm Hg before treatment to decrease the risk of hemorrhagic transformation of the stroke.[13] Patients who are outside the window for thrombolytics but going for mechanical thrombectomy likely also benefit from these blood pressure

Table 1
National institutes of health stroke scale score

1a. Level of consciousness	0. Alert, responsive 1. Not alert, but arousable by minor stimulation 2. Not alert, requires repeated stimulation 3. Unresponsive or responds only with reflex
1b. Level of consciousness questions (month? age?)	0. Both answers correct 1. Answers one question correctly 2. Answers neither question correctly
1c. Level of consciousness commands (open/close eyes, grip and release hand)	0. Performs both tasks correctly 1. Performs one task correctly 2. Performs neither task correctly
2. Best gaze	0. Normal 1. Partial gaze palsy 2. Forced deviation
3. Visual	0. No visual loss 1. Partial hemianopia 2. Complete hemianopia 3. Bilateral hemianopia
4. Facial palsy	0. Normal symmetric movements 1. Minor paralysis 2. Partial paralysis 3. Complete paralysis of one or both sides
5. *Motor arm* 5a. Left arm 5b. Right arm	0. No drift 1. Drift 2. Some effort against gravity 3. No effort against gravity 4. No movement
6. *Motor leg* 6a. Left leg 6b. Right leg	0. No drift 1. Drift 2. Some effort against gravity 3. No effort against gravity 4. No movement
7. Limb ataxia	0. Absent 1. Present in 1 limb 2. Present in 2 limbs
8. Sensory	0. Normal, no sensory loss 1. Mild-to-moderate sensory loss 2. Severe-to-total sensory loss
9. Best language	0. Normal, no aphasia 1. Mild-to-moderate aphasia 2. Severe aphasia 3. Mute, global aphasia
10. Dysarthria	0. Normal 1. Mild-to-moderate dysarthria 2. Severe dysarthria
11. Extinction and inattention	0. No abnormality 1. Visual, tactile, auditory, spatial, or personal inattention 2. Profound hemi-inattention or extinction
Total score—0–42	

parameters.[14] Blood pressure control for these patients can be accomplished by any medications that the patient will tolerate, most commonly used antihypertensives are the beta-adrenergic and calcium-channel blockers labetalol and nicardipine, respectively. All efforts should be made to avoid hyperthermia and hyperglycemia because these are both associated with worse outcomes after AIS.[15]

After receiving thrombolytics, patients should be monitored for adverse effects, including bleeding complications and angioedema.

Indications for mechanical thrombectomy with a stent retriever include prestroke modified ranking scale (mRS) score of 0 to 1, causative occlusion of the internal carotid artery or MCA segment 1, age greater than or equal to 18 years, NIHSS score of greater than or equal to 6, ASPECTS score of greater than or equal to 6, and initiation within 6 hours of symptom onset.[16] Direct aspiration thrombectomy was found to be noninferior to stent retriever in patients meeting the same criteria.[17] For patients with lesions in the more distal MCA territory, anterior cerebral artery, vertebral arteries, basilar arteries, posterior cerebral arteries and/or worse mRS and ASPECTS scores, mechanical thrombectomy with stent retriever is also a reasonable option within 6 hours of symptom onset but the data is not as strong as that of the initially proposed criteria. Mechanical thrombectomy is also recommended for patients with AIS at 6 to 16 hours after symptom onset if they have anterior circulation occlusions or meet the DAWN or DEFUSE 3 (Endovascular Therapy Following Imaging Evaluation for Ischemic Stroke) trial criteria. It is reasonable to pursue mechanical thrombectomy up to 24 hours from last known well.[18]

The goal of mechanical thrombectomy is to achieve reperfusion of the infarcted territory, defined by a modified Thrombolysis in Cerebral Infarction score of 2B or 3 (**Table 2**).

Intraoperative Considerations

In patients presenting with LVO in the anterior circulation, the standard of care incorporates mechanical thrombectomy along with medical management if all eligibility requirements are met.[19] Despite this notion, the anesthetic management for patients undergoing mechanical thrombectomy remains unsettled.

General anesthesia and monitored anesthesia care each have unique advantages and disadvantages (**Table 3**). General anesthesia ensures a secured airway reducing aspiration risk and better control of patient movement during the procedure. Advantages of monitored anesthetic care include the potential for direct neurologic assessment of the patient, shorter time period to intervention, and less anesthetic-induced hemodynamic fluctuations. Main disadvantages of general anesthesia are the increased time from door-puncture time and intraprocedural hemodynamic lability, specifically hypotensive episodes. However, disadvantages of monitored anesthetic care include increased patient discomfort, respiratory compromise (eg, aspiration

Table 2	
Modified thrombolysis in cerebral infarction scale	
0	No Reperfusion
1	Flow beyond occlusion but not to distal branches
2a	Reperfusion of less than half of downstream territory
2b	Reperfusion of more than half of downstream territory
3	Complete reperfusion of territory distally

Table 3		
Advantages and disadvantages of general anesthesia and conscious sedation		
	General Anesthesia	**Conscious Sedation**
Pros	Ensures a secured airway reducing aspiration risk Better control of patient movement during the procedure	Direct neurologic assessment of the patient Shorter time period to intervention Less anesthetic-induced hemodynamic fluctuations
Cons	Increased time from door-puncture time Intraprocedural hemodynamic lability, specifically hypotensive episodes Inability to directly assess patients neurologically	Increased patient discomfort Potential for respiratory compromise (eg, aspiration risk, hypoxia) Patient movement leading to increased intraprocedural time

risk, hypoxia), and patient movement leading to increased intraprocedural time. In these regards, the ramifications of anesthetic choice on patient outcomes remain a point of ongoing evaluation.

To date, the medical literature offers mixed results regarding this question. Initial retrospective, cohort studies showed general anesthesia to be inferior to conscious sedation resulting in worse neurologic outcomes and mortality.[20–22] In contrast, 4 subsequent single-centered randomized trials comparing general anesthesia to conscious sedation and its effects on functional outcome concluded that general anesthesia was not inferior to conscious sedation with functional outcome either the same or improved in the patients undergoing general anesthesia.[23–26] General anesthesia did lend to longer times until groin puncture but neither the door-to-reperfusion time nor the duration of the thrombectomy procedure was adversely affected.[27]

It is not definite as to why these polar differences in outcome between the retrospective cohort studies and the prospective randomized trials exist but several deductions can be made. In the randomized controlled trials, there was explicit protocolized management implemented by specialized anesthesia teams where anesthetic drug regimens and cardiopulmonary parameters were reported. Hemodynamic parameters among both the general anesthesia and conscious sedation arms in the randomized trials maintained SBP greater than 140 mm Hg.[28] This adheres to consensus guidelines where the recommendation is for SBP to be maintained between 140 and 180 mm Hg with mean arterial pressure (MAP) greater than or equal to 70 mm Hg (**Table 4**).[29] In contrast, neither there were formal protocols specifying anesthetics and analgesics nor was documented intraprocedural hemodynamics within the retrospective cohort studies.

Subsequent meta-analyses have revealed mixed conclusions as well. Several meta-analyses evaluating the results of the cohort studies and randomized controlled trials concluded that patients undergoing nongeneral anesthesia for mechanical thrombectomy had both better functional outcomes at 3 months and lower 3-month mortality compared with those undergoing general anesthesia.[24,30] Inclusion of the nonrandomized trials is likely the reason for this. However, 3 meta-analyses isolated the randomized controlled trials and concluded that patients undergoing general anesthesia compared with conscious sedation had significantly less disability at 3 months and more functional independence.[29,31,32] Additionally, general anesthesia was also associated with higher rates of successful recanalization and no significant differences in mortality were appreciated.[32,33]

Most recently, a 2022 multicentered randomized controlled trial with the focus on standardized anesthetic management and intraoperative hemodynamic control was

Table 4		
Hemodynamic management of patients presenting for mechanical thrombectomy		
Preprocedural Management	Intraprocedural Management	Postprocedural Management
Goal <185/110 mm Hg for tPA and MT candidates[36] Avoidance of hypotension a. Potential reduction in functional outcome with reductions of SBP >50 mm Hg and abrupt reductions >30 mm Hg[42] b. Increased mortality associated with SBP <110 mm Hg[43]	Goal SBP 140–180 mm Hg[31] Ensure MAP >70 mm Hg[31]	TICI 2 b/3 SBP <160 mm Hg If intracerebral hemorrhage present SBP <140 mm Hg[44,45] TICI 0-2a SBP <180/105 mm Hg for ≥24 h[36]

conducted. The primary outcome was 3-month functional outcomes.[33] Patients were randomized to either general anesthesia or conscious sedation. Patients in the general anesthesia arm were induced with etomidate (0.25–0.4 mg/kg) and then a target-controlled propofol infusion (maximum target 4 µg/mL) and remifentanil (0.5–4 ng/mL) and succinylcholine (1 mg/kg). Patients in the conscious sedation group received target-controlled infusions of remifentanil (max target, 2 ng/mL) and local anesthesia with lidocaine 10 mg/mL (max 10 mL). In both arms, blood pressure management was standardized using norepinephrine for a goal SBP range of 140 to 185 mm Hg and DBP less than 110 mm Hg. Postoperatively, blood pressure targets were again followed and maintained. The primary outcome of functional outcome evaluated at 3 months was similar between the general anesthesia and conscious sedation groups. Again appreciated was the higher hemodynamic lability in the general anesthesia group with more episodes of hypotension but the total duration of hypotension was no different. Technical failure of endovascular therapy was higher in the conscious sedation group. Interestingly, neither the increased incidence of hypotension in the general anesthesia group or the increased failure rate of endovascular therapy in the conscious sedation group altered outcomes at 3 months. Conversion from conscious sedation to general anesthesia occurred in about 5% of cases, with excessive agitation being the primary reason (38%). This is in comparison to prior observed conversion rates of 11.5% with the primary culprit being excessive agitation (43%).[29]

Whether the choice of anesthetic and analgesic agents during LVO thrombectomy has any impact on patient outcome is also unclear. There currently is no evidence or recommendation to support one drug over another. In looking at the randomized controlled trials, the majority used a combination of propofol and remifentanil for both the conscious sedation group and general anesthesia group with the exceptions of AnStroke, which used sevoflurane in the general anesthesia arm, and Goliath, which used fentanyl in the conscious sedation arm. Of note, patients undergoing mechanical thrombectomy typically are older, present with multiple comorbidities, and display some degree of depressed neurologic status with or without aphasia. As a result, the anesthetic doses required for either conscious sedation or general anesthesia have the potential to be less than other situations. This is supported by the dosages used in the randomized trials (**Table 5**).

To date, there is no definite conclusion as to the best anesthetic technique to implement in managing patients with AIS presenting for mechanical thrombectomy.

Table 5
Anesthetic doses utilized in the randomized controlled trials[30]

Trial	General Anesthesia	Conscious Sedation
Siesta	Propofol 49 ± 15 µg/kg/min Remifentanil 0.1 ± 0.06 µg/kg/min	Propofol 14 ± 14 µg/kg/min Remifentanil 0.03 ± 0.03 µg/kg/min
AnStroke	Sevoflurane 0.7 (0.6–0.7) MAC Remifentanil TCI 6 (5–6) ng/mL	Remifentanil TCI 1.3 (1.0–1.7) ng/mL
Goliath	Propofol 56 ± 29 µg/kg/min Remifentanil 0.26 ± 0.13 µg/kg/min	Propofol 35 ± 33 µg/kg/min Fentanyl 0.9 ± 0.5 µg/kg
Canvas Pilot[26]	Sufentanil 0.2 µg/kg bolus Propofol TCI (1–4 µg/mL) Remifentanil 0.1–0.2 µg/kg/min	Sufentanil 0.1 µg/kg bolus Propofol TCI (0.5–1 µg/mL)
GASS Trial[33]	Etomidate 0.25–0.4 mg/kg Propofol TCI Max target 4 µg/mL Remifentanil TCI 2.6 ± 1.1 (0.5–4 ng/mL)	Remifentanil TCI 1.4 ± 0.7 (Max target 2 ng/mL)

The likelihood that patient outcomes following mechanical thrombectomy are reliant on one variable alone (eg, general anesthesia vs conscious sedation) is rather unlikely but instead a multitude of factors are likely responsible. Based on the current data, anesthesiologists can implement general anesthesia without concern for causing detrimental effects on patient outcomes if strict adherence to intraprocedural blood pressure management with an SBP goal of greater than 140 mm Hg is maintained. In the end, the anesthetic must be tailored individually, being mindful of the clinical characteristics of each patient, location of the stroke, and difficulty of the procedure.[34]

Postoperative Considerations

Postthrombectomy in-hospital management includes early institution of essential secondary prevention measures. Aspirin should be administered to patients with AIS within 24 to 48 hours of symptoms, or 24 hours after fibrinolytics.[35] It can be administered rectally or via nasogastric tube in patients who are intubated or are deemed unsafe to swallow. The CHANCE (Clopidogrel in High-Risk Patients with Acute Non-disabling Cerebrovascular Events) and POINT (Platelet-Oriented Inhibition in New TIA and Minor Ischemic Stroke) trials have demonstrated the efficacy of dual antiplatelet therapy with aspirin and clopidogrel for 21 days to reduce recurrence of ischemic stroke for up to 90 days after the initial event in patients with NIHSS less than 3 who did not receive thrombolytics but are at high risk for ischemic events.[36,37]

Although the exact parameters for patient optimization are unknown, hypotension, hypovolemia, and hypoxemia should be avoided and often corrected in patients with AIS.[38] Hypertension should also be avoided. Acute correction of hypertension may be necessary in patients with certain preexisting or comorbid conditions, such as heart failure, preeclampsia, or dissection. For those without these conditions, hypertension should be treated slowly to avoid compromising cerebral perfusion to ischemic areas of the brain. Hyperthermia and hyperglycemia should also be treated as both are associated with worse outcome after AIS.[17] With the goal of starting nutrition within 7 days of admission, patients with AIS should be screened for dysphagia to determine if they are at risk for aspiration.[39]

Cerebral edema can be significant in patients with large territorial cerebral and cerebellar infarcts, leading to herniation. Goals of care conversations should be held early with patients or their next of kin or legal representative in case emergent decompressive surgery is needed.[40] For patients with malignant cerebral edema due to an MCA infarction, decompressive hemicraniectomy decreases mortality and disability at 12 months. For cerebellar infarctions causing obstructive hydrocephalus, ventriculostomy can be considered before suboccipital decompressive hemicraniectomy.[41] Recurrent seizures after AIS should be treated with antiepileptic agents but they are not required for prophylaxis.

SUMMARY

In summary, the management of patients with stroke can be complex and is best performed through multidisciplinary collaboration. On arrival to the hospital, initial neurologic assessment, resuscitation, and stabilization are essential to optimize perfusion to affected areas of the brain, and treatment with IV tissue-type plasminogen activator can improve survival if initiated early and up to 4.5 hours after onset of symptoms. Beyond this initial window, mechanical thrombectomy may improve disability outcomes of patients with clinical deficits that are disproportionately severe relative to the infarct volume. To date, there is no definite conclusion as to the best anesthetic technique to implement in managing patients presenting for mechanical thrombectomy. Both general anesthesia and monitored anesthetic care have advantages and disadvantages and the anesthetic technique should be tailored to the individual being mindful of the clinical characteristics of each patient, the location of the stroke, and difficulty of the procedure. General anesthesia can be implemented without concern for causing detrimental effects on patient outcomes if strict adherence to intraprocedural blood pressure management with SBP goals greater than 140 mm Hg is maintained. Postoperative optimization of physiology is crucial and hypotension, hypovolemia, hypoxemia, hyperthermia, and hyperglycemia should be treated aggressively. Despite best efforts, cerebral edema can occur during the postoperative period and may require emergent decompressive surgery.

DISCLOSURE

Neither author has any disclosures

CLINICS CARE POINTS

- Treatment of AIS with IV tissue-type plasminogen activator has proven to be beneficial for select patients up to 4.5 hours after onset of symptoms. The greatest benefits, including reduced in-hospital mortality, reduced symptomatic intracerebral hemorrhage, and increased independent ambulation at discharge, occur when the drug is administered early after stroke onset, and decline with time.

- In patients receiving thrombolytics, systolic blood pressure (SBP) should be lowered to less than 185 mm Hg and diastolic blood pressure (DBP) should be lowered to less than 110 mmHg prior to treatment to decrease the risk of hemorrhagic transformation of the stroke.

- In patients presenting with large vessel occlusion in the anterior circulation, the standard of care incorporates mechanical thrombectomy along with medical management if all eligibility requirements are met.

- General anesthesia and monitored anesthesia care each have unique advantages and disadvantages. To date, there is no definite conclusion as to the best anesthetic technique to implement in managing patients with AIS presenting for mechanical thrombectomy.

- Though the exact parameters for patient optimization are unknown, hypotension, hypovolemia, and hypoxemia should be avoided and often corrected in patients with AIS.

REFERENCES

1. Virani SS, Alonso A, Benjamin EJ, et al. on behalf of the American Heart Association Council on Epidemiology and Prevention Statistics Committee and Stroke Statistics Subcommittee. Heart disease and stroke statistics–2020 update: a report from the American Heart Association. Circulation 2020;141: e139–596.
2. Powers WJ, Rabinstein AA, Ackerson T, et al. Guidelines for the Early Management of Patients with Acute Ischemic Stroke: 2019 Update to the 2018 Guidelines for the Early Management of Acute Ischemic Stroke. A Guideline for Healthcare Professionals From the American Heart Association/American Stroke Association. Stroke 2019;50:e344–418.
3. Hacke W, Kaste M, Bluhmki E, et al. ECASS Investigators. Thrombolysis with alteplase 3 to 4.5 hours after acute ischemic stroke. N Engl J Med 2008;359: 1317–29.
4. Nogueira RG, Jadhav AP, Haussen DC, et al. DAWN Trial Investigators. Thrombectomy 6 to 24 hours after stroke with a mismatch between deficit and infarct. N Engl J Med 2018;378:11–21.
5. Adams HP Jr, Davis PH, Leira EC, et al. Baseline NIH Stroke Scale score strongly predicts outcome after stroke: a report of the Trial of Org 10172 in Acute Stroke Treatment (TOAST). Neurology 1999;53:126–31.
6. Wardlaw JM, Seymour J, Cairns J, et al. Immediate computed tomography scanning of acute stroke is cost-effective and improves quality of life. Stroke 2004;35: 2477–83.
7. Thomalla G, Simonsen CZ, Boutitie F, et al. WAKE-UP Investigators. MRI-guided thrombolysis for stroke with unknown time of onset. N Engl J Med 2018;379: 611–22.
8. Bash S, Villablanca JP, Jahan R, et al. Intracranial vascular stenosis and occlusive disease: evaluation with CT angiography, MR angiography, and digital subtraction angiography. AJNR Am J Neuroradiol 2005;26:1012–21.
9. Mokin M, Primiani CT, Siddiqui AH, et al. ASPECTS (alberta stroke program early ct score) measurement using hounsfield unit values when selecting patients for stroke thrombectomy. Stroke 2017;48:1574–9.
10. Campbell BC, Mitchell PJ, Kleinig TJ, et al, EXTEND-IA Investigators. Endovascular therapy for ischemic stroke with perfusion-imaging selection. N Engl J Med 2015;372:1009–18.
11. Bracard S, Ducrocq X, Mas JL, et al. Mechanical thrombectomy after intravenous alteplase versus alteplase alone after stroke (THRACE): a randomised controlled trial. Lancet Neurol 2016;15:1138–47.
12. Wohlfahrt P, Krajcoviechova A, Jozifova M, et al. Low blood pressure during the acute period of ischemic stroke is associated with decreased survival. J Hypertens 2015;33:339–45.
13. Mazya M, Egido JA, Ford GA, et al, for the SITS Investigators. Predicting the risk of symptomatic intracerebral hemorrhage in ischemic stroke treated with

intravenous alteplase: Safe Implementation of Treatments in Stroke (SITS) symptomatic intracerebral hemorrhage risk score. Stroke 2012;43:1524–31.

14. Goyal M, Demchuk AM, Menon BK, et al. ESCAPE Trial Investigators. Randomized assessment of rapid endovascular treatment of ischemic stroke. N Engl J Med 2015;372:1019–30.

15. Saxena M, Young P, Pilcher D, et al. Early temperature and mortality in critically ill patients with acute neurological diseases: trauma and stroke differ from infection. Intensive Care Med 2015;41:823–32.

16. Goyal M, Menon BK, van Zwam WH, et al, HERMES Collaborators. Endovascular thrombectomy after large-vessel ischaemic stroke: a meta-analysis of individual patient data from five randomised trials. Lancet 2016;387:1723–31.

17. Turk AS 3rd, Siddiqui A, Fifi JT, et al. Aspiration thrombectomy versus stent retriever thrombectomy as first-line approach for large vessel occlusion (COMPASS): a multicentre, randomised, open label, blinded outcome, non-inferiority trial. Lancet 2019;393:998–1008.

18. Albers GW, Marks MP, Kemp S, et al. DEFUSE 3 Investigators. Thrombectomy for stroke at 6 to 16 hours with selection by perfusion imaging. N Engl J Med 2018; 378:708–18.

19. Mokin M, Ansari SA, McTaggart RA, et al. Indications for thrombectomy in acute ischemic stroke from emergent large vessel occlusion (ELVO): report of the SNIS Standards and Guidelines Committee. J Neurointerv Surg 2019; 11(3):215–20.

20. Abou-Chebl A, Lin R, Hussain MS, et al. Conscious sedation versus general anesthesia during endovascular therapy for acute anterior circulation stroke: preliminary results from a retrospective, multicenter study. Stroke 2010;41(6):1175–9.

21. Abou-Chebl A, Yeatts SD, Yan B, et al. Impact of General Anesthesia on Safety and Outcomes in the Endovascular Arm of Interventional Management of Stroke (IMS) III Trial. Stroke 2015;46(8):2142–8.

22. Campbell BCV, van Zwam WH, Goyal M, et al. Effect of general anaesthesia on functional outcome in patients with anterior circulation ischaemic stroke having endovascular thrombectomy versus standard care: a meta-analysis of individual patient data. Lancet Neurol 2018;17(1):47–53.

23. Schonenberger S, Uhlmann L, Hacke W, et al. Effect of conscious sedation vs general anesthesia on early neurological improvement among patients with ischemic stroke undergoing endovascular thrombectomy: a randomized clinical trial. JAMA 2016;316(19):1986–96.

24. Lowhagen Henden P, Rentzos A, Karlsson JE, et al. General anesthesia versus conscious sedation for endovascular treatment of acute ischemic stroke: the anstroke trial (anesthesia during stroke). Stroke 2017;48(6):1601–7.

25. Simonsen CZ, Yoo AJ, Sorensen LH, et al. Effect of general anesthesia and conscious sedation during endovascular therapy on infarct growth and clinical outcomes in acute ischemic stroke: a randomized clinical trial. JAMA Neurol 2018;75(4):470–7.

26. Sun J, Liang F, Wu Y, et al. Choice of anesthesia for endovascular treatment of acute ischemic stroke (canvas): results of the canvas pilot randomized controlled trial. J Neurosurg Anesthesiol 2020;32(1):41–7.

27. Schonenberger S, Henden PL, Simonsen CZ, et al. Association of general anesthesia vs procedural sedation with functional outcome among patients with acute ischemic stroke undergoing thrombectomy: a systematic review and meta-analysis. JAMA 2019;322(13):1283–93.

28. Hindman BJ, Dexter F. Anesthetic Management of Emergency Endovascular Thrombectomy for Acute Ischemic Stroke, Part 2: Integrating and Applying Observational Reports and Randomized Clinical Trials. Anesth Analg 2019; 128(4):706–17.

29. Talke PO, Sharma D, Heyer EJ, et al. Society for Neuroscience in Anesthesiology and Critical Care Expert consensus statement: anesthetic management of endovascular treatment for acute ischemic stroke*: endorsed by the Society of Neuro-Interventional Surgery and the Neurocritical Care Society. J Neurosurg Anesthesiol 2014;26(2):95–108.

30. Goyal N, Malhotra K, Ishfaq MF, et al. Current evidence for anesthesia management during endovascular stroke therapy: updated systematic review and meta-analysis. J Neurointerv Surg 2019;11(2):107–13.

31. Campbell D, Diprose WK, Deng C, et al. General anesthesia versus conscious sedation in endovascular thrombectomy for stroke: a meta-analysis of 4 randomized controlled trials. J Neurosurg Anesthesiol 2021;33(1):21–7.

32. Zhang Y, Jia L, Fang F, et al. General anesthesia versus conscious sedation for intracranial mechanical thrombectomy: a systematic review and meta-analysis of randomized clinical trials. J Am Heart Assoc 2019;8(12):e011754.

33. Maurice A, Eugene F, Ronziere T, et al. General Anesthesia versus Sedation, Both with Hemodynamic Control, during Intraarterial Treatment for Stroke: The GASS Randomized Trial. Anesthesiology 2022;136(4):567–76.

34. Powers WJ, Rabinstein AA, Ackerson T, et al. 2018 Guidelines for the early management of patients with acute ischemic stroke: a guideline for healthcare professionals from the american heart association/american stroke association. Stroke 2018;49(3):e46–110.

35. Sandercock PA, Counsell C, Tseng MC, et al. Oral antiplatelet therapy for acute ischaemic stroke. Cochrane Database Syst Rev 2014;CD000029.

36. Wang Y, Wang Y, Zhao X, et al. CHANCE Investigators. Clopidogrel with aspirin in acute minor stroke or transient ischemic attack. N Engl J Med 2013;369:11–9.

37. Johnston SC, Easton JD, Farrant M, et al, Clinical Research Collaboration. Neurological emergencies treatment trials network, and the POINT Investigators. Clopidogrel and aspirin in acute ischemic stroke and high-risk TIA. N Engl J Med 2018; 379:215–25.

38. Lee M, Ovbiagele B, Hong KS, et al. Effect of blood pressure lowering in early ischemic stroke: meta-analysis. Stroke 2015;46:1883–9.

39. Miles A, Zeng IS, McLauchlan H, et al. Cough reflex testing in Dysphagia following stroke: a randomized controlled trial. J Clin Med Res 2013;5:222–33.

40. Vahedi K, Hofmeijer J, Juettler E, et al, Decimal, Destiny, and Hamlet Investigators. Early decompressive surgery in malignant infarction of the middle cerebral artery: a pooled analysis of three randomised controlled trials. Lancet Neurol 2007;6:215–22.

41. Mostofi K. Neurosurgical management of massive cerebellar infarct outcome in 53 patients. Surg Neurol Int 2013;4:28.

42. Silver B, Lu M, Morris DC, et al. Blood pressure declines and less favorable outcomes in the NINDS tPA stroke study. J Neurol Sci 2008;271(1–2):61–7.

43. Maier B, Gory B, Taylor G, et al. Mortality and disability according to baseline blood pressure in acute ischemic stroke patients treated by thrombectomy: a collaborative pooled analysis. J Am Heart Assoc 2017;6(10). https://doi.org/10.1161/JAHA.117.006484silv.

44. Jovin TG, Saver JL, Ribo M, et al. Diffusion-weighted imaging or computerized tomography perfusion assessment with clinical mismatch in the triage of wake up and late presenting strokes undergoing neurointervention with Trevo (DAWN) trial methods. Int J Stroke 2017;12(6):641–52.

45. Goyal N, Tsivgoulis G, Pandhi A, et al. Blood pressure levels post mechanical thrombectomy and outcomes in large vessel occlusion strokes. Neurology 2017;89(6):540–7.

Traumatic Brain Injury
Intraoperative Management and Intensive Care Unit Multimodality Monitoring

Krassimir Denchev, MD[a], Jonathan Gomez, MD, MS[b],
Pinxia Chen, MD[c], Kathryn Rosenblatt, MD, MHS[b,d],*

KEYWORDS

- Traumatic brain injury • Multimodality neuromonitoring • Intracranial pressure
- Cerebral autoregulation • Brain tissue oxygen monitoring • Transcranial doppler
- Near-infrared spectroscopy • Cerebral microdialysis

KEY POINTS

- Management of patients with traumatic brain injury (TBI) entails the trauma triage, cardio-pulmonary stabilization, and diagnostic imaging with targeted interventions, which may consist of decompressive hemicraniectomy, intraventricular or intraparenchymal monitors or drains, and pharmacologic agents to reduce intracranial pressure.
- Anesthesia and intensive care of patients with TBI requires control of multiple systems and physiologic variables and incorporates evidence-based practices to reduce secondary brain injury.
- Advances in biomedical engineering and technology have enhanced assessments of intracranial pressure and cerebral oxygenation, blood flow, metabolism, and autoregulation and many specialized centers currently use multimodality neuromonitoring for targeted therapies with the hope to improve TBI recovery.

INTRODUCTION

Traumatic brain injury (TBI) is heterogeneous, effects all populations worldwide, and spares no age groups.[1] Identifying and halting ongoing effects of the primary trauma, preventing secondary brain injury, and managing extracranial complications related to TBI require multidisciplinary and interdisciplinary efforts. A clear and organized

[a] Department of Anesthesiology, Wayne State University, 44555 Woodward Avenue, SJMO Medical Office Building, Suite 308, Pontiac, MI 48341, USA; [b] Department of Anesthesiology & Critical Care Medicine, Johns Hopkins University School of Medicine, 600 North Wolfe Street, Phipps 455, Baltimore, MD 21287, USA; [c] Department of Anesthesiology and Critical Care Medicine, St. Luke's University Health Network, 801 Ostrum Street, Bethlehem, PA 18015, USA; [d] Department of Neurology, Johns Hopkins University School of Medicine, 600 North Wolfe Street, Phipps 455, Baltimore, MD 21287, USA
* Corresponding author.
E-mail address: krosenb3@jhmi.edu

Anesthesiology Clin 41 (2023) 39–78
https://doi.org/10.1016/j.anclin.2022.11.003
1932-2275/23/© 2022 Elsevier Inc. All rights reserved.

approach is essential in all aspects of management. Early anesthesiologist and intensivist involvement in the care of the acute traumatic brain-injured patient is not uncommon and may begin in the emergency department, with resuscitation continuing in the operating room and intensive care unit.[2] Knowledge of the physiologic principles of acute brain injury is essential to understanding current evidence-supported treatment guidelines and allows for sound clinical judgment in areas where current evidence is lacking. This article reviews the best practices of intraoperative management and current recommendations for intensive care monitoring of TBI patients, hence focusing on moderate and severe TBI. First, the epidemiology, pathophysiology, and classification of TBI are discussed, followed by the key elements of early stabilization and intraoperative anesthesia care during decompressive hemicraniectomy and/or extracranial surgery. Finally, noninvasive and invasive intervention-based monitoring modalities and targeted physiologic variables are reviewed.

EPIDEMIOLOGY

TBI is a leading cause of death and disability worldwide with a global prevalence of over 50 million annually and 69 million new cases each year.[3] In 2020, there were over 64,000 TBI-related deaths in the United States.[4] TBI is defined as an alteration in brain function or other evidence of brain pathology caused by an external force.[5] This force may be blunt (closed head) or penetrating. Most of the civilian TBI is caused by falls or motor vehicle collisions, with the burden of TBI from falls in elderly people on the rise in high-income countries and the number of TBI from traffic accidents increasing in low- and middle-income countries.[6,7] In combat areas, TBI mainly results from violent impact, ballistic penetration, or explosive device exposure.[8] Although penetrating TBI and blast injuries are less common than closed head and non-blast injuries in the civilian population, they are often more lethal and have different pathophysiologic mechanisms of injury and clinical courses.

Clinical Classification

Classifying TBI etiologically by its physical mechanism (ie, causative force) is popular in the prevention and public health fields. Alternatively, TBI can be stratified by pathoanatomic type, pathophysiological process (primary vs secondary injury), or by clinical indices of severity at presentation.[9,10] The latter symptom-based system stratifies patients based on neurologic injury severity and is used most often in clinical research for trial inclusion criteria and to compare patients among centers. Owing to its simplicity, rapidity, relatively high interobserver reliability, and generally good prognostic capabilities, the Glasgow Coma Scale (GCS) is the most recognized and widely used neurologic injury severity scale for adult TBI patients[11–14] (Table 1). Patients are divided into the broad categories of mild (GCS 13–15), moderate (GCS 9–12), and severe (GCS 3–8) injury, which represents the total sum of the component subscale scores. Reporting of the GCS component subscale scores is important in detecting changes in consciousness and may better predict morbidity and functional outcome at the individual level.

Pathophysiological Classification

The pathophysiology-based classification of TBI into primary and secondary injury is important when directing therapy. Primary injury refers to the initial insult, and the processes set in motion by the immediate parenchymal damage occurring at the time of injury. Primary brain injury consists of focal contusions; intraparenchymal, intraventricular, or extra-axial hemorrhage; focal or global cerebral edema; and shearing of white

Table 1 Glasgow coma scale		
Behavior	**Response**	**Score**
Eye opening	Spontaneously	4
	To speech	3
	To pain	2
	No response	1
Best verbal response	Oriented	5
	Confused	4
	Inappropriate	3
	Incomprehensible	2
	No response	1
Best motor response	Obeys commands	6
	Localizes to pain	5
	Withdraws from pain	4
	Flexes to pain (decorticate)	3
	Extends to pain (decerebrate)	2
	No response	1
Total	Severe	3–8
	Moderate	9–12
	Mild	13–15

A multidimensional consciousness assessment scale based on three different aspects of response; examiners rate patients' best eye opening, verbal, and motor responses at presentation and subsequent assessments.

matter tracts leading to diffuse axonal injury. The primary injury incites a cascade of biomolecular changes related to the body's inflammatory response to the initial trauma, termed secondary injury, which may begin within seconds and can last for days but is potentially avoidable. Disruption of intracranial or extracranial blood vessel endothelium causes hemorrhage, swelling, and subsequent thrombosis and vasospasm, which decreases cerebral perfusion and leads to ischemia.[15] This also increases blood brain barrier (BBB) permeability for cytokine-releasing inflammatory cells, which promote apoptosis. In addition, cellular membrane disruption leads to ionic dysregulation, free radial production, necrosis, mitochondrial dysfunction, and release of glutamate, which has an excitotoxic effect on neurons and glial cells. The release of tissue factor and phospholipids into the systemic circulation leads to consumptive coagulopathy, hemorrhage expansion, and intravascular thromboses.[16,17] These mechanisms all contribute to cerebral edema and increased intracranial pressure (ICP), which further exacerbate ischemia and brain injury.

Systemic effects contributing to secondary injury include hypertension and hypercarbia, which increases ICP due to impaired cerebrovascular autoregulation; hypotension or hypoxia, which prevents delivery of oxygen and glucose, further contributing to ischemia and acidosis; hyperthermia and seizures, which increase metabolic demands; hyperglycemia, which further leads to acidosis in setting of ischemia and anaerobic metabolism; and infections. Neurosurgical intervention to halt or relieve effects of the primary injury may be part of the initial management or occur later in response to secondary injury. Although the main focus of intensive care is the prevention, identification, and management of secondary brain injury, similar measures must be taken in the perioperative period.

Owing to the heterogeneity of TBI, current classification schemes lack the detailed characterization necessary for precise treatment choices and accurate prognostic modeling in all patients. Recent focus on developing noninvasive blood-based biomarkers,[18] unified TBI phenotyping,[19] improved neuroimaging classification systems,[20] and advanced neuroimaging techniques[21] for rapid assessment of TBI severity and pathophysiology may change current practices and improve prognostication.

PERIOPERATIVE MANAGEMENT

Management of TBI is multifold, interdisciplinary and begins immediately at the time of injury. National and international guidelines support a standardized approach to management of severe TBI which begins in the prehospital setting and continues through the intensive care unit stay in efforts to improve outcomes. The Advanced Trauma Life Support (ATLS) protocols and Emergency Neurologic Life Support guide initial diagnostic assessments and early management of TBI, whereas the fourth and latest edition of evidence-based guidelines released by the Brain Trauma Foundation (BTF) provide recommendations for subsequent interventions, clinical thresholds for treatment, and monitoring.[22–24]

When presenting for emergent intracranial or extracranial surgery, neurologically targeted interventions should coincide with relentless resuscitation of the circulatory and respiratory systems because hypotension and hypoxia are the key systemic insults associated with secondary brain injury and worse outcomes.[25,26] If time allows, hemodynamic stability should be obtained and preoxygenation initiated before induction and airway manipulation.

Airway

Patients sustaining TBI may require tracheal intubation for a variety of factors.[27] Depression of consciousness is associated with an inability to protect the airway and lungs from aspiration, maintain airway patency, and ensure adequate ventilatory drive.[28] The BTF guidelines recommend intubation in all TBI patients with GCS less than 9 as well as those with GCS of 9 or greater if there is rapid deterioration, concomitant severe body injury, or impending procedures that necessitate airway protection and mechanical ventilation.[22] Up to 30% of TBI patients have associated facial and neck injuries with the potential for disturbing both airway patency and protection.[29,30]

For patients with acute TBI and suspected cervical spine injury who require intubation, the standard of care is rapid sequence intubation (RSI) with in-line spinal immobilization.[23] These patients will have a semirigid cervical collar in place, which follows ATLS guidelines, and a properly performed jaw thrust may be used to maintain airway patency during mask ventilation.[23] Of note, the reverse Trendelenburg position or elevation of the head of the bed to 30° to 45° is a routine maneuver initiated in the care of TBI patients and is often essential in those with known elevated ICP and impending cerebral herniation to permit adequate venous drainage from the brain without compromising cerebral perfusion. This position, however, may worsen hypotension in patients with high spinal cord injury. The removal of a cervical collar may also assist in venous drainage and reduction of ICP. Manual in-line cervical spine immobilization with an assistant standing at the head of the bed or reaching across the chest can be performed with the anterior portion of a rigid collar removed and is associated with less movement of the spine during intubation than collar immobilization alone. Video laryngoscopy may provide better views of the glottis in less time than conventional laryngoscopy when performed in a neutral neck position unless blood or secretions compromise image clarity.[31]

Breathing

Nearly every organ and organ system can be affected after TBI, yet lungs may be the most vulnerable. Mechanisms of lung injury in TBI include neurogenic pulmonary edema, autonomic dysfunction, inflammation, neurotransmitter dysregulation, and immune suppression.[32] Direct injury to the chest in multi-organ trauma victims and initiation of mechanical ventilation insight further lung damage.

In the absence of cerebral herniation and ICP crisis, BTF guidelines recommend tight regulation of oxygenation and ventilation with the goal of normalizing physiologic parameters (oxygen saturation [SpO_2] > 90%; arterial partial pressure of carbon dioxide [$PaCO_2$] 35–45 mm Hg).[22] Carbon dioxide is a potent mediator of vasomotor tone. The relationship between $PaCO_2$ and cerebral blood flow (CBF) is nearly linear in normal physiologic ranges (ie, $PaCO_2$ 20 mm Hg to 80 mm Hg); for each 1 mm Hg increase or decrease in $PaCO_2$, there is a 2% to 4% increase or decrease in CBF.[33,34] Respiratory hypercapnia or hypocapnia leads to relaxation or contraction of the cerebral vasculature through associated changes in cerebrospinal fluid (CSF) pH and also directly by PCO_2 within CSF and arterial blood.[35] Nitric oxide, prostaglandins, cyclic nucleotides, intracellular calcium, and potassium channel activity are also important mediators of cerebrovascular reactivity to carbon dioxide.[33] In patients with limited intracranial compliance, increased CBF results in increased cerebral blood volume and elevation in ICP.

Unlike $PaCO_2$, arterial partial pressure of oxygen (PaO_2) has little influence on CBF in normal physiologic ranges (ie, 60 mm Hg to 300 mm Hg). Severe hypoxemia (PaO_2 < 60 mm Hg), however, can precipitate a dramatic increase in CBF.[36] A reduction in arterial oxygen content increases CBF through hypoxia-induced release of nitric oxide and its metabolites, opening of ATP-dependent K^+ channels in vascular smooth muscle leading to hyperpolarization and vasodilation and stimulation of the rostral ventrolateral medulla.[36] Thus, hypoxia contributes to not just ischemia but also hyperemia, which commonly coexist in TBI patients and is compounded by abnormal flow-metabolism and disturbed autoregulation.[37]

Therefore, targeting oxygen saturations greater than 90% ensures a PaO_2 greater than 60 mm Hg, which reduces secondary brain injury from both hypoxia and hyperemia. Likewise, maintaining normocapnia ($PaCO_2$ 35–45 mm Hg) avoids cerebral ischemia and hyperemia. In the operating room, continuous capnography is a good surrogate for measuring $PaCO_2$ with the caveat that the $PaCO_2$ and end-tidal CO_2 ($EtCO_2$) gradient [P(a-Et)CO_2] is increased from its normal gradient of 2 to 5 mm Hg with increased physiologic dead space.[38] Discordance between $PaCO_2$ and $EtCO_2$ is a concern in TBI patients with severe chest trauma, hypotension, and metabolic acidosis.[39]

Therapeutic hyperventilation, a commonly used maneuver in the practice of neuro-anesthesia, reduces brain volume and elevated ICP by manipulating autoregulatory functions connected to cerebrovascular CO_2 reactivity. If there are clinical signs of imminent cerebral herniation (eg, new unilaterally or bilaterally dilated pupils) or refractory intracranial hypertension (eg, ICP sustained > 22 mm Hg for > 5 min), hyperventilation can be initiated as a temporary measure until the ICP crisis resolves. However, this maneuver may not influence the likelihood of neurologic recovery and instead may elicit or augment cerebral ischemia.[40] Hypocapnia-induced vasoconstriction reduces CBF and volume and thus ICP but also oxygen supply. Oxygen delivery to the brain is also reduced because of hypocapnia-induced leftward shift of the oxyhemoglobin dissociation curve. To compound this, hyperventilation effects metabolic activity. Hypocapnia increases neuronal excitability, which increases oxygen and glucose consumption.[41,42] Such imbalance of supply and demand of oxygen can substantially increase the risk of cerebral ischemia.[43] Furthermore, in patients with impaired CO_2 reactivity, as can be seen in severe TBI, hyperventilation may have less predictable effects on ICP reduction.[44]

Therefore, BTF guidelines do not recommend prophylactic hyperventilation below a $PaCO_2$ of 25 mm Hg, especially in the first 24 to 48 hours after TBI when CBF is often critically reduced.[22] A reduction of $EtCO_2$ to 25 to 30 mm Hg ($PaCO_2$ 28–35 mm Hg) is a reasonable temporizing measure during an ICP crisis, although there is limited evidence to support even very short durations (less than 30 minutes) of therapeutic hyperventilation. Finally, although high-quality evidence is lacking, BTF recommends the use of multimodality monitoring (MMM) of cerebral oxygenation and metabolism, such as jugular venous oxygen saturation or brain tissue oxygen partial pressure, during therapeutic hyperventilation to prevent ischemia.[22]

Optimal ventilatory strategies in TBI patients have not yet been established, likely related to the exclusion of this population from the major trials investigating the effect of lung-protective ventilation. The traditional approach with low positive end-expiratory pressures (PEEP) and high tidal volumes for tight CO_2 control in TBI patients has recently been reevaluated given the improved outcomes seen with lung-protective strategies (ie, low tidal volumes, moderate-to-high PEEP) in both acute respiratory distress syndrome (ARDS) and non-ARDS patients.[45,46] Although PEEP reduces atelectasis and improves PaO_2 and lung compliance, PEEP may induce lung overdistension in patients with normal lung compliance, thus reducing cerebral venous return and increasing ICP.[47,48] Elevated PEEP may also reduce systemic venous return and consequently cerebral perfusion pressure (CPP), especially in the setting of impaired autoregulation.[49]

An international survey investigating ventilatory management of TBI patients found that low tidal volumes with a $PaCO_2$ target of 36 to 40 mm Hg and a PaO_2 target of 81 to 100 mm Hg are frequently used with lower levels of PEEP used in cases of elevated ICP.[45] Despite limited scientific evidence, recent guidelines from the European Society of Intensive Care Medicine (ESICM) on mechanical ventilation settings for patients with acute brain injury concur with this practice. ESICM recommends that in patients without significant ICP elevation (and with or without concurrent ARDS), the same lung-protective strategies and the level of PEEP should be used as in patients without brain injury.[50] In patients with clinically significant ICP elevation, ESICM recommends the same level of PEEP be used as in patients without acute brain injury if ICP is PEEP-insensitive (ie, if ICP does not increase after a trial of increased PEEP). ESICM further recommends an optimal target PaO_2 of 80 to 120 mm Hg in acute brain injured patients with or without clinically significant ICP elevation and to target a $PaCO_2$ of 35 to 45 mm Hg in the latter scenario but short-term therapeutic hyperventilation is recommended in the former scenario of elevated ICP (**Table 2**).

Circulation

In TBI patients, the circulatory system can be affected either directly via trauma (eg, chest injury, acute blood loss) or indirectly via a neurogenic phenomenon (stress-induced catecholamine surge), inflammatory process affecting cardiac myocytes, coronary hypoperfusion from trauma-related hypotension, or consumptive coagulopathy from BBB breakdown with release of brain tissue factor, phospholipids, and tissue-type plasminogen activator into the systemic circulation.[17,51] Clinical manifestations of cardiovascular dysfunction in TBI patients include, but are not limited to, neurogenic stress cardiomyopathy, arrhythmias, left ventricular dysfunction, subendocardial ischemia, intravascular microthrombosis and hypocoagulability akin to disseminated intravascular coagulation (DIC), and persistent autonomic dysregulation. The latter often presents as paroxysmal sympathetic hyperactivity or "storming," a phenomenon characterized by paroxysms of hyperthermia, tachycardia, tachypnea, hypertension, diaphoresis, and posturing and is seen in up to 33% of TBI patients.[52]

Table 2
Recommendations of the European Society of Intensive Care Medicine consensus of mechanical ventilation in patients with acute brain injury

Domain	Consensus Recommendation	Level of Recommendation	Level of Evidence
Should we use specific mechanical ventilation settings (eg, tidal volume/PBW; PEEP; FiO_2) and target-specific respiratory physiologic parameters (eg, Pplat) in patients with ABI?	We recommend that in mechanically ventilated patients with ABI who do not have clinically significant ICP elevation, the same level of PEEP should be used as in patients without brain injury	Strong recommendation	Very low evidence in favor
	We recommend that in mechanically ventilated patients with ABI who have clinically significant ICP elevation that is PEEP-insensitive, the same level of PEEP should be used as in patients without ABI	Strong recommendation	No evidence
	We recommend that in mechanically ventilated patients with concurrent ABI and ARDS who do not have clinically significant ICP elevation, a strategy of lung-protective mechanical ventilation should be used	Strong recommendation	No evidence
	We suggest that in mechanically ventilated patients with ABI without clinically significant ICP elevation, a strategy of lung-protective mechanical ventilation should be considered	Weak recommendation	No evidence
	We are unable to provide a recommendation regarding lung-protective mechanical ventilation in mechanically ventilated patients with ABI who have clinically significant ICP elevation	No recommendation	No evidence

(continued on next page)

Table 2
(continued)

Domain	Consensus Recommendation	Level of Recommendation	Level of Evidence
Should we target specific values of pH, PaO_2 and $PaCO_2$ in patients with ABI?	We are unable to provide a recommendation regarding lung-protective mechanical ventilation in mechanically ventilated patients who have concurrent ABI, ARDS, and clinically significant ICP elevation	No recommendation	No evidence
	We recommend that the optimal target range of PaO_2 in patients with ABI who do not have clinically significant ICP elevation is 80–120 mm Hg	Strong recommendation	Contradictory low-quality evidence
	We recommend that the optimal target range of PaO_2 in patients with ABI who have clinically significant ICP elevation is 80–120 mm Hg	Strong recommendation	No evidence
	We recommend that the optimal target range of $PaCO_2$ in patients with ABI who do not have clinically significant ICP elevation is 35–45 mm Hg	Strong recommendation	Low-quality evidence
	We recommend hyperventilation as a therapeutic option in patients with ABI who have brain herniation	No recommendation	No evidence
	We are unable to provide a recommendation regarding the use of hyperventilation as a therapeutic option in patients with ABI who have clinically significant ICP elevation	Weak recommendation	No evidence

Abbreviations: ABI, acute brain injury; ARDS, acute respiratory distress syndrome; ICP, intracranial pressure; PaO_2, partial pressure of oxygen; PBW, predicted body weight; PEEP, positive end-expiratory pressure; $PaCO_2$, partial pressure of carbon dioxide; PaO_2, partial pressure of oxygen.
From Robba C, Poole D, McNett M, et al. Mechanical ventilation in patients with acute brain injury: recommendations of the European Society of Intensive Care Medicine consensus. Intensive Care Med. 2020;46(12):2397-2410; with permission from Springer.

Hypotension of all etiologies contributes to secondary brain injury and is a major determinate of poor clinical outcome after TBI.[25,26] Anesthesiologists may consider point-of-care ultrasound in TBI patients to evaluate cardiopulmonary function in their approach to treatment of hypotension.[53] This can be especially helpful in elucidating acute neurogenic stress cardiomyopathy (low ejection fraction, basal hypokinesis),[54–56] neurogenic pulmonary edema (diffuse bilateral B lines),[57] and intravascular volume depletion (inferior vena cava distensibility index, left ventricle collapse).[58,59]

In health, cerebral autoregulation maintains constant cerebral perfusion in the face of fluctuating blood pressure through arteriolar vasodilation or vasoconstriction. Blood flow further adapts to changes in energy consumption, cardiac output, carbon dioxide and oxygen levels in the blood, neuronal activity, pressure inside the skull, and other factors. These myogenic, neurogenic, endothelial, and metabolic response-mechanisms are absent or impaired in many patients after TBI.[60,61] When autoregulation is impaired, CBF becomes passive to changes in arterial pressure. Decreases in systemic blood pressure and CPP result in decreases in CBF that may reach ischemic levels, further exacerbating secondary injury.

The updated BTF guidelines, therefore, suggest maintaining systolic blood pressure (SBP) greater than or equal to 100 mm Hg for patients 50 to 69 year old or greater than or equal to 110 mm Hg for patients 15 to 49 or over 79 year old[22] to maintain CPP and reduce the risk of secondary brain injury from hypotension. Although these updated SBP goals are only supported by indirect Class 2 evidence from one large retrospective cohort study and direct albeit low-quality Class 3 evidence from two studies,[26,62,63] even one episode of SBP less than 90 mm Hg in the acute setting has been associated with increased mortality and worse functional outcomes.[64] Performing a large randomized controlled trial to provide Class 1 evidence in this vulnerable patient population would clearly be unethical.

If the TBI patient presenting for surgery has an ICP monitor in situ or one is being placed in the operating room, mean arterial pressure (MAP) should be maintained to achieve a CPP goal of 60 to 70 mm Hg with volume resuscitation followed by vasopressors if necessary (**Fig. 1**).

Hypotensive TBI patients should be administered rapid infusions of isotonic fluids with avoidance of hypotonic and hyponatremic fluids, such as lactated ringers, half normal saline, and glucose-containing solutions, as they may exacerbate cerebral edema. Aggressive fluid administration is especially indicated in TBI patients with shock. Although normal saline is the preferred solution for initial resuscitation in TBI, hypertonic saline (HTS) is also acceptable even in polytrauma TBI patients because it simultaneously reduces cerebral edema and expands intravascular volume.

Hypotensive hemorrhaging TBI patients should be transfused accordingly until bleeding is controlled. Although several studies have demonstrated an association between anemia and poor outcome after TBI,[65,66] transfusion thresholds have not been clearly defined.[67] It is generally recommended to transfuse packed red blood cells to maintain Hb greater than 7 g/dL.[68–70] A large randomized controlled trial showed an association between higher rate of thromboembolic events without improvement in outcomes using a higher Hb threshold of 10 g/dL.[71] However, certain guidelines recommend transfusing to a target of 9 g/dL in patients with TBI who have evidence of cerebral ischemia to improve oxygen delivery.[68]

Treatment of coagulopathy is also essential with rapid reversal of therapeutic anticoagulation when present and supplementing platelets and clotting factors where needed. The antifibrinolytic, tranexamic acid, given as a loading dose (1 g over 10 minutes) and then infusion (1 g over 8 hours), has also been shown to improve survival

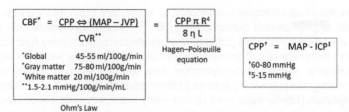

Ohm's Law

Fig. 1. Derivation of cerebrovascular hemodynamic targets. Ohm's law states that flow is proportional to the difference in inflow and outflow pressure divided by the resistance to flow. In the brain, ΔP is cerebral perfusion pressure (CPP), the difference between arterial pressure (ie, inflow pressure) and the pressure in veins (ie, outflow pressure or jugular venous pressure [JVP]). Venous pressure is normally low (2–5 mm Hg). In traumatic brain injury, the intracranial pressure (ICP) surrounding cerebral vessels may be elevated and higher than the JVP. Therefore, ΔP or CPP is calculated as the difference in mean arterial pressure (MAP) and either JVP or ICP, whichever is greater. Cerebral blood flow (CBF) can also be estimated using the Hagen–Poiseuille equation, which describes the relationship between pressure, fluidic resistance, and flow rate and is analogous to Ohm's law. It states that flow is directly related to ΔP, blood viscosity (η), and the length of the vessel (L) and inversely related to radius (R) to the fourth power. Therefore, radius is the most powerful determinant of blood flow, and even small changes in lumen diameter have significant effects on CBF. It is by this mechanism that vascular resistance can change rapidly to alter regional and global CBF. Global CBF averages 50 mL/100 g/min with more blood flow in gray matter than in subcortical white matter. In the face of a declining CBF and therefore oxygen supply, neuronal function deteriorates progressively and a CPP less than 60 mm Hg leads to a rapid decrease in jugular venous bulb saturations representing an increase in oxygen extraction by brain tissue. ICP is normally less than 15 mm Hg in supine adults, and at this ICP, a MAP of 75 mm Hg will provide a CPP of 60 mm Hg.

and outcome in trauma patients as well as in a subgroup of moderate and severe TBI patients when treatment is initiated within 3 hours of injury.[72]

Pharmacologic sedation of any kind may blunt the systemic physiologic protective vasoconstriction that occurs in trauma, which could lead to fluid-unresponsive vasodilation. Severe tissue damage with release of pro-inflammatory mediators also incites vasoplegia.[73,74] Persistent bleeding and hemorrhagic shock in a polytrauma patient may benefit from vasopressors to maintain organ perfusion before attaining surgical hemorrhage control even with early and rapid blood product transfusion. Although early vasopressor use has been associated with increased mortality in trauma patients,[75] its use in certain scenarios, including TBI, is consistent with guidelines on management of major bleeding following trauma.[76]

Evidence to support an optimal vasopressor in TBI is limited. Cerebrovascular α_1 and α_2 adrenoreceptors mediate vasoconstriction and β_1 and β_2 adrenoreceptors mediate vasodilation.[77] Historically, phenylephrine, a selective α_1-adrenergic agonist, has been the most commonly used vasopressor for treatment of hypotension in TBI patients and to maintain CPP.[78] Phenylephrine has a direct vasoconstrictive effect on cerebral precapillary arterioles. Given that cerebrovascular reactivity is believed to occur at the precapillary arteriole level, the impact of phenylephrine on cerebrovascular reactivity and autoregulation may be significant.[78] These interactions may vary based on bolus versus continuous phenylephrine dosing and the patient's autoregulatory capacity.

Norepinephrine is commonly used to restore organ perfusion in hemorrhagic and septic shock yet its value in TBI in contrast to phenylephrine is not clear. Compared with dopamine, norepinephrine use in TBI patients had more predictable and consistent effect on CPP augmentation in one small yet prospective randomized crossover trial.[79] A large single-center retrospective study of severe TBI patients found that patients receiving phenylephrine had a greater increase in MAP and CPP than patients who received norepinephrine or dopamine.[80] In a more recent large multicenter retrospective cohort study of TBI patients who received any vasopressor during the first 2 days of hospital admission, the use of norepinephrine compared with phenylephrine was associated with an increased risk of in-hospital mortality in propensity-matched analysis.[81] This study must be interpreted with caution due to its many limitations; type of shock state and dose effect were not ascertained, and lack of randomization introduced confounding by indication (patients who received norepinephrine were more critically ill).

Vasopressin is also commonly used in trauma patients but is used less frequently and has been studied less in brain-injured patients. There is concern about safety of vasopressin use in TBI from cerebral vasoconstriction via its action on V_1 receptors and water resorption via renal V_2 receptors, which can lead to cerebral ischemia and cerebral edema, respectively. However, small studies in severe TBI patients have not demonstrated increases in ICP or edema with its use.[82,83]

Treating hemodynamic instability in the setting of left ventricular dysfunction and cardiogenic shock related to neurogenic stress cardiomyopathy may require inotropes such as dobutamine or milrinone to maintain CPP.[51,54] An immediate rescue with norepinephrine may be most effective in acute cardiogenic shock scenarios.[53,84,85] In settings when there is little time, equipment, or available expertise to evaluate cardiac function, as is often the case during emergency surgical management of TBI patients with hemorrhagic shock, myocardial dysfunction and left ventricular compromise from increased afterload should be suspected if there is poor response to fluid expansion and norepinephrine administration.[76] In this scenario, inotropic support with dobutamine or epinephrine may be indicated.

Management of dysautonomia related to paroxysmal sympathetic hyperactivity intraoperatively involves symptom elimination in the form of opioids, short-acting benzodiazepines, antipyretics, fluid hydration, beta-blockers, and cooling (removing OR warming devices).[86] Symptom prevention with bromocriptine, gabapentin, baclofen, and long-acting benzodiazepines may be initiated in the intensive care unit and refractory treatment with continuous infusions of propofol, benzodiazepines, opioids, or dexmedetomidine is not uncommon.

Induction

Laryngoscopy and the subsequent reflex sympathetic response can increase ICP during intubation. Fentanyl or lidocaine may be useful in blocking this reflex sympathetic response and increase in ICP that occurs during laryngoscopy, with lidocaine having a lower incidence of hypotension at the cost of decreasing the seizure threshold at higher doses.[87] Propofol's favorable neurologic properties (anticonvulsant, reduced cerebral metabolism) must be weighed against its cardiovascular effects (reduced systemic vascular resistance, venous return, and inotropy) as hypotension may exacerbate a decline in CBF leading to ischemia in TBI patients with impaired autoregulation.[25,88] Etomidate is an alternate choice for induction as it maintains stable hemodynamics and is believed to reduce cerebral oxygen demand and ICP while maintaining CPP. This favorable hemodynamic profile must be weighed against the predilection to lower the seizure threshold and its potential for adrenal insufficiency.[89] Historically, ketamine was avoided in patients with intracranial hypertension due to its sympathomimetic activity, as the resulting hypertension, tachycardia, increased CBF, and increased myocardial and cerebral oxygen consumption were thought to increase ICP. However, this has more recently come into question with data suggesting that CPP may be preserved or improved and that ICP may be unchanged especially when ketamine is delivered in conjunction with GABA agonists.[90–93] Non-depolarizing neuromuscular blocking medications such as rocuronium are preferred over depolarizing agents because they are associated with less increase in ICP. Although the transient increase in ICP with depolarizing agents may not be clinically significant,[94] succinylcholine has been associated with increased mortality if used for RSI in severe TBI patients[95] and can induce an exaggerated and potentially life-threatening intracellular potassium efflux if the TBI patient has been immobile for longer than 24 hours due to upregulation of extra-junctional acetylcholine receptors.[96]

Anesthesia Maintenance

Administration of most anesthetics results in a dose-related reduction in neuronal activity and thus the cerebral metabolic rate of oxygen ($CMRO_2$). Anesthetics modulate cerebral vessel diameter and CBF through such indirect metabolic effects as well through direct effects on vasoactivity. Drugs such as pentobarbital are commonly used anesthetic agents to reduce ICP in cases of refractory intracranial hypertension, as can be seen in severe TBI. The maximum reduction of $CMRO_2$ and cerebral blood volume, and thus ICP, occurs with the dose that results in electrophysiologic silence. At this point, the energy utilization associated with electrophysiologic activity is reduced to zero, but the energy utilization for cellular homeostasis persists unchanged. Additional barbiturates cause no further decrease in CBF or $CMRO_2$. Anesthetics also affect ICP by altering the speed of production and reabsorption of CSF (**Table 3**).

In general, intravenous anesthetics decrease $CMRO_2$ and CBF in parallel, whereas most inhalational anesthetics decrease $CMRO_2$ with an increase in CBF.[97] Despite the evidence of preserved flow-metabolism coupling with both intravenous and inhalational anesthetics, the latter are potent cerebral vasodilators and this direct

Table 3
Anesthetic effects on cerebrovascular physiology and cerebrospinal fluid dynamics

	MAP	CBF	ICP	$CMRO_2$	Direct Cerebral Vasodilation	CSF Reabsorption	CSF Production
Nitrous Oxide (N_2O)	NC	↑↑	↑	↑/NC	No	NC	NC
Isoflurane	↓	↑	↑/NCa	↓↓	Yes	↓/↑	NC
Sevoflurane	↓	↑	↑/NCa	↓↓	Yes	↓	NC
Desflurane	↓	↑	↑/NCa	↓↓	Yes	NC	NC/↑
Benzodiazepines	↓/NC	↓	↓/NC	↓	No	NC/↓	NC/↓
Barbiturates	↓	↓↓↓	↓↓	↓↓↓	No	NC	NC
Propofol	↓	↓↓	↓↓	↓↓	No	NC	NC
Etomidate	NC	↓↓	↓↓	↓↓	No	NC/↑	NC/↓
Ketamine	↑	↑	↑/NC	↑/NC	No	↓	NC
Dexmedetomidine	↓/NC	↓	NC	↓/NC	No	ND	ND

Abbreviations: ↑, increase; ↓, decrease; CBF, cerebral blood flow; $CMRO_2$, cerebral metabolic rate of oxygen; CSF, cerebrospinal fluid; MAP, mean arterial pressure; NC, no change; ND, not determined.
a Cerebral vasculature remains responsive to changes in $PaCO_2$. Therefore, hypocapnia mitigates increases in ICP.

vasodilation surpasses indirect metabolism-induced vasoconstriction, resulting in a higher ratio of $CBF/CMRO_2$ with inhaled agents.[98] Thus, all inhalational agents can theoretically increase ICP, even though they depress oxidative metabolism.

Although nitrous oxide (N_2O) seems to have no direct vasodilating effects,[99] the addition of N_2O to volatile anesthetics seems to increase CBF with no[100] or only a slight increase[101] in $CMRO_2$. When N_2O is paired with intravenous agents, it seems to counteract CBF and $CMRO_2$ reductions typically expected.[101] Overall, N_2O and volatile anesthetics increase ICP, although this effect can be attenuated by hypocapnia.[97]

Among the intravenous anesthetics, ketamine is unique because it increases CBF, which seems to be a result of metabolic stimulation, direct vasodilation, and cholinergic effects.[102,103] Ketamine in isolation can markedly increase ICP. However, its effects on CBF and $CMRO_2$ are attenuated with coadministration of propofol, and in a study of TBI patients sedated with propofol, low- and high-doses of ketamine decreased ICP.[104] When elevations in ICP must be averted and CPP maintained such as often the case in TBI, propofol in combination with opioids or ketamine may be preferable to inhaled anesthetics.[105]

Intraoperative Anesthesia Interventions to Reduce Intracranial Hypertension

Anesthesiologists possess several instruments to achieve ICP reduction and brain relaxation in the intraoperative management of TBI patients. The best treatment of elevated ICP is to address its underlying cause. Yet, even during definitive decompressive hemicraniectomy, TBI patients may suffer additional harm from transcalvarial herniation if the brain is not optimally relaxed before bone removal. TBI patients may present to the OR for emergent, urgent, and even elective extracranial surgery. In all scenarios, an anesthesiologist should assess for signs and symptoms of elevated ICP. These include pupillary changes, vomiting, depressed level of consciousness unrelated to sedation, and Cushing's triad (widened pulse pressure with increasing systolic and decreasing diastolic pressure, bradycardia, irregular breathing). Performing a brief clinical examination and reviewing previously documented neurologic assessments will help guide necessary interventions. No matter what the indication for surgery, a series of steps should be instituted to lessen harm from elevated ICP in TBI patients.

Management can begin with simple maneuvers to reduce iatrogenic causes of intracranial hypertension. Ventilator synchrony reduces intrathoracic pressure, increases preload, reduces the volume of venous blood and CSF in the skull, and enhances CBF. Muscle relaxation may assist in reducing intrathoracic pressure and should be considered if it does not interfere with intraoperative neuromonitoring. Likewise, compression of the internal jugular vein should be avoided because failure of venous outflow to match arterial inflow will result in a progressive rise in intracranial volume and ICP.

The most popular pharmacologic agent to decrease ICP in the intraoperative period is mannitol. Hypertonic solutions like mannitol and HTS work by increasing osmolarity in blood and withdrawing extravascular fluid to the intravascular compartment whereby it is excreted by the kidneys, thus dehydrating brain parenchyma.[106] A study comparing equiosmolar concentrations of mannitol and 3% saline demonstrated comparable effects on ICP reduction.[107] However, HTS had a statistically significant reduction in ICP at 15 and 20 minutes compared with mannitol but the effect on ICP eventually equalized.[107]

Mannitol has two properties: it initially acts as a volume expander and then serves as an osmotic agent. On administration, intravascular volume expands and blood viscosity decreases, which results in augmentation of CBF. Once volume expansion has occurred, osmotic movement of fluid from the cellular compartment to the intravascular compartment begins and results in a decrease in ICP. There are reports of rebound increases in ICP, perhaps when mannitol enters the brain through a disrupted BBB and reverses the osmotic gradient.[108]

Mannitol can be given at doses of 0.25 to 1 g/kg as a bolus dose every 2 to 6 hours as needed or routinely to reduce ICP; the half-life ranges from 90 minutes to 6 hours. Of note, the effect of mannitol on ICP is transient; repeated doses lose their ability to decrease ICP over time. The osmotic effect usually occurs within 15 minutes and peaks at approximately 1 hour. Mannitol can cause a precipitous drop in blood pressure (and CPP) in hypovolemic patients. Therefore, mannitol is relatively contraindicated in hypotensive patients. It also may cause renal damage as serum osmolarity increases.

HTS in bolus doses can also acutely lower ICP and is a good alternative to mannitol in patients who are hypotensive. In the critical care environment, the use of HTS in place of mannitol is increasing. Theoretically, HTS is an ideal resuscitation fluid for patients with head injury and hemorrhagic shock because it can effectively expand intravascular volume while causing osmotic diuresis of the brain.

Importantly, CSF diversion in the operating room is an effective mechanism to reduce ICP. If a TBI patient presents to the OR with an external ventricular drain (EVD) (ie, intraventricular catheter, ventriculostomy) or one is placed in the OR, the anesthesiologist should be familiar with managing the device and draining CSF (Fig. 2). Briefly, EVDs are temporary devices placed into the frontal horn of the lateral ventricle near the foramen of Monro to facilitate external CSF drainage and to monitor ICP and CSF composition.[109]

The Society for Neuroscience in Anesthesiology and Critical Care (SNACC) Task Force for Perioperative Management of External Ventricular Drains and Lumbar Drains set forth guidelines for management and the Neurocritical Care Society offers similar recommendations.[109,110] We refer the readers to the free EVD tutorial available on the SNACC Website www.snacc.org for further guidance and found here: https://snacc.org/wp-content/uploads/2017/03/MARCH_27_2017_EVD_LD_SNACC_Education_Document.pdf.

INTENSIVE CARE UNIT MULTIMODALITY MONITORING

MMM in TBI serves to augment the bedside neurologic examination by integrating specialized brain-monitoring technology with traditional monitoring devices. The goal is to provide clinicians a holistic assessment of brain health, yet sufficient granular time-sensitive information to intervene before irreversible damage occurs. Mitigating the effects of secondary brain injury may require accurate measures of ICP, CPP, CBF, brain tissue oxygenation, cerebral metabolism, and cerebrovascular autoregulation. Intensivists may visualize these physiologic variables at the bedside using invasive, noninvasive, single, or multiparametric devices and real-time data acquisition software that allows both integration and analysis of these parameters, such as ICM+ (University of Cambridge, Cambridge, UK),[111] CNS Monitor (Moberg Solutions, Inc, Ambler, PA),[112] Sickbay (Medical Informatics Corp, Houston, TX),[113] Bedmaster (Excel Medical Electronics, Jupiter, FL),[114] and Root + IRIS + Patient SafetyNet (Masimo, Irvine, CA).[115,116] Several monitoring devices may be inserted in the operating room or be in situ in patients presenting to the operating room. Thus, it is important for both anesthesiologists and intensivists to understand the physiologic principles behind their use and the variables targeted.

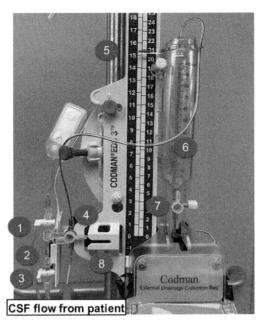

CSF flow from patient

Fig. 2. Components of an external ventricular drain (EVD) collecting system. (1) Stopcock between transducer and air filter. (2) Flushless transducer. (3) Stopcock between pressure tubing and transducer. (4) 3-way stopcock between patient's EVD, pressure tubing, and drip chamber. (5) EVD set at +15 mm Hg "pop-off". (6) Graduated drip chamber (burette) for collecting cerebrospinal fluid. (7) Stopcock between drip chamber and collecting bag. (8) Laser holder for leveling.

Intracranial Pressure

ICP is the most commonly measured cerebral physiologic parameter in TBI management and its elevation, or intracranial hypertension, is an independent predictor of mortality and poor outcome.[117–119] ICP is normally less than 15 mm Hg in supine adults. Elevations of ICP reach clinical significance when they are sustained longer than at least 5 minutes. Pathologic intracranial hypertension is present at pressures greater than or equal to 20 mm Hg, and targeting a goal ICP of less than or equal to 22 mm Hg is recommended for a more favorable outcome after TBI.[22,120] However, a single ICP threshold for all severe TBI may be an oversimplification of a heterogeneous and multifaceted pathophysiological process.[121]

BTF guidelines recommend placement of an ICP monitor for management in TBI patients who remain comatose after resuscitation with a GCS of 3 to 8 and have either (1) abnormalities on cranial CT scan *or* (2) meet at least two of the following three criteria: age greater than 40 years; SBP less than 90 mm Hg; or abnormal posturing.[22] In addition, ICP monitoring is indicated when clinical suspicion of intracranial hypertension exists, when patients worsen to GCS less than 9, or in patients who have moderate TBI without a reliable neurologic examination due to sedation requirements (eg, alternative indications for sedation/anesthesia/analgesia).

Intracranial pressure monitors

Invasive ICP monitoring of TBI patients is classified into two groups: fluid-filled catheter systems, such as the EVD, and microtransducer-tipped catheters.

The EVD connects a catheter whose tip sits in the lateral ventricle to an external strain-gauged fluid-coupled device, which is calibrated at the external auditory meatus, the anatomic landmark of the foramen of Monro. The EVD allows for in-line continuous ICP monitoring as well as simultaneous drainage, although a true and uniformly distributed ICP can only be measured when CSF circulates freely between all ventricles and when the EVD is temporarily clamped off to drainage to facilitate an accurate measure of the pressure in the fluid column.

Alternatively, ICP can be measured with intraparenchymal devices, which consist of a fiberoptic (Camino, Camino Laboratories, San Diego, CA, USA),[122] a piezoelectric strain gauze (Codman, Johnson & Johnson Professional, Inc, Raynham, MA, USA[123]; Raumedic Neurovent-P and S type, Raumedic AG, Helmbrechts, Germany[124]; Pressio, Sophysa, Orsay, France[125]), or a pneumatic (Spiegelberg ICP sensor, Spiegelberg GmbH & Co KG, Hamburg, Germany[126]) transducer at the tip of a thin cable. The monitor is typically inserted into the white matter of the nondominant frontal hemisphere at a depth of around 2 cm through a standard twist-drill craniostomy or through a coronal burr hole. Alternatively, it may be inserted using a tunneling technique intraoperatively during a craniotomy. One advantage over EVD monitoring is that intraparenchymal monitors do not require fluid coupling for pressure transduction, which provides less opportunity for contamination and infection and also avoids inaccuracy from waveform dampening and artifacts. However, intraparenchymal monitors reflect only local, compartmentalized pressure[124,127] and cannot generally be re-zeroed after insertion and therefore have a shorter dwell time with substantial drift, or inaccuracy, after 7 to 10 days.[128]

In TBI, multiple physiologic and anatomic perturbations may lead to hydrocephalus from obstruction of CSF flow or CSF reabsorption. An EVD is favored over intraparenchymal monitors when there is acute hydrocephalus to reduce ICP with CSF diversion. Because intracranial compliance decreases as the combined volume of the intracranial contents increase, even small increases in the volume of the CSF compartment may lead to exponentially increased ICP. For that reason, small reductions in CSF volume via drainage from even normally sized ventricles may off-load an increase in ICP from brain tissue edema or mass effect from intra-axial or extra-axial hematomas. Consequently, an EVD is used to both diagnose and treat elevated ICP, whereas an ICP-monitoring device is used only for diagnosis and to guide alternative methods of brain relaxation. Furthermore, CSF diversion may also help clear inflammatory mediators that contribute to secondary brain injury in TBI.

Despite modern ventricular and intraparenchymal systems that reduce infection rate and improve accuracy, the role of ICP monitoring in TBI remains controversial. Ongoing investigations by groups such as the NINDS-funded, multicenter Transforming Research and Clinical Knowledge in Traumatic Brain Injury initiative and the Collaborative European NeuroTrauma Effectiveness Research project seek to resolve controversies surrounding appropriate patient selection for ICP monitoring, optimal therapies, and thresholds for treatment.[129] The only randomized controlled trial examining ICP monitoring—the Benchmark Evidence from South American Trials: Treatment of Intracranial Pressure—failed to show any benefit in functional outcome or mortality than care based on imaging and clinical examination.[130] However, a more recent large multicenter international prospective, albeit observational, cohort study found that ICP monitoring was associated with significantly lower 6-month mortality in severe TBI cases.[131] In the latter study, clinicians applied a more aggressive therapeutic approach in ICP-monitored patients, contrary to the former trial, in which clinicians more aggressively treated the patients without ICP monitors. In both studies, however, aggressive treatment was associated with reduced mortality. If more aggressive care improves outcome as these studies suggest, perhaps ICP-related or alternative markers of injury should be monitored and targeted in lieu of, or in concert with, ICP.

Additional elements derived from ICP monitoring have indeed shown to be valuable in assessing brain health and preventing secondary brain injury in TBI.[132] ICP waveform morphology has guided clinical interventions in TBI management for decades and despite the availability of modern analytical processing of waveform characteristics, a mere inspection is required to make use of this modality in its simplest form. Likewise, the easily calculated ICP-derived measure, CPP, has long been a therapeutic target in management of TBI. Several other ICP-derived indices may also help guide therapy in TBI but require time-synchronized capture of multiple physiologic dynamics at high sampling frequency, not often collected by commercial devices, and automated computation of algorithms using software tools not routinely available.[133]

Intracranial pressure waveform morphology

Waveform inspection and analysis attempts to assess intracranial compliance and determine whereby the patient is along the pressure–volume curve. This may involve simple inspection of the three classical peaks within the individual pulsatile tracing: P1—percussion wave, reflecting arterial pulses of the carotid plexus into the CSF; P2—tidal wave, representing arterial pulses reflected off brain parenchyma with elevations indicating poor compliance; P3—dicrotic notch, reflecting aortic valve closure. Normally, the three peaks of the ICP pulsatile waveform, which correlates with the propagation of the arterial pulse, appear in descending height (P1 > P2 > P3). However, when intracranial compliance diminishes, the second peak becomes higher than the first (P1 < P2 > P3) (**Fig. 3**). Compliance can also be assessed by inspection of the tracing over time for slow and semi-periodic alterations in mean ICP, that is, Lundberg's A, B, and C waves.[134] Lundberg A waves are plateau or vasogenic waves during very high ICP (>50 mm Hg lasting 5–20 min) and signify reduced compliance and impending herniation. B waves are short-duration elevations to 30 to 50 mm Hg with 0.5 to 2 waves per minute, whose appearance has indeterminate clinical implications but may represent decreased compliance.[135,136] C waves are frequent elevations up to 30 mm Hg with 4 to 8 cycles per minute and are thought to reflect physiologic interactions between the cardiac and pulmonary cycles (**Fig. 4**).

Intracranial pressure-derived measures of cerebral perfusion pressure and autoregulation

The ICP-derived score, CPP, is simply the calculated difference between MAP and mean ICP and reflects the pressure gradient across the intracranial vascular bed that drives CBF and thus oxygen and nutrients. Optimal CPP targets in the care of TBI patients have been debated for years and remain controversial because the effectiveness of most interventions to reduce ICP and optimize CPP often depends on intact intracerebral homeostatic mechanisms. The target CPP currently recommended by the BTF for survival and favorable outcomes based on a Level IIB (low-quality) body of evidence is between 60 and 70 mm Hg.[22] The BTF acknowledges that this minimum optimal threshold may depend on the autoregulatory status of the patient.

In a TBI patient with functional autoregulation, increased ICP resulting in reduced CPP is met by cerebral arteriolar relaxation. In parallel, MAP is increased through a rise in cardiac output mediated by a systemic autonomic response. As cerebral vessel relaxation increases cerebral blood volume, a vicious cycle may ensue, further raising ICP. In this fashion, an acute reduction in CPP or MAP may acutely increase ICP, which is termed the vasodilatory cascade[137] (**Fig. 5**). In the presence of elevated

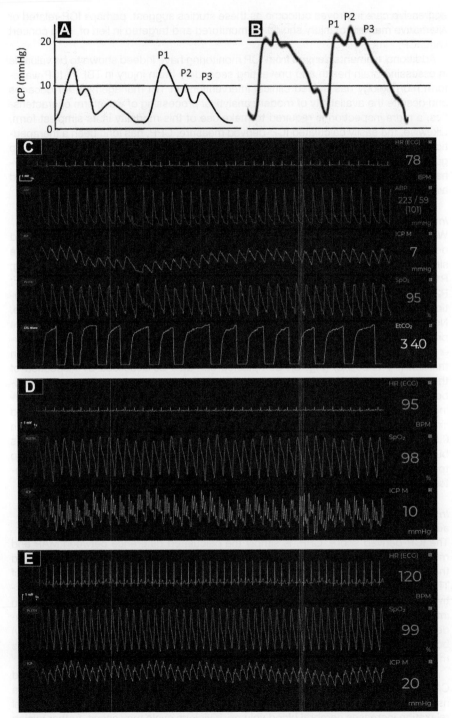

Fig. 3. Intracranial pressure waveform morphology. Depicted by artistic rendering (*A*, *B*) and real-time clinical surveillance of external ventricular drain ICP monitoring in three patients (*C–E*) using the data acquisition software platform Sickbay (Medical Informatics Corp,

ICP beyond the ability for compensation through elevation of MAP, CPP will be compromised and cerebral ischemia may follow. Ischemia results at levels of CBF below 20 mL/100 g/min unless CPP is restored, (either by increasing MAP or decreasing ICP) or cerebral metabolic demand is reduced (eg, through deepened anesthesia).

Aggressive efforts to elevate MAP in the setting of high ICP to achieve CPP targets using fluids and vasopressors may increase the risk of acute hypoxic respiratory failure and may worsen cerebral edema when autoregulation is impaired (due to pressure passive hyperemia).[138] With intact autoregulation, an increase in MAP induces vasoconstriction with a subsequent fall in ICP[139] (see case example in **Fig. 3**C). When autoregulation is disrupted, ICP increases with increases in MAP. Thus, strategies to lower ICP should take precedent and assessing ICP responses to MAP challenges may be useful because increasing CPP can lower ICP if autoregulation is found to be intact.[61,139,140] Higher CPP targets (>70 mm Hg) may thus be indicated to assist in reducing ICP in patients with intact autoregulation, whereas lower CPP may better serve patients with dysfunctional autoregulation.[141]

In fact, the three-tier comprehensive algorithm developed by the Seattle International Severe Traumatic Brain Injury Consensus Conference (SIBICC) for ICP-monitor-based management includes a simplified method of testing autoregulation based on that of Rosenthal and colleagues.[142,143] By initiating a vasopressor-induced 10-mm Hg increase in MAP, the vasoconstriction associated with active autoregulation will decrease cerebral blood volume and ICP. If this trial of augmenting MAP (ie, "MAP challenge") is successful in reducing ICP, judgment should be rendered as to whether the benefit of ICP reduction outweighs the risks associated with pharmacological augmentation of MAP. Caution should be taken in applying the results of this MAP challenge to clinical practice, as the results may not be simple to interpret, especially in the operating room, given the dynamic influence of pathological, physiologic, and pharmacologic mediators of functional autoregulation and its limits.[144]

Enhanced intracranial pressure-derived indices of autoregulation and optimal cerebral perfusion pressure

Given that failure of autoregulation is associated with worse outcome after TBI,[145,146] there is much interest in continuous monitoring of autoregulation to aid in prognostication and to assist in individualizing CPP targets. Additional mean ICP waveform-derived scores, such as the RAP (moving correlation coefficient [R] between ICP wave amplitude and ICP)[147] and pulsatile ICP waveform-derived scores,[148,149] such as the pressure amplitude index (correlation between ICP wave amplitude and arterial blood pressure source signals),[150] are more sophisticated ways to assess cerebral autoregulation.[151] The most commonly used autoregulation index, pressure reactivity

---

Houston, TX). Arterial pulsations transmit to the intracranial compartment with three characteristic peaks: P1, percussion wave (systolic peak); P2, tidal wave (proxy for intracranial compliance); P3, dicrotic notch (aortic valve closure peak). (A, C, D) In normal physiology, the three peaks appear in descending height (P1 > P2 > P3). (B, E) In pathologic states of reduced intracranial compliance or raised ICP, P2 is highest. Recording in (E) demonstrates a case of permissive hypertension; ICP is improved with elevated blood pressure due to functional autoregulatory mechanisms. ABP, arterial blood pressure; BPM, beats per minute; ECG, electrocardiogram; EtCO₂, end-tidal partial pressure of carbon dioxide measured in mm Hg; HR, heart rate; ICP M, mean intracranial pressure; PLETH, plethysmography.

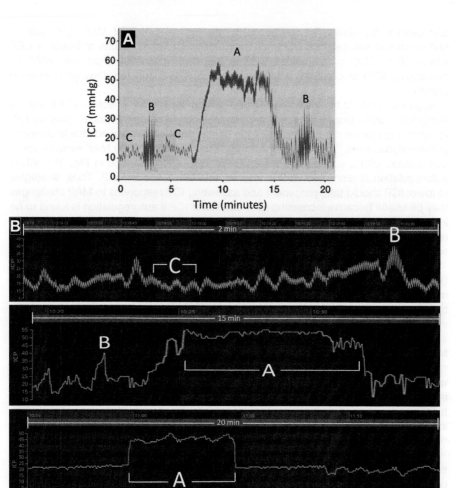

Fig. 4. Mean intracranial pressure wave patterns. Depicted by computer-assisted artistic rendering (*A*) and real-time clinical surveillance of external ventricular drain ICP monitoring in one patient (*B*) over time using the data acquisition software platform Sickbay (Medical Informatics Corp, Houston, TX). Lundberg A waves (or plateau waves) reflect reduced intra-cranial compliance and impending herniation. B waves (or slow vasogenic waves) may reflect diminishing compliance. Lundberg C waves are physiologic ICP fluctuations in response to the cardiac and respiratory cycles. ABP, arterial blood pressure; BPM, beats per minute; ECG, electrocardiogram; $EtCO_2$, end-tidal partial pressure of carbon dioxide measured in mm Hg; HR, heart rate; ICP M, mean intracranial pressure; PLETH, plethysmography.

index (PRx), is a moving Pearson correlation coefficient between mean ICP and sys-temic MAP, assuming ICP strictly reflects changes in blood volume without compen-satory pressure–volume responses from the other two intracranial components (brain tissue and CSF) within a closed cranial vault.[146] Positive PRx values indicate impaired pressure reactivity with pressure-passive blood flow, and consequently, worse outcome and negative values indicate intact cerebrovascular reactivity.[120,146,152] One management approach uses PRx and biomedical engineering principles of signal processing and computational methods to determine the optimal CPP (CPPopt) that

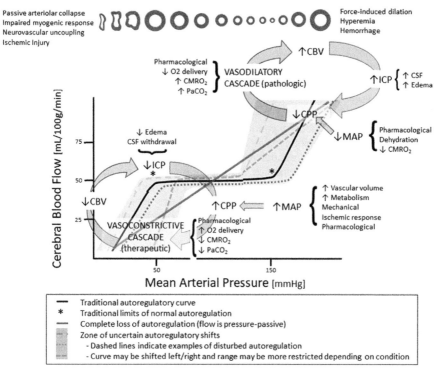

Fig. 5. Cerebral autoregulation and the vasodilatory cascade. CBV, cerebral blood volume; CMRO$_2$, cerebral metabolic rate of oxygen consumption; CPP, cerebral perfusion pressure; CSF, cerebrospinal fluid; ICP, intracranial pressure; MAP, mean arterial pressure; Paco$_2$, arterial partial pressure of carbon dioxide. Bush B, Sam K, Rosenblatt K. The Role of Near-infrared Spectroscopy in Cerebral Autoregulation Monitoring. J Neurosurg Anesthesiol. 2019;31(3):269-270; with permission from Wolters Kluwer Health, Inc.

corresponds to the lowest, most favorable PRx values in an individual patient. Several retrospective studies have demonstrated that deviations of CPP from CPPopt are associated with worse outcome after TBI[153–155] and the prospective CPPopt-Guided Therapy: Assessment of Target Effectiveness trial confirmed the feasibility and safety of TBI management using this technique, although it was not powered to detect differences in clinical outcome.[156]

Noninvasive measures of raised intracranial pressure and autoregulation
As the patient-customized approach to management of TBI grows in momentum, so does the exploration of noninvasive surrogate markers of ICP and cerebral autoregulation as part of the multimodality armamentarium of TBI management. Several noninvasive brain monitors may confirm the presence or absence of ICP without providing a specific numerical value, such as electroencephalography (EEG) and cerebral ultrasound. EEG patterns associated with elevated ICP include generalized slowing, focal slowing of underlying rhythms, or global EEG suppression progressing to burst suppression. Although optic nerve sheath diameter (ONSD) using ocular ultrasound has relatively high sensitivity and specificity for diagnosing intracranial hypertension with ONSD greater than 5 mm representing an ICP greater than 20 mm Hg, its use is still in its infancy compared with transcranial Doppler (TCD) ultrasonography measures

of increased ICP, such as a low diastolic flow velocity (<20 cm/s) and a high pulsatility index (>1.3).[157-160] Cerebral ultrasound may also be used to diagnosis intracranial hematomas, midline shift, and hydrocephalus.[161]

Several noninvasive methods exist to assess cerebral autoregulation. Some use mathematical algorithms similar to the calculation of PRx to compute autoregulation indices, like the TCD-derived mean flow velocity index (Mx) and systolic flow velocity index (Sx), which correlate middle cerebral artery blood flow velocity with CPP or with MAP (Mxa, Sxa),[145,162] and the near-infrared spectroscopy (NIRS)-derived cerebral oximetry index (COx), tissue oxygenation index (TOx), and hemoglobin volume index (HVx), which correlate regional oxygen saturation, tissue oxygenation, and relative total hemoglobin with MAP, respectively.[163-165] Similar to PRx, positive values of Mx, COx, TOx, and HVx above specific thresholds denote impaired autoregulation and have been associated with unfavorable outcome in brain-injured patients.[120] These indices may be more reliable than PRx in settings where the pressure–volume compensatory reserve is not finite, such as after a decompressive craniectomy or in those undergoing CSF diversion with an EVD.[166,167] TCD- and NIRS-based techniques can also be extrapolated to estimate optimal blood pressure targets, or the CPP or MAP at which autoregulation is most robust.[165,168]

Electroencephalography

After ICP, continuous EEG monitoring of TBI patients is reportedly the next most commonly applied neuromonitor and in some advanced neurocritical care units is incorporated into a multimodality neuromonitoring platform.[169] EEG records spontaneous excitatory impulses of the cerebral cortex and is therefore tightly linked to cerebral metabolism and sensitive to cerebral ischemia and hypoxia. Because it exposes changes in neuronal function before structural damage, EEG is used to detect cerebral ischemia in the operating room during cerebrovascular surgery, in the emergency department in acute stroke diagnosis,[170,171] and in the intensive care unit in subarachnoid hemorrhage management.[172] EEG may also detect impending deterioration due to intracranial hypertension[173,174] and specific EEG features, if present early after TBI, may assist with prognostication.[175,176] EEG is necessary when measuring high-dose barbiturate-induced burst suppression for the control of elevated ICP refractory to maximum standard medical and surgical treatment. However, its most common application in the management of TBI is to detect nonconvulsive seizures, which occurs in up to 25% of patients post-traumatically and if prolonged can cause excitotoxicity, enhance metabolic demand, and raise ICP.[177]

Extracellular cortical current fluctuations detected by EEG may be recorded from electrodes placed either on the scalp or directly on the brain (electrocorticography). Subdural strips and intracortical depth electrodes eliminate contamination from muscle artifact and the poor spatial resolution of scalp EEG and can detect seizures and cortical spreading depression that cannot be seen on scalp EEG.[177-179] Insertion involves six or eight electrode contacts distributed over both gray and white matter through a dedicated burr hole or may be part of a multi-lumen catheter or multi-port bolt system for simultaneous parametric measurements.[180]

Cerebral Blood Flow

Directly assessing alterations in CBF has long been an attractive objective in management of TBI. Modern imaging techniques such as CT perfusion, Xenon-CT, positron emission tomography, and perfusion-weighted MRI have enhanced the ability to monitor CBF.[181] However, these imaging modalities provide only a snapshot of the injured brain and most require transportation outside of the ICU. TCD ultrasonography is a noninvasive bedside tool that can detect inadequate CBF by measuring flow velocities in insonated vessels. Although it lacks the spatial resolution of techniques such as MRI, it benefits from high temporal resolution but due to technical difficulties with probe dislodgement is limited to brief periods of data acquisition.

Thermal diffusion flowmetry is an invasive bedside tool that can detect regional changes in CBF in real time continuously.[143,182] It consists of a 1-mm diameter catheter with two in-line thermistor probes at its tip inserted into white matter either through a dedicated burr hole or as part of a multiparametric bolt system. The temperature difference between the two probes after heating the distal probe approximate 2°C above tissue temperature reflects the power dissipated by the tissue's ability to carry heat through both thermal conduction within the tissue and through thermal convection due to tissue blood flow. Perfusion, as indicated by the latter, is calculated by subtracting the thermal conduction (the initial rate of propagation) from the total dissipated power and is converted to an absolute measurement of blood flow in mL/100 g/min. Although thermal diffusion flowmetry has been validated by Xenon perfusion neuroimaging,[182] treatment thresholds for values of CBF have not been well established.[182] There is interest, however, in using thermal diffusion-based computational signal processing methods, similar to calculations of PRx, to provide an index of autoregulation (rCBFx), which is the moving Pearson correlation between CPP and regional CBF.[143,183] This method may provide a more direct measure of autoregulation than ICP-based PRx and is not constrained to intact skulls. Unfortunately, data acquisition from thermal diffusion probes is limited by safety concerns when brain temperature is intrinsically elevated, such as in pyrexia, which is common in TBI. In addition, if the probe tip is near a thermally significant vessel that produces substantial pulsatility, the monitor will produce an error message and prevent regional CBF measures. In our experience, thermal diffusion probes provide data in less than 50% of the TBI patients monitored, which is similar to other reports.[184,185]

Cerebral Oxygenation

Because of the brain's high oxygen consumption and near total dependence on aerobic glucose metabolism, modern MMM in TBI includes assessment of cerebral oxygenation to identify brain tissue at risk for ischemia. Continuous bedside assessment of cerebral oxygenation can be performed noninvasively with NIRS-based cerebral oximeters or invasively with parenchymal extracellular oxygen partial pressure ($PbtO_2$) and jugular venous oxygen saturation ($SjvO_2$) monitoring.

Near-infrared spectroscopy

NIRS determines the relative concentrations of oxyhemoglobin and deoxyhemoglobin within the frontal lobe tissue in the path of emitted light using their differential light absorption spectra. NIRS measures of regional cerebral oxygenation saturation (rSO2) assume that absorption from other biological chromophores is minimal, proportional scattering of infrared light from the tissues remains constant, and the hemoglobin measured is contained in a fixed mixture of venous and arterial blood vessels.[186,187] The presence of cerebral edema, hematomas, and subarachnoid blood nullify some of these assumptions. Further, equations used to account for variability are manufacturer-specific, limiting use of discrete measures of rSO_2 especially among different oximeters.[188–191] Therefore, relative changes in rSO_2 may have more meaning than the absolute value. However, thresholds for actionable decrements in NIRS-measured rSO_2 have not been established in the TBI population nor have rSO_2 thresholds predicting secondary brain injury.

Changes in rSO_2 can even be considered a surrogate of CBF when other determinants, such as hemoglobin, tissue diffusivity of oxygen, $CMRO_2$, and arterial oxygen saturation, are held constant. This drives the popularity of continuous NIRS-based techniques in the multimodal management of TBI, such as time-synchronized correlation of arterial pressure with NIRS-derived surrogates of CBF to monitor cerebral autoregulation and define its limits, as was mentioned previously.[192]

Brain tissue oxygen partial pressure

The direct measurement of brain tissue oxygenation is considered by some authors to be the gold standard of bedside cerebral oxygenation monitoring and is an important component of invasive multimodality neuromonitoring.[193] Brain tissue oxygen partial pressure ($PbtO_2$) monitors are microcatheters that measure local interstitial and capillary oxygen tension using a modified Clark polarographic electrode or a fluorescent fiberoptic sensor. They are inserted in subcortical white matter in a manner similar to an intraparenchymal fiberoptic ICP monitor via a tunneling technique during a craniotomy or through a single or multiple lumen bolt.[194] Measurements after insertion may be unreliable for a variable period of time while the monitor calibrates, and an oxygen challenge may also need to be performed to assess functionality. This involves increasing the fraction of inspired oxygen (FiO_2) to 1.0. The probe should respond with a $PbtO_2$ reading of 200% or more from baseline if it is performing properly.

$PbtO_2$ monitoring provides regional measures, which obviously are affected by the multiple determinants of oxygen delivery as well as oxygen diffusivity, probe placement, ICP, autoregulatory status, and metabolism.[195–197] Normal $PbtO_2$ values range from 20 to 40 mm Hg, with values less than 15 to 20 mm Hg indicating cerebral ischemia, below 10 mm Hg indicating severe ischemia, and above 40 mm Hg indicating hyperemia or hyperoxia.[198,199] Similar to ICP thresholds, injury may occur when abnormal values are sustained over time.[198] Also like ICP management, more than one intervention may be used to remedy low $PbtO_2$, such as optimizing hemoglobin concentration, MAP, $PaCO_2$, or PaO_2[193,196,200]; sole reliance on increasing FiO_2 may lead to harmful cerebral and systemic effects of hyperoxia.[201,202]

Evidence from a large retrospective study that outcomes after TBI were no different after treatments in response to $PbtO_2$ monitoring[203] and equipoise among a group of smaller studies prompted the treatment threshold of $PbtO_2$ less than 15 mm Hg to be removed from the most recent BTF guidelines.[22,204] However, the strong association between low $PbtO_2$ and poor outcome[205,206] drives ongoing randomized trials comparing ICP-directed therapies versus ICP combined with $PbtO_2$-directed therapies[207](p3).[208] Moreover, the 42 TBI clinical experts of the SIBICC consensus working group combined formal evidence with practical experience and developed two separate comprehensive three-tier algorithms for treatment of intracranial hypertension—an ICP-only[142] and an ICP plus PbtO2-guided[209] approach—in response to the newest BTF guidelines' omission of what was considered non-evidence-based treatment.

Jugular venous oxygen saturation

Jugular venous oximetry was the earliest method of monitoring cerebral oxygenation, though its contribution to MMM in TBI is declining, especially compared with $PbtO_2$ monitoring.[169] $SjvO_2$ can be intermittently sampled from an indwelling catheter or continuously measured from a fiberoptic catheter sited in the jugular bulb through retrograde cannulation of the dominant internal jugular vein independent from, or simultaneously with, central venous catheterization. The cerebral venous sinuses drain intracranial blood through the sigmoid sinuses into the internal jugular veins via the jugular foramina. The bulbous dilatation of the jugular vein just below the base of the skull contains cerebral venous blood free of contamination from the numerous extracranial veins that join the internal jugular vein in its caudal passage through the neck. Therefore, to monitor the SjvO2 of cerebral blood correctly, the catheter tip must be placed high in the bulb with its position confirmed radiographically: ideally, cranial to the line extending from the atlanto-occipital joint space just medial to the mastoid process and caudal to the lower margin of the orbit. With careful insertion technique and appropriate placement, $SjvO_2$ monitoring can be safely performed in TBI patients without causing venous insufficiency or obstruction and without aggravating intracranial hypertension.[210]

Unlike the regional data provided by $PbtO_2$ monitoring, $SjvO_2$ monitoring provides global information on the balance of cerebral perfusion and metabolism. When $CMRO_2$ is greater than the oxygen supply, cerebral oxygen extraction from the blood will increase, resulting in a decrease in $SjvO_2$. This increased cerebral oxygen extraction is reflected by a wide arteriovenous difference of oxygen ($AVDO_2$), which is calculated by the difference between arterial oxygen saturation (SaO_2) and $SjvO_2$. If oxygen supplied by CBF is substantially reduced, anaerobic metabolism ensues with production of lactic acid. When cerebral oxygen supply is larger than consumption, $SjvO_2$ will increase and $AVDO_2$ will be narrow. This occurs in severe TBI when there is defective metabolic autoregulation, such that CBF exceeds metabolic demands, and has been termed "luxury perfusion." The normal range of $SjVO_2$ is approximately 55% to 75%[211] and normal $AVDO_2$ values are between 4 vol% and 8 vol%.[212,213] Although jugular desaturation reliably indicates cerebral hypoperfusion or ischemia and is strongly associated with poor neurologic outcome after TBI, high values of $SjvO_2$ have also been associated with poor outcome.[214,215] Elevated $SjvO_2$ may represent hyperemia, which is a common sequela of TBI, or decreased $CMRO_2$, which may occur with coma or cerebral infarction. Thus, the BTF recommends jugular bulb monitoring of SjvO2 and $AVDO_2$ to identify and treat jugular desaturation events and to inform management strategies that help normalize flow-metabolism coupling, such as hyperventilation.[22,216]

Cerebral Metabolism and Biochemistry

A cerebral microdialysis catheter is an intraparenchymal monitor inserted in a manner similar to a $PbtO_2$ probe that allows sampling of extracellular interstitial fluid through a semipermeable dialysis membrane incorporated in its tip. Compounds at high concentration with a molecular weight less than 20 kDa, such as glucose, lactate, pyruvate, glycerol, and glutamate, diffuse across the microdialysis membrane along their concentration gradient from brain extracellular fluid into the isotonic dialysis fluid, which circulates through the catheter at a rate of 0.3 μL/min.[217] Macromolecules such as inflammatory mediators, brain injury biomarkers, and cytokines may also be sampled using a higher molecular weight cutoff microdialysis membrane (100 kDa). A semiautomated calorimetric bedside analyzer measures the concentration of accumulated clinically relevant compounds at set hourly intervals, with more frequent sampling possible.[218]

By providing real-time bedside information about substrate delivery and metabolism at the cellular level, microdialysis uniquely enhances ICP and $PbtO_2$ monitoring and has increased our understanding of the pathophysiology of TBI. Metabolic changes may precede impending ICP crises and therefore microdialysis may be used as an early warning system of secondary insults.[219,220] Disordered glycemic control with imbalance in the supply and demand for glucose after brain injury can lead to a cerebral metabolic crisis from ischemic and nonischemic causes.[177,221] Furthermore, brain glucose may fall to levels that are insufficient to meet metabolic demand even with normal serum glucose levels, termed neuroglycopenia. In oxidative conditions metabolism of glucose via glycolysis to pyruvate feeds into the tricarboxylic acid cycle. In hypoxic conditions, or if mitochondrial function is disturbed, pyruvate is metabolized to lactate. Therefore, an elevated lactate:pyruvate ratio (LPR) in the setting of low pyruvate indicates anaerobic metabolism and a reduction in substrate in the setting of ischemia while an elevated LPR with normal or high pyruvate suggests mitochondrial dysfunction or hyperglycolysis in the absence of ischemia. In the former scenario, when pyruvate is low and LPR is greater than 35 to 40, increasing CPP or $PbtO_2$ is recommended. When cerebral extracellular glucose concentration is very low (0.2 mmol/L), a trial of increasing serum glucose concentration intravenously or enterally and/or loosening glycemic control is recommended even if serum glucose concentration is within a normal range.[222] Both low brain glucose concentration (<0.7–1 mmol/L) and elevated LPR (>25) are associated with poor outcome.[223–225] Glutamate is measured as a marker of hypoxia/ischemia and excitotoxicity.[226] Glycerol is also a nonspecific marker of hypoxia/ischemia-related cell membrane breakdown.[227] In diffuse TBI, a microdialysis catheter may be placed in the right (nondominant) frontal lobe; however, in focal TBI, catheter placement is based on whether the goal is to monitor areas of brain most vulnerable to ischemia (ipsilateral to a focal lesion) or to guide systemic glucose treatment in normal brain (contralateral to a lesion).[222]

SUMMARY

Patients benefit from comprehensive, interdisciplinary perioperative, and intensive care to monitor for secondary brain insults and to manage the potentially devastating multisystem sequelae of TBI. The growing understanding of the pathophysiology of TBI has led to a surge of research in mitigating secondary injury through advanced monitoring. Although early delivery of specialized medical and surgical care of the TBI patient is routine, multiple obstacles restrict implementation of the full complement of multimodality neuromonitoring in many centers. The ongoing development of integrated physiologic data monitoring platforms drive the evolution of TBI management toward individualize care with the hope of improving survival and long-term outcomes.

CLINICS CARE POINTS

- When patients with traumatic brain injury (TBI) present for emergent intracranial or extracranial surgery, neurologically-targeted interventions should coincide with relentless resuscitation of the circulatory and respiratory systems because hypotension and hypoxia are key systemic insults associated with secondary brain injury and worse outcomes.

- The updated Brain Trauma Foundation (BTF) guidelines suggest maintaining systolic blood pressure (SBP) greater than or equal to 100 mmHg for patients 50 to 69 years old or greater than or equal to 110 mmHg for patients 15 to 49 or over 79 years old to maintain cerebral perfusion pressure (CPP) and reduce the risk of secondary brain injury from hypotension. If the TBI patient presenting for surgery has an intracranial pressure (ICP) monitor in situ or one is being placed in the operating room, mean arterial pressure (MAP) should be maintained to achieve a CPP goal of 60 to 70 mmHg with volume resuscitation followed by vasopressors if necessary. Hypotensive TBI patients should be administered rapid infusions of isotonic fluids with avoidance of hypotonic and hyponatremic fluids, such as lactated ringers, ½ normal saline, and glucose containing solutions, as they may exacerbate cerebral edema.

- Point-of-care ultrasound in TBI patients may be used to evaluate cardiopulmonary function in the approach to treatment of hypotension and can be especially helpful in elucidating acute neurogenic stress cardiomyopathy (low ejection fraction, basal hypokinesis), neurogenic pulmonary edema (diffuse bilateral B lines), and intravascular volume depletion (inferior vena cava distensibility index, left ventricle collapse).

- Pathologic intracranial hypertension is present at pressures greater than or equal to 20 mmHg and targeting a goal ICP of less than or equal to 22 mmHg is recommended for a more favorable outcome after TBI. However, a single ICP threshold for all severe TBI may be an oversimplification of a heterogenous and multifaceted pathophysiological process.

- In the absence of cerebral herniation and ICP crisis, BTF guidelines recommend tight regulation of oxygenation and ventilation in TBI patients who require intubation with the goal of normalizing physiologic parameters [oxygen saturation (SpO_2) > 90%; arterial partial pressure of carbon dioxide ($PaCO_2$) 35-45 mm Hg.

- If there are clinical signs of imminent cerebral herniation or refractory intracranial hypertension, hyperventilation can be initiated as a temporary measure until the ICP crisis resolves. However, this maneuver may not influence the likelihood of neurological recovery and instead may elicit or augment cerebral ischemia.

- If a TBI patient presents to the operating room (OR) with an external ventricular drain or one is placed in the OR, the anesthesiologist should be familiar with managing the device and draining cerebrospinal fluid.

DISCLOSURE

K. Rosenblatt receives research funding from the Foundation for Anesthesia Education and Research, United States. K. Rosenblatt received honoraria for educational activities from Medical Informatics Corp.

REFERENCES

1. Rubiano AM, Carney N, Chesnut R, et al. Global neurotrauma research challenges and opportunities. Nature 2015;527(7578):S193–7.
2. McCunn M, Dutton RP, Dagal A, et al. Trauma, critical care, and emergency care anesthesiology: a new paradigm for the "acute care" anesthesiologist? Anesth Analg 2015;121(6):1668–73.
3. Dewan MC, Rattani A, Gupta S, et al. Estimating the global incidence of traumatic brain injury. J Neurosurg 2018;130(4):1080–97.
4. Get the Facts About TBI | Concussion | Traumatic Brain Injury | CDC Injury Center. Available at: https://www.cdc.gov/traumaticbraininjury/get_the_facts.html. Published March 21, 2022. Accessed August 19, 2022.
5. Menon DK, Schwab K, Wright DW, et al. Demographics and clinical assessment working group of the international and interagency initiative toward common data elements for research on traumatic brain injury and psychological health. position statement: definition of traumatic brain injury. Arch Phys Med Rehabil 2010;91(11):1637–40.
6. Maas AIR, Menon DK, Adelson PD, et al. Traumatic brain injury: integrated approaches to improve prevention, clinical care, and research. Lancet Neurol 2017;16(12):987–1048.
7. Brazinova A, Rehorcikova V, Taylor MS, et al. Epidemiology of traumatic brain injury in europe: a living systematic review. J Neurotrauma 2021;38(10): 1411–40.

8. Kong LZ, Zhang RL, Hu SH, et al. Military traumatic brain injury: a challenge straddling neurology and psychiatry. Mil Med Res 2022;9(1):2.

9. Saatman KE, Duhaime AC, Bullock R, et al. Classification of Traumatic Brain Injury for Targeted Therapies. J Neurotrauma 2008;25(7):719–38.

10. Marshall LF, Marshall SB, Klauber MR, et al. The diagnosis of head injury requires a classification based on computed axial tomography. J Neurotrauma 1992;9(Suppl 1):S287–92.

11. Teasdale G, Jennett B. Assessment of coma and impaired consciousness. A practical scale. Lancet Lond Engl 1974;2(7872):81–4.

12. Marmarou A, Lu J, Butcher I, et al. Prognostic value of the glasgow coma scale and pupil reactivity in traumatic brain injury assessed pre-hospital and on enrollment: an impact analysis. J Neurotrauma 2007;24(2):270–80.

13. Fischer M, Rüegg S, Czaplinski A, et al. Inter-rater reliability of the full outline of unresponsiveness score and the glasgow coma scale in critically ill patients: a prospective observational study. Crit Care Lond Engl 2010;14(2):R64.

14. Teasdale G, Maas A, Lecky F, et al. The glasgow coma scale at 40 years: standing the test of time. Lancet Neurol 2014;13(8):844–54.

15. Kaur P, Sharma S. Recent advances in pathophysiology of traumatic brain injury. Curr Neuropharmacol 2018;16(8):1224–38.

16. Maegele M, Schöchl H, Menovsky T, et al. Coagulopathy and haemorrhagic progression in traumatic brain injury: advances in mechanisms, diagnosis, and management. Lancet Neurol 2017;16(8):630–47. https://doi.org/10.1016/S1474-4422(17)30197-7.

17. Wada T, Shiraishi A, Gando S, et al. Pathophysiology of coagulopathy induced by traumatic brain injury is identical to that of disseminated intravascular coagulation with hyperfibrinolysis. Front Med 2021;8. Available at: https://www.frontiersin.org/articles/10.3389/fmed.2021.767637. Accessed August 20, 2022.

18. Thomas I, Dickens AM, Posti JP, et al. Serum metabolome associated with severity of acute traumatic brain injury. Nat Commun 2022;13(1):2545. https://doi.org/10.1038/s41467-022-30227-5.

19. Pugh MJ, Kennedy E, Prager EM, et al. Phenotyping the Spectrum of Traumatic Brain Injury: A Review and Pathway to Standardization. J Neurotrauma 2021;38(23):3222–34.

20. Wilson MH, Ashworth E, Hutchinson PJ, British Neurotrauma Group. A proposed novel traumatic brain injury classification system - an overview and inter-rater reliability validation on behalf of the Society of British Neurological Surgeons. Br J Neurosurg 2022;36(5):633–8.

21. Smith LGF, Milliron E, Ho ML, et al. Advanced neuroimaging in traumatic brain injury: an overview. Neurosurg Focus 2019;47(6):E17.

22. Carney N, Totten AM, O'Reilly C, et al. Guidelines for the management of severe traumatic brain injury. Neurosurgery 2017;80(1):6–15. Fourth Edition.

23. American College of Surgeons, Committee on Trauma. Advanced trauma life support: student course manual. 10th. Chicago, IL: American College of Surgeons; 2018.

24. Garvin R, Mangat HS. Emergency neurological life support: severe traumatic brain injury. Neurocrit Care 2017;27(Suppl 1):159–69.

25. McHugh GS, Engel DC, Butcher I, et al. Prognostic value of secondary insults in traumatic brain injury: results from the IMPACT study. J Neurotrauma 2007;24(2):287–93.

26. Brenner M, Stein DM, Hu PF, et al. Traditional systolic blood pressure targets underestimate hypotension-induced secondary brain injury. J Trauma Acute Care Surg 2012;72(5):1135–9.

27. Sharrock MF, Rosenblatt K. Acute airway management and ventilation in the neurocritical care unit. In: Nelson SE, Nyquist PA, editors. Neurointensive care unit: clinical practice and organization. Cham, Switzerland: Springer International Publishing; 2020. p. 31–47.

28. Bronchard R, Albaladejo P, Brezac G, et al. Early onset pneumonia: risk factors and consequences in head trauma patients. Anesthesiology 2004;100(2): 234–9.

29. Fujii T, Faul M, Sasser S. Risk factors for cervical spine injury among patients with traumatic brain injury. J Emerg Trauma Shock 2013;6(4):252–8.

30. Grant AL Ranger A, Young GB, Yazdani A. Incidence of major and minor brain injuries in facial fractures. J Craniofac Surg 2012;23(5):1324–8.

31. Brown CA, Bair AE, Pallin DJ, et al. Improved glottic exposure with the video macintosh laryngoscope in adult emergency department tracheal intubations. Ann Emerg Med 2010;56(2):83–8.

32. Ziaka M, Exadaktylos A. Brain–lung interactions and mechanical ventilation in patients with isolated brain injury. Crit Care 2021;25(1):358.

33. Brian JE. Carbon dioxide and the cerebral circulation. Anesthesiology 1998; 88(5):1365–86.

34. Buxton RB. The thermodynamics of thinking: connections between neural activity, energy metabolism and blood flow. Philos Trans R Soc B Biol Sci 2021; 376(1815):20190624.

35. Yoon S, Zuccarello M, Rapoport RM. pCO2 and pH regulation of cerebral blood flow. Front Physiol 2012;3:365.

36. Hoiland RL, Bain AR, Rieger MG, et al. Hypoxemia, oxygen content, and the regulation of cerebral blood flow. Am J Physiol Regul Integr Comp Physiol 2016;310(5):R398–413.

37. Launey Y, Fryer TD, Hong YT, et al. Spatial and temporal pattern of ischemia and abnormal vascular function following traumatic brain injury. JAMA Neurol 2020; 77(3):339–49.

38. Nunn JF, Hill DW. Respiratory dead space and arterial to end-tidal carbon dioxide tension difference in anesthetized man. J Appl Physiol 1960;15:383–9.

39. Lee SW, Hong YS, Han C, et al. Concordance of end-tidal carbon dioxide and arterial carbon dioxide in severe traumatic brain injury. J Trauma 2009;67(3): 526–30.

40. Gouvea Bogossian E, Peluso L, Creteur J, et al. Hyperventilation in Adult TBI Patients: How to Approach It? Front Neurol 2021;11. Available at: https://www.frontiersin.org/articles/10.3389/fneur.2020.580859. Accessed August 22, 2022.

41. Curley G, Kavanagh BP, Laffey JG. Hypocapnia and the injured brain: more harm than benefit. Crit Care Med 2010;38(5):1348–59.

42. Laffey JG, Kavanagh BP. Hypocapnia. N Engl J Med 2002;347(1):43–53.

43. Marion DW, Puccio A, Wisniewski SR, et al. Effect of hyperventilation on extracellular concentrations of glutamate, lactate, pyruvate, and local cerebral blood flow in patients with severe traumatic brain injury. Crit Care Med 2002;30(12): 2619–25.

44. Lee JH, Kelly DF, Oertel M, et al. Carbon dioxide reactivity, pressure autoregulation, and metabolic suppression reactivity after head injury: a transcranial Doppler study. J Neurosurg 2001;95(2):222–32.

45. Picetti E, Pelosi P, Taccone FS, et al. VENTILatOry strategies in patients with severe traumatic brain injury: the VENTILO survey of the european society of intensive care medicine (ESICM). Crit Care 2020;24(1):158.

46. Walkey AJ, Goligher EC, Del Sorbo L, et al. Low tidal volume versus non-volume-limited strategies for patients with acute respiratory distress syndrome. a systematic review and meta-analysis. Ann Am Thorac Soc 2017; 14(Supplement_4):S271–9.

47. Caricato A, Conti G, Della Corte F, et al. Effects of PEEP on the intracranial system of patients with head injury and subarachnoid hemorrhage: the role of respiratory system compliance. J Trauma 2005;58(3):571–6.

48. Robba C, Bragazzi NL, Bertuccio A, et al. Effects of prone position and positive end-expiratory pressure on noninvasive estimators of ICP: a pilot study. J Neurosurg Anesthesiol 2017;29(3):243–50.

49. Muench E, Bauhuf C, Roth H, et al. Effects of positive end-expiratory pressure on regional cerebral blood flow, intracranial pressure, and brain tissue oxygenation. Crit Care Med 2005;33(10):2367–72.

50. Robba C, Poole D, McNett M, et al. Mechanical ventilation in patients with acute brain injury: recommendations of the European Society of Intensive Care Medicine consensus. Intensive Care Med 2020;46(12):2397–410.

51. El-Menyar A, Goyal A, Latifi R, et al. Brain-heart interactions in traumatic brain injury. Cardiol Rev 2017;25(6):279–88.

52. Meyfroidt G, Baguley IJ, Menon DK. Paroxysmal sympathetic hyperactivity: the storm after acute brain injury. Lancet Neurol 2017;16(9):721–9.

53. Krishnamoorthy V, Sharma D, Prathep S, et al. Myocardial dysfunction in acute traumatic brain injury relieved by surgical decompression. Case Rep Anesthesiol 2013;2013:e482596.

54. Piliponis L, Neverauskaitė-Piliponienė G, Kazlauskaitė M, et al. Neurogenic stress cardiomyopathy following aneurysmal subarachnoid haemorrhage: a literature review. Semin Cardiovasc Med 2018;25(1):44–52.

55. Ancona F, Bertoldi LF, Ruggieri F, et al. Takotsubo cardiomyopathy and neurogenic stunned myocardium: similar albeit different. Eur Heart J 2016;37(37): 2830–2.

56. Kenigsberg BB, Barnett CF, Mai JC, et al. Neurogenic stunned myocardium in severe neurological injury. Curr Neurol Neurosci Rep 2019;19(11):90.

57. Blanco P, Volpicelli G. Common pitfalls in point-of-care ultrasound: a practical guide for emergency and critical care physicians. Crit Ultrasound J 2016; 8(1):15.

58. Li L, Yong RJ, Kaye AD, et al. Perioperative point of care ultrasound (POCUS) for anesthesiologists: an overview. Curr Pain Headache Rep 2020;24(5):20.

59. Gunst M, Ghaemmaghami V, Sperry J, et al. Accuracy of cardiac function and volume status estimates using the bedside echocardiographic assessment in trauma/critical care. J Trauma 2008;65(3):509–16.

60. Bouma GJ, Muizelaar JP, Bandoh K, et al. Blood pressure and intracranial pressure-volume dynamics in severe head injury: relationship with cerebral blood flow. J Neurosurg 1992;77(1):15–9.

61. Rangel-Castilla L, Gasco J, Nauta HJW, et al. Cerebral pressure autoregulation in traumatic brain injury. Neurosurg Focus 2008;25(4):E7.

62. Berry C, Ley EJ, Bukur M, et al. Redefining hypotension in traumatic brain injury. Injury 2012;43(11):1833–7.

63. Murray GD, Butcher I, McHugh GS, et al. Multivariable prognostic analysis in traumatic brain injury: results from the IMPACT study. J Neurotrauma 2007; 24(2):329–37.

64. Chesnut RM, Marshall LF, Klauber MR, et al. The role of secondary brain injury in determining outcome from severe head injury. J Trauma 1993;34(2):216–22.

65. Salim A, Hadjizacharia P, DuBose J, et al. Role of anemia in traumatic brain injury. J Am Coll Surg 2008;207(3):398–406.

66. Van Beek JGM, Mushkudiani NA, Steyerberg EW, et al. Prognostic value of admission laboratory parameters in traumatic brain injury: results from the IMPACT Study. J Neurotrauma 2007;24(2):315–28.

67. Mirski MA, Frank SM, Kor DJ, et al. Restrictive and liberal red cell transfusion strategies in adult patients: reconciling clinical data with best practice. Crit Care Lond Engl 2015;19:202.

68. Retter A, Wyncoll D, Pearse R, et al. Guidelines on the management of anaemia and red cell transfusion in adult critically ill patients. Br J Haematol 2013;160(4): 445–64.

69. Napolitano LM, Kurek S, Luchette FA, et al. Clinical practice guideline: red blood cell transfusion in adult trauma and critical care. Crit Care Med 2009;37(12): 3124–57.

70. American Society of Anesthesiologists Task Force on Perioperative Blood Management. Practice guidelines for perioperative blood management: an updated report by the American Society of Anesthesiologists Task Force on Perioperative Blood Management. Anesthesiology 2015;122(2):241–75.

71. Robertson CS, Hannay HJ, Yamal JM, et al. Effect of erythropoietin and transfusion threshold on neurological recovery after traumatic brain injury: a randomized clinical trial. JAMA 2014;312(1):36–47.

72. CRASH-3 trial collaborators. Effects of tranexamic acid on death, disability, vascular occlusive events and other morbidities in patients with acute traumatic brain injury (CRASH-3): a randomised, placebo-controlled trial. Lancet Lond Engl 2019;394(10210):1713–23.

73. Richards JE, Harris T, Dünser MW, et al. Vasopressors in Trauma: A Never Event? Anesth Analg 2021;133(1):68–79.

74. Lambden S, Creagh-Brown BC, Hunt J, et al. Definitions and pathophysiology of vasoplegic shock. Crit Care 2018;22(1):174.

75. Sperry JL, Minei JP, Frankel HL, et al. Early use of vasopressors after injury: caution before constriction. J Trauma 2008;64(1):9–14.

76. Spahn DR, Bouillon B, Cerny V, et al. The European guideline on management of major bleeding and coagulopathy following trauma: fifth edition. Crit Care 2019; 23(1):98.

77. Guimarães S, Moura D. Vascular adrenoceptors: an update. Pharmacol Rev 2001;53(2):319–56.

78. Froese L, Dian J, Gomez A, et al. Cerebrovascular response to phenylephrine in traumatic brain injury: a scoping systematic review of the human and animal literature. Neurotrauma Rep 2020;1(1):46–62.

79. Steiner LA, Johnston AJ, Czosnyka M, et al. Direct comparison of cerebrovascular effects of norepinephrine and dopamine in head-injured patients. Crit Care Med 2004;32(4):1049–54.

80. Sookplung P, Siriussawakul A, Malakouti A, et al. Vasopressor use and effect on blood pressure after severe adult traumatic brain injury. Neurocrit Care 2011; 15(1):46–54.

81. Toro C, Ohnuma T, Komisarow J, et al. Early vasopressor utilization strategies and outcomes in critically ill patients with severe traumatic brain injury. Anesth Analg.:10.1213/ANE.0000000000005949.
82. Allen CJ, Subhawong TK, Hanna MM, et al. Does vasopressin exacerbate cerebral edema in patients with severe traumatic brain injury? Am Surg 2018;84(1): 43–50.
83. Van Haren RM, Thorson CM, Ogilvie MP, et al. Vasopressin for cerebral perfusion pressure management in patients with severe traumatic brain injury: preliminary results of a randomized controlled trial. J Trauma Acute Care Surg 2013; 75(6):1024–30, discussion 1030.
84. van Diepen S, Katz JN, Albert NM, et al. Contemporary management of cardiogenic shock: a scientific statement from the american heart association. Circulation 2017;136(16):e232–68.
85. van Diepen S. Norepinephrine as a first-line inopressor in cardiogenic shock: oversimplification or best practice? J Am Coll Cardiol 2018;72(2):183–6.
86. Zheng RZ, Lei ZQ, Yang RZ, et al. Identification and management of paroxysmal sympathetic hyperactivity after traumatic brain injury. Front Neurol 2020;11:81.
87. Lin CC, Yu JH, Lin CC, et al. Postintubation hemodynamic effects of intravenous lidocaine in severe traumatic brain injury. Am J Emerg Med 2012;30(9):1782–7.
88. Volpi PC, Robba C, Rota M, et al. Trajectories of early secondary insults correlate to outcomes of traumatic brain injury: results from a large, single centre, observational study. BMC Emerg Med 2018;18(1):52.
89. Cuthbertson BH, Sprung CL, Annane D, et al. The effects of etomidate on adrenal responsiveness and mortality in patients with septic shock. Intensive Care Med 2009;35(11):1868–76.
90. Filanovsky Y, Miller P, Kao J. Myth: Ketamine should not be used as an induction agent for intubation in patients with head injury. CJEM 2010;12(2):154–7.
91. Cohen L, Athaide V, Wickham ME, et al. The effect of ketamine on intracranial and cerebral perfusion pressure and health outcomes: a systematic review. Ann Emerg Med 2015;65(1):43–51, e2.
92. Strebel S, Kaufmann M, Maître L, et al. Effects of ketamine on cerebral blood flow velocity in humans. Influence of pretreatment with midazolam or esmolol. Anaesthesia 1995;50(3):223–8.
93. Sakai K, Cho S, Fukusaki M, et al. The effects of propofol with and without ketamine on human cerebral blood flow velocity and CO(2) response. Anesth Analg 2000;90(2):377–82.
94. Kovarik WD, Mayberg TS, Lam AM, et al. Succinylcholine does not change intracranial pressure, cerebral blood flow velocity, or the electroencephalogram in patients with neurologic injury. Anesth Analg 1994;78(3):469–73.
95. Patanwala AE, Erstad BL, Roe DJ, et al. Succinylcholine is associated with increased mortality when used for rapid sequence intubation of severely brain injured patients in the emergency department. Pharmacotherapy 2016;36(1): 57–63.
96. Martyn JAJ, Richtsfeld M. Succinylcholine-induced hyperkalemia in acquired pathologic statesetiologic factors and molecular mechanisms. Anesthesiol J Am Soc Anesthesiol 2006;104(1):158–69.
97. Matsumoto M, Sakabe T. Effects of Anesthetic Agents and Other Drugs on Cerebral Blood Flow, Metabolism, and Intracranial Pressure. In: Cottrell JE, Patel P, Warner DS, editors. Cottrell and Patel's Neuroanesthesia. 6th edition. Edinburgh, Scotland: Elsevier; 2017. p. 74–90.

98. Matta BF, Heath KJ, Tipping K, et al. Direct cerebral vasodilatory effects of sevoflurane and isoflurane. Anesthesiology 1999;91(3):677–80.
99. Reinstrup P, Ryding E, Algotsson L, et al. Effects of nitrous oxide on human regional cerebral blood flow and isolated pial arteries. Anesthesiology 1994; 81(2):396–402.
100. Algotsson L, Messeter K, Rosén I, et al. Effects of nitrous oxide on cerebral haemodynamics and metabolism during isoflurane anaesthesia in man. Acta Anaesthesiol Scand 1992;36(1):46–52.
101. Kaisti KK, Långsjö JW, Aalto S, et al. Effects of sevoflurane, propofol, and adjunct nitrous oxide on regional cerebral blood flow, oxygen consumption, and blood volume in humans. Anesthesiology 2003;99(3):603–13.
102. Oren RE, Rasool NA, Rubinstein EH. Effect of ketamine on cerebral cortical blood flow and metabolism in rabbits. Stroke 1987;18(2):441–4.
103. Slupe AM, Kirsch JR. Effects of anesthesia on cerebral blood flow, metabolism, and neuroprotection. J Cereb Blood Flow Metab 2018;38(12):2192–208.
104. Albanese J, Arnaud S, Rey M, et al. Ketamine decreases intracranial pressure and electroencephalographic activity in traumatic brain injury patients during propofol sedation. Anesthesiology 1997;87(6):1328–34.
105. Godoy DA, Badenes R, Pelosi P, et al. Ketamine in acute phase of severe traumatic brain injury "an old drug for new uses?". Crit Care 2021;25(1):19.
106. Ropper AH. Hyperosmolar therapy for raised intracranial pressure. N Engl J Med 2012;367(8):746–52.
107. Sokhal N, Rath GP, Chaturvedi A, et al. Comparison of 20% mannitol and 3% hypertonic saline on intracranial pressure and systemic hemodynamics. J Clin Neurosci 2017;42:148–54.
108. Chen H, Song Z, Dennis JA. Hypertonic saline versus other intracranial pressure–lowering agents for people with acute traumatic brain injury. Cochrane Database Syst Rev 2020;2020(1):CD010904.
109. Fried HI, Nathan BR, Rowe AS, et al. The insertion and management of external ventricular drains: an evidence-based consensus statement : a statement for healthcare professionals from the neurocritical care society. Neurocrit Care 2016;24(1):61–81.
110. Lele AV, Hoefnagel AL, Schloemerkemper N, et al. Perioperative management of adult patients with external ventricular and lumbar drains: guidelines from the society for neuroscience in anesthesiology and critical care. J Neurosurg Anesthesiol 2017;29(3):191.
111. Smielewski P, Czosnyka M, Steiner L, et al. ICM+: software for on-line analysis of bedside monitoring data after severe head trauma. Acta Neurochir Suppl 2005; 95:43–9.
112. MOBERG® CNS Monitor. Micromed Group. Available at: https://micromedgroup.com/products/moberg/cns-monitor/. Accessed September 24, 2022.
113. Sickbay™ Platform | Virtual Care and Healthcare Data Analytics. Available at: https://michealthcare.com/sickbay/. Accessed September 24, 2022.
114. Hu PF, Yang S, Li HC, et al. Reliable collection of real-time patient physiologic data from less reliable networks: a "monitor of monitors" system (MoMs). J Med Syst 2016;41(1):3.
115. Baldassano SN, Roberson SW, Balu R, et al. IRIS: a modular platform for continuous monitoring and caretaker notification in the intensive care unit. IEEE J Biomed Health Inform 2020;24(8):2389–97.

116. Masimo - Patient SafetyNet. Available at: https://www.masimo.com/products/hospital-automation/surveillance/safetynet/. Accessed September 25, 2022.

117. Balestreri M, Czosnyka M, Hutchinson P, et al. Impact of intracranial pressure and cerebral perfusion pressure on severe disability and mortality after head injury. Neurocrit Care 2006;4(1):8–13.

118. Vik A, Nag T, Fredriksli OA, et al. Relationship of "dose" of intracranial hypertension to outcome in severe traumatic brain injury. J Neurosurg 2008;109(4):678–84.

119. Badri S, Chen J, Barber J, et al. Mortality and long-term functional outcome associated with intracranial pressure after traumatic brain injury. Intensive Care Med 2012;38(11):1800–9.

120. Sorrentino E, Diedler J, Kasprowicz M, et al. Critical thresholds for cerebrovascular reactivity after traumatic brain injury. Neurocrit Care 2012;16(2):258–66.

121. Helbok R, Meyfroidt G, Beer R. Intracranial pressure thresholds in severe traumatic brain injury: Con. Intensive Care Med 2018;44(8):1318–20.

122. Gelabert-González M, Ginesta-Galan V, Sernamito-García R, et al. The camino intracranial pressure device in clinical practice. Assessment in a 1000 cases. Acta Neurochir (Wien) 2006;148(4):435–41.

123. Koskinen LOD, Olivecrona M. Clinical experience with the intraparenchymal intracranial pressure monitoring Codman MicroSensor system. Neurosurgery 2005;56(4):693–8, discussion 693-698.

124. Citerio G, Piper I, Chambers IR, et al. Multicenter clinical assessment of the Raumedic Neurovent-P intracranial pressure sensor: a report by the BrainIT group. Neurosurgery 2008;63(6):1152–8, discussion 1158.

125. Allin D, Czosnyka M, Czosnyka Z. Laboratory testing of the Pressio intracranial pressure monitor. Neurosurgery 2008;62(5):1158–61 ; discussion 1161.

126. Lang JM, Beck J, Zimmermann M, et al. Clinical evaluation of intraparenchymal Spiegelberg pressure sensor. Neurosurgery 2003;52(6):1455–9, discussion 1459.

127. Wolfla CE, Luerssen TG, Bowman RM, et al. Brain tissue pressure gradients created by expanding frontal epidural mass lesion. J Neurosurg 1996;84(4):642–7.

128. Al-Tamimi YZ, Helmy A, Bavetta S, et al. Assessment of zero drift in the codman intracranial pressure monitor: a study from 2 neurointensive care units. Neurosurgery 2009;64(1):94–9.

129. Zeiler FA, Ercole A, Cabeleira M, et al. Patient-specific ICP Epidemiologic Thresholds in Adult Traumatic Brain Injury: A CENTER-TBI Validation Study. J Neurosurg Anesthesiol 2021;33(1):28–38.

130. Chesnut RM, Temkin N, Carney N, et al. A trial of intracranial-pressure monitoring in traumatic brain injury. N Engl J Med 2012;367(26):2471–81.

131. Robba C, Graziano F, Rebora P, et al. Intracranial pressure monitoring in patients with acute brain injury in the intensive care unit (SYNAPSE-ICU): an international, prospective observational cohort study. Lancet Neurol 2021;20(7):548–58.

132. Evensen KB, Eide PK. Measuring intracranial pressure by invasive, less invasive or non-invasive means: limitations and avenues for improvement. Fluids Barriers CNS 2020;17(1):34.

133. Foreman B, Lissak IA, Kamireddi N, et al. Challenges and opportunities in multimodal monitoring and data analytics in traumatic brain injury. Curr Neurol Neurosci Rep 2021;21(3):6.

134. Lundberg N. Continuous recording and control of ventricular fluid pressure in neurosurgical practice. J Neuropathol Exp Neurol 1962;21(3):489.

135. Martinez-Tejada I, Arum A, Wilhjelm JE, et al. B waves: a systematic review of terminology, characteristics, and analysis methods. Fluids Barriers CNS 2019; 16(1):33.

136. Droste DW, Krauss JK, Berger W, et al. Rhythmic oscillations with a wavelength of 0.5–2 min in transcranial Doppler recordings. Acta Neurol Scand 1994;90(2): 99–104.

137. Rosner MJ, Rosner SD, Johnson AH. Cerebral perfusion pressure: management protocol and clinical results. J Neurosurg 1995;83(6):949–62.

138. Robertson CS, Valadka AB, Hannay HJ, et al. Prevention of secondary ischemic insults after severe head injury. Crit Care Med 1999;27(10):2086–95.

139. Rosner MJ. Introduction to cerebral perfusion pressure management. Neurosurg Clin N Am 1995;6(4):761–73.

140. Lang EW, Chesnut RM. A bedside method for investigating the integrity and critical thresholds of cerebral pressure autoregulation in severe traumatic brain injury patients. Br J Neurosurg 2000;14(2):117–26.

141. Howells T, Elf K, Jones PA, et al. Pressure reactivity as a guide in the treatment of cerebral perfusion pressure in patients with brain trauma. J Neurosurg 2005; 102(2):311–7.

142. Hawryluk GWJ, Aguilera S, Buki A, et al. A management algorithm for patients with intracranial pressure monitoring: the Seattle International Severe Traumatic Brain Injury Consensus Conference (SIBICC). Intensive Care Med 2019;45(12): 1783–94.

143. Rosenthal G, Sanchez-Mejia RO, Phan N, et al. Incorporating a parenchymal thermal diffusion cerebral blood flow probe in bedside assessment of cerebral autoregulation and vasoreactivity in patients with severe traumatic brain injury. J Neurosurg 2011;114(1):62–70.

144. Goettel N, Patet C, Rossi A, et al. Monitoring of cerebral blood flow autoregulation in adults undergoing sevoflurane anesthesia: a prospective cohort study of two age groups. J Clin Monit Comput 2016;30(3):255–64.

145. Czosnyka M, Smielewski P, Kirkpatrick P, et al. Monitoring of cerebral autoregulation in head-injured patients. Stroke 1996;27(10):1829–34.

146. Czosnyka M, Smielewski P, Kirkpatrick P, et al. Continuous assessment of the cerebral vasomotor reactivity in head injury. Neurosurgery 1997;41(1):11–7, discussion 17-19.

147. Zeiler FA, Donnelly J, Menon DK, et al. A description of a new continuous physiological index in traumatic brain injury using the correlation between pulse amplitude of intracranial pressure and cerebral perfusion pressure. J Neurotrauma 2018;35(7):963–74.

148. Eide PK, Park EH, Madsen JR. Arterial blood pressure vs intracranial pressure in normal pressure hydrocephalus. Acta Neurol Scand 2010;122(4):262–9.

149. Evensen KB, Eide PK. Mechanisms behind altered pulsatile intracranial pressure in idiopathic normal pressure hydrocephalus: role of vascular pulsatility and systemic hemodynamic variables. Acta Neurochir (Wien) 2020;162(8): 1803–13.

150. Aries MJH, Czosnyka M, Budohoski KP, et al. Continuous monitoring of cerebrovascular reactivity using pulse waveform of intracranial pressure. Neurocrit Care 2012;17(1):67–76.

151. Zeiler FA, Ercole A, Cabeleira M, et al. Univariate comparison of performance of different cerebrovascular reactivity indices for outcome association in adult TBI: a CENTER-TBI study. Acta Neurochir (Wien) 2019;161(6):1217–27.

152. Steiner LA, Czosnyka M, Piechnik SK, et al. Continuous monitoring of cerebrovascular pressure reactivity allows determination of optimal cerebral perfusion pressure in patients with traumatic brain injury. Crit Care Med 2002;30(4):733–8.

153. Aries MJH, Czosnyka M, Budohoski KP, et al. Continuous determination of optimal cerebral perfusion pressure in traumatic brain injury. Crit Care Med 2012;40(8):2456–63.

154. Liu X, Maurits NM, Aries MJH, et al. Monitoring of optimal cerebral perfusion pressure in traumatic brain injured patients using a multi-window weighting algorithm. J Neurotrauma 2017;34(22):3081–8.

155. Zeiler FA, Ercole A, Cabeleira M, et al. Comparison of performance of different optimal cerebral perfusion pressure parameters for outcome prediction in adult traumatic brain injury: a collaborative european neurotrauma effectiveness research in traumatic brain injury (CENTER-TBI) study. J Neurotrauma 2019; 36(10):1505–17.

156. Tas J, Beqiri E, van Kaam RC, et al. Targeting autoregulation-guided cerebral perfusion pressure after traumatic brain injury (COGiTATE): a feasibility randomized controlled clinical trial. J Neurotrauma 2021;38(20):2790–800.

157. Bouzat P, Almeras L, Manhes P, et al. Transcranial doppler to predict neurologic outcome after mild to moderate traumatic brain injury. Anesthesiology 2016; 125(2):346–54.

158. Cardim D, Robba C, Donnelly J, et al. Prospective study on noninvasive assessment of intracranial pressure in traumatic brain-injured patients: comparison of four methods. J Neurotrauma 2016;33(8):792–802.

159. Bellner J, Romner B, Reinstrup P, et al. Transcranial Doppler sonography pulsatility index (PI) reflects intracranial pressure (ICP). Surg Neurol 2004;62(1): 45–51, discussion 51.

160. Robba C, Cardim D, Tajsic T, et al. Ultrasound non-invasive measurement of intracranial pressure in neurointensive care: A prospective observational study. PLOS Med 2017;14(7):e1002356.

161. Robba C, Goffi A, Geeraerts T, et al. Brain ultrasonography: methodology, basic and advanced principles and clinical applications. A narrative review. Intensive Care Med 2019;45(7):913–27.

162. Zeiler FA, Donnelly J, Cardim D, et al. ICP versus laser doppler cerebrovascular reactivity indices to assess brain autoregulatory capacity. Neurocrit Care 2018; 28(2):194–202.

163. Highton D, Ghosh A, Tachtsidis I, et al. Monitoring cerebral autoregulation after brain injury: multimodal assessment of cerebral slow-wave oscillations using near-infrared spectroscopy. Anesth Analg 2015;121(1):198–205.

164. Roldán M, Kyriacou PA. Near-Infrared Spectroscopy (NIRS) in Traumatic Brain Injury (TBI). Sensors 2021;21(5):1586.

165. Zweifel C, Castellani G, Czosnyka M, et al. Noninvasive Monitoring of Cerebrovascular Reactivity with Near Infrared Spectroscopy in Head-Injured Patients. J Neurotrauma 2010;27(11):1951–8.

166. Timofeev I, Czosnyka M, Nortje J, et al. Effect of decompressive craniectomy on intracranial pressure and cerebrospinal compensation following traumatic brain injury. J Neurosurg 2008;108(1):66–73.

167. Zweifel C, Lavinio A, Steiner LA, et al. Continuous monitoring of cerebrovascular pressure reactivity in patients with head injury. Neurosurg Focus 2008;25(4):E2.

168. Zeiler FA, Czosnyka M, Smielewski P. Optimal cerebral perfusion pressure via transcranial Doppler in TBI: application of robotic technology. Acta Neurochir (Wien) 2018;160(11):2149–57.

169. Sivakumar S, Taccone FS, Rehman M, et al. Hemodynamic and neuro-monitoring for neurocritically ill patients: An international survey of intensivists. J Crit Care 2017;39:40–7.

170. Ajčević M, Furlanis G, Miladinović A, et al. Early EEG Alterations Correlate with CTP Hypoperfused Volumes and Neurological Deficit: A Wireless EEG Study in Hyper-Acute Ischemic Stroke. Ann Biomed Eng 2021;49(9):2150–8.

171. Sutcliffe L, Lumley H, Shaw L, et al. Surface electroencephalography (EEG) during the acute phase of stroke to assist with diagnosis and prediction of prognosis: a scoping review. BMC Emerg Med 2022;22(1):29.

172. Yu Z, Wen D, Zheng J, et al. Predictive accuracy of alpha-delta ratio on quantitative electroencephalography for delayed cerebral ischemia in patients with aneurysmal subarachnoid hemorrhage: meta-analysis. World Neurosurg 2019; 126:e510–6.

173. Newey CR, Sarwal A, Hantus S. Continuous electroencephalography (cEEG) changes precede clinical changes in a case of progressive cerebral edema. Neurocrit Care 2013;18(2):261–5.

174. Sheikh ZB, Maciel CB, Dhakar MB, et al. Nonepileptic Electroencephalographic Correlates of Episodic Increases in Intracranial Pressure. J Clin Neurophysiol 2022;39(2):149–58.

175. Lee H, Mizrahi MA, Hartings JA, et al. Continuous Electroencephalography after Moderate to Severe Traumatic Brain Injury. Crit Care Med 2019;47(4):574–82.

176. Haveman ME, Van Putten MJAM, Hom HW, et al. Predicting outcome in patients with moderate to severe traumatic brain injury using electroencephalography. Crit Care Lond Engl 2019;23(1):401.

177. Vespa P, Tubi M, Claassen J, et al. Metabolic crisis occurs with seizures and periodic discharges after brain trauma. Ann Neurol 2016;79(4):579–90.

178. Waziri A, Claassen J, Stuart RM, et al. Intracortical electroencephalography in acute brain injury. Ann Neurol 2009;66(3):366–77.

179. Hartings JA, Bullock MR, Okonkwo DO, et al. Spreading depolarisations and outcome after traumatic brain injury: a prospective observational study. Lancet Neurol 2011;10(12):1058–64.

180. Mikell CB, Dyster TG, Claassen J. Invasive seizure monitoring in the critically-Ill brain injury patient: Current practices and a review of the literature. Seizure 2016;41:201–5.

181. Rostami E, Engquist H, Enblad P. Imaging of Cerebral Blood Flow in Patients with Severe Traumatic Brain Injury in the Neurointensive Care. Front Neurol 2014;5. Available at: https://www.frontiersin.org/articles/10.3389/fneur.2014.00114. Accessed September 21, 2022.

182. Vajkoczy P, Roth H, Horn P, et al. Continuous monitoring of regional cerebral blood flow: experimental and clinical validation of a novel thermal diffusion microprobe. J Neurosurg 2000;93(2):265–74.

183. Tackla R, Hinzman JM, Foreman B, et al. Assessment of Cerebrovascular Autoregulation Using Regional Cerebral Blood Flow in Surgically Managed Brain Trauma Patients. Neurocrit Care 2015;23(3):339–46.

184. Hinzman JM, Andaluz N, Shutter LA, et al. Inverse neurovascular coupling to cortical spreading depolarizations in severe brain trauma. Brain J Neurol 2014;137(Pt 11):2960–72.

185. Akbik OS, Carlson AP, Krasberg M, et al. The Utility of Cerebral Blood Flow Assessment in TBI. Curr Neurol Neurosci Rep 2016;16(8):72.
186. Rolfe P. In Vivo near-infrared spectroscopy. Annu Rev Biomed Eng 2000;2(1): 715–54.
187. Ghosh A, Elwell C, Smith M. Cerebral near-infrared spectroscopy in adults: a work in progress. Anesth Analg 2012;115(6):1373–83.
188. Steppan J, Hogue CW. Cerebral and tissue oximetry. Best Pract Res Clin Anaesthesiol 2014;28(4):429–39.
189. Yoshitani K, Kawaguchi M, Miura N, et al. Effects of hemoglobin concentration, skull thickness, and the area of the cerebrospinal fluid layer on near-infrared spectroscopy measurements. Anesthesiology 2007;106(3):458–62.
190. Robertson CS, Gopinath SP, Chance B. A new application for near-infrared spectroscopy: detection of delayed intracranial hematomas after head injury. J Neurotrauma 1995;12(4):591–600.
191. Gill AS, Rajneesh KF, Owen CM, et al. Early optical detection of cerebral edema in vivo. J Neurosurg 2011;114(2):470–7.
192. Bush B, Sam K, Rosenblatt K. The Role of Near-infrared Spectroscopy in Cerebral Autoregulation Monitoring. J Neurosurg Anesthesiol 2019;31(3):269–70.
193. Kirkman MA, Smith M. Brain oxygenation monitoring. Anesthesiol Clin 2016; 34(3):537–56.
194. Purins K, Enblad P, Sandhagen B, et al. Brain tissue oxygen monitoring: a study of in vitro accuracy and stability of Neurovent-PTO and Licox sensors. Acta Neurochir (Wien) 2010;152(4):681–8.
195. Oddo M, Nduom E, Frangos S, et al. Acute lung injury is an independent risk factor for brain hypoxia after severe traumatic brain injury. Neurosurgery 2010;67(2):338–44.
196. Oddo M, Levine JM, Kumar M, et al. Anemia and brain oxygen after severe traumatic brain injury. Intensive Care Med 2012;38(9):1497–504.
197. Menon DK, Coles JP, Gupta AK, et al. Diffusion limited oxygen delivery following head injury. Crit Care Med 2004;32(6):1384–90.
198. Van Den Brink WA, Van Santbrink H, Steyerberg EW, et al. Brain oxygen tension in severe head injury. Neurosurgery 2000;46(4):868–78.
199. Johnston AJ, Steiner LA, Coles JP, et al. Effect of cerebral perfusion pressure augmentation on regional oxygenation and metabolism after head injury. Crit Care Med 2005;33(1):189–95.
200. Oddo M. Bösel J, and the participants in the international multidisciplinary consensus conference on multimodality monitoring. monitoring of brain and systemic oxygenation in neurocritical care patients. Neurocrit Care 2014;21(2): 103–20.
201. Quintard H, Patet C, Suys T, et al. Normobaric hyperoxia is associated with increased cerebral excitotoxicity after severe traumatic brain injury. Neurocrit Care 2015;22(2):243–50.
202. Damiani E, Adrario E, Girardis M, et al. Arterial hyperoxia and mortality in critically ill patients: a systematic review and meta-analysis. Crit Care 2014;18(1). https://doi.org/10.1186/s13054-014-0711-x.
203. Martini RP, Deem S, Yanez ND, et al. Management guided by brain tissue oxygen monitoring and outcome following severe traumatic brain injury. J Neurosurg 2009;111(4):644–9.
204. Brain Trauma Foundation, American Association of Neurological Surgeons, Congress of Neurological Surgeons. Guidelines for the management of severe traumatic brain injury. J Neurotrauma 2007;24(Suppl 1):S1–106.

205. Spiotta AM, Stiefel MF, Gracias VH, et al. Brain tissue oxygen-directed management and outcome in patients with severe traumatic brain injury. J Neurosurg 2010;113(3):571–80.

206. Oddo M, Levine JM, Mackenzie L, et al. Brain hypoxia is associated with short-term outcome after severe traumatic brain injury independently of intracranial hypertension and low cerebral perfusion pressure. Neurosurgery 2011;69(5): 1037–45 ; discussion 1045.

207. Bernard F, Barsan W, Diaz-Arrastia R, et al. Brain Oxygen Optimization in Severe Traumatic Brain Injury (BOOST-3): a multicentre, randomised, blinded-endpoint, comparative effectiveness study of brain tissue oxygen and intracranial pressure monitoring versus intracranial pressure alone. BMJ Open 2022;12(3): e060188.

208. Okonkwo DO, Shutter LA, Moore C, et al. Brain Tissue Oxygen Monitoring and Management in Severe Traumatic Brain Injury (BOOST-II): a Phase II Randomized Trial. Crit Care Med 2017;45(11):1907–14.

209. Chesnut R, Aguilera S, Buki A, et al. A management algorithm for adult patients with both brain oxygen and intracranial pressure monitoring: the Seattle International Severe Traumatic Brain Injury Consensus Conference (SIBICC). Intensive Care Med 2020;46(5):919–29.

210. Goetting MG, Preston G. Jugular bulb catheterization does not increase intracranial pressure. Intensive Care Med 1991;17(4):195–8.

211. Nims LF, Gibbs EL, Lennox WG. Arterial and cerebral venous blood. J Biol Chem 1942;145(1):189–95.

212. Obrist WD, Langfitt TW, Jaggi JL, et al. Cerebral blood flow and metabolism in comatose patients with acute head injury: Relationship to intracranial hypertension. J Neurosurg 1984;61(2):241–53.

213. Kety SS, Schmidt CF. The nitrous oxide method for the quantitative determination of cerebral blood flow in man: theory, procedure and normal values. J Clin Invest 1948;27(4):476–83.

214. Cormio M, Valadka AB, Robertson CS. Elevated jugular venous oxygen saturation after severe head injury. J Neurosurg 1999;90(1):9–15.

215. Robertson CS, Gopinath SP, Goodman JC, et al. SjvO2 monitoring in head-injured patients. J Neurotrauma 1995;12(5):891–6.

216. Cruz J. The first decade of continuous monitoring of jugular bulb oxyhemoglobin saturation: Management strategies and clinical outcome. Crit Care Med 1998; 26(2):344–51.

217. Carpenter KLH, Young AMH, Hutchinson PJ. Advanced monitoring in traumatic brain injury: microdialysis. Curr Opin Crit Care 2017;23(2):103–9.

218. Rogers ML, Feuerstein D, Leong CL, et al. Continuous online microdialysis using microfluidic sensors: dynamic neurometabolic changes during spreading depolarization. ACS Chem Neurosci 2013;4(5):799–807.

219. Adamides AA, Rosenfeldt FL, Winter CD, et al. Brain tissue lactate elevations predict episodes of intracranial hypertension in patients with traumatic brain injury. J Am Coll Surg 2009;209(4):531–9.

220. Belli A, Sen J, Petzold A, et al. Metabolic failure precedes intracranial pressure rises in traumatic brain injury: a microdialysis study. Acta Neurochir (Wien) 2008; 150(5):461–70.

221. Larach DB, Kofke WA, Le Roux P. Potential non-hypoxic/ischemic causes of increased cerebral interstitial fluid lactate/pyruvate ratio: a review of available literature. Neurocrit Care 2011;15(3):609–22.

222. Hutchinson PJ, Jalloh I, Helmy A, et al. Consensus statement from the 2014 International Microdialysis Forum. Intensive Care Med 2015;41:1517–28.

223. Timofeev I, Carpenter KLH, Nortje J, et al. Cerebral extracellular chemistry and outcome following traumatic brain injury: a microdialysis study of 223 patients. Brain 2011;134(2):484–94.

224. Oddo M, Schmidt JM, Carrera E, et al. Impact of tight glycemic control on cerebral glucose metabolism after severe brain injury: a microdialysis study. Crit Care Med 2008;36(12):3233–8.

225. Vespa PM, McArthur D, O'Phelan K, et al. Persistently low extracellular glucose correlates with poor outcome 6 months after human traumatic brain injury despite a lack of increased lactate: a microdialysis study. J Cereb Blood Flow Metab 2003;23(7):865–77.

226. Chamoun R, Suki D, Gopinath SP, et al. Role of extracellular glutamate measured by cerebral microdialysis in severe traumatic brain injury. J Neurosurg 2010;113(3):564–70.

227. Clausen T, Alves OL, Reinert M, et al. Association between elevated brain tissue glycerol levels and poor outcome following severe traumatic brain injury. J Neurosurg 2005;103(2):233–8.

Update on Mechanical Circulatory Support

Suzanne Bennett, MD, FCCM[a],*, Lauren Sutherland, MD[b,1], Promise Ariyo, MD, MPH[c,2], Frank M. O'Connell, MD, FACP, FCCP, FCCM[d,3]

KEYWORDS

- Mechanical circulatory devices • Venovenous extracorporeal life support
- Extracorporeal membrane oxygenation • Venoarterial extracorporeal life support
- Intra-aortic balloon pump • Impella • Left ventricular assist device

KEY POINTS

- Mechanical circulatory support technology and understanding have driven a tremendous growth in its use.
- Mechanical circulatory support provides both short-term and intermediate- to long-term support for acute cardiopulmonary failure.
- Several types of mechanical circulatory support devices exist on patients with refractory acute respiratory failure and/or cardiogenic shock.
- Patient selection, cannulation strategy, and prevention of complications play a critical role in patient outcomes.
- Establishing an exit strategy (bridge to decision, transplant, recovery, or destination therapy) must be delineated before initiation of mechanical circulatory support.

INTRODUCTION

Since the development of mechanical circulatory support (MCS) in the 1950s, these pumps have continued to develop at a rapid pace, especially in the last 15 years. With the advances in technology, improved patient selection and understanding of the mechanics of the circuit and flow, patient outcomes have improved, resulting in an increased use of this technology. The first successful use of extracorporeal membrane oxygenation (ECMO)/extracorporeal life support (ECLS) occurred in the 1950s.[1,2] The advent of the first heart lung bypass machine laid the foundation for

[a] Department of Anesthesiology, University of Cincinnati College of Medicine, 2139 Albert Sabin Way, Cincinnati, OH 45267-0531, USA; [b] Columbia University Irving Medical Center, 622 W 168th Street, New York, NY 10032, USA; [c] Johns Hopkins University, 1800 Orleans Street, Baltimore, MD 21287, USA; [d] Anesthesiology, Atlanticare Regional Medical Center, 65 W Jimmie Leeds Road, Pomona, NJ 08240, USA
[1] Present address. 47 James Street, Hastings on Hudson, NY 10706.
[2] Present address. 2013 Holly Ridge Ct, Lutherville, MD 21093.
[3] Present address. 1150 Colts Lane, Yardley, PA 19067.
* Corresponding author.
E-mail address: suzanne.bennett@uc.edu

Anesthesiology Clin 41 (2023) 79–102
https://doi.org/10.1016/j.anclin.2022.08.019
1932-2275/23/© 2022 Elsevier Inc. All rights reserved.
anesthesiology.theclinics.com

the advancement of MCS with the first successful pneumatic left ventricular assist device (LVAD) implant in the 1960s.[3] The first successful use of ECMO in both adults and pediatrics occurred in the 1970s.[4]

Between the 1980s and 2000s, temporary MCS use and development were limited due to poor outcomes. However, durable MCS exploration and development continued, resulting in the approval of the first pulsatile flow LVAD pump in 1986.[3] As technology evolved and clinical trials demonstrated the safety and use of LVADs, clinical trials and efforts evaluating LVADs as a long-term therapy increased, resulting in more options available to patients suffering from heart failure today.

The use of MCS for acute respiratory failure (ARF) remained stagnant between the 1980s and 2000s. However, the improvements in circuits and oxygenators, coupled with the high mortality associated with ARF related to the 2009 H1N1 pandemic, fueled the use of ECLS for ARF.[5] Simultaneously, a paradigm shift in the application of MCS before end-organ damage for acute cardiogenic shock (CS) occurred, resulting in increased use of ECLS for acute CS.[6] Over the last 20 to 30 years, the use of MCS has grown (**Figs. 1–3**)[7]

MECHANICAL CIRCULATORY SUPPORT OVERVIEW

Primarily, MCS provides support for patients with exhausted physiologic reserve either as a temporary form of support or for more long-term use. Some MCS devices are used for respiratory support only, whereas others function for gas exchange as well as circulatory support. The decision to initiate such support is usually multidisciplinary and depends on several patient-related factors, such as severity of physiologic derangement, overall prognosis as well as institution-related resources, such as technical skills and other resources to support the MCS system. For the short-term support devices, an "exit strategy" should be a major consideration both at the time of initiation and for continuation of support.

TEMPORARY MECHANICAL CIRCULATORY SUPPORT
Mechanical Circulatory Support for Pulmonary Failure: Venovenous Extracorporeal Life Support

Brief description
The use of venovenous (VV) ECLS for ARF in adults continues to grow rapidly with a focus on minimizing ongoing lung injury and improving oxygenation/ventilation in patients in whom conventional therapies for acute respiratory distress syndrome (ARDS) have been exhausted. ARDS, which represents about a tenth of all intensive care unit admissions, portends a high mortality despite evidence demonstrating that lung protection strategies improves outcomes.[8] Although outcome data from prospective randomized clinical trials on the use of ECLS for ARDS are lacking, recent trials have demonstrated survival benefit with the use of ECLS in adults with severe ARDS treated at experienced centers.[5,9,10] Advances in technology and supportive multidisciplinary care, increasing literature with improved outcome trends, and the broader understanding of ECLS as a rescue therapy have driven the increase in the use of ECLS for ARF.[10–13] By the end of 2021, the ELSO registry had documented greater than 28,000 ECMO runs for ARF among greater than 500 centers internationally.[14]

The role of ECLS in severe ARDS is primarily gas exchange support while allowing for lung rest with healing, and reduction in inflammation and tissue injury. ECLS refers to the removal of blood from a central vein via a cannula, pumped through a semipermeable membrane (often called "membrane oxygenator") where carbon dioxide (CO_2) is removed and oxygen is delivered, and then the blood is returned to the patient via a

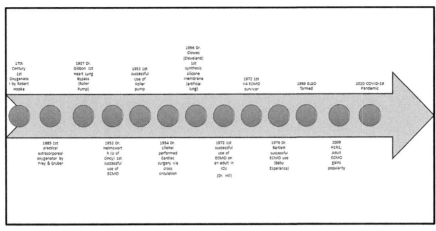

Fig. 1. MCS therapy timeline. ICU, intensive care unit.

central vein. ECLS consists of 2 different types of support: VV ECLS and extracorporeal carbon dioxide removal ($ECCO_2R$). During VV ECLS, blood flow rates are high, enabling both oxygenation and co_2 removal. After conventional therapies for severe ARDS have been exhausted, VV ECLS may be considered. $ECCO_2R$, which uses lower blood flow rates and smaller cannulas, permits effective co_2 removal but limited oxygenation improvement. $ECCO_2R$ use in ARDS exits when ventilation is the primary concern and other disease states where primarily ventilation is compromised (ie, status asthmaticus, chronic obstructive pulmonary disease [COPD]).

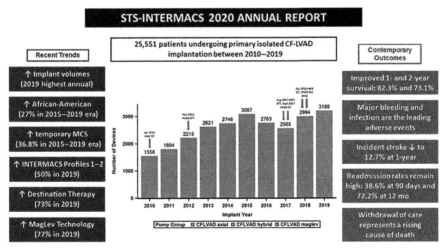

Fig. 2. MCS volumes in the Society of Thoracic Surgeons Interagency Registry for Mechanically Assisted Circulatory Support for all durable device types implanted between January 1, 2010 and December 31, 2019. CFLVAD, continuous flow left ventricular assist device; HVAD, HeartWare ventricular assist device; STS, society of thoracic surgeons. (Reprinted with permission of Elsevier7Molina EJ, Shah P, Kiernan MS, et al. The Society of Thoracic Surgeons Intermacs 2020 Annual Report. *The Annals of Thoracic Surgery.* 2021/03/01/ 2021;111(3):778 to 792. https://doi.org/10.1016/j.athoracsur.2020.12.038)

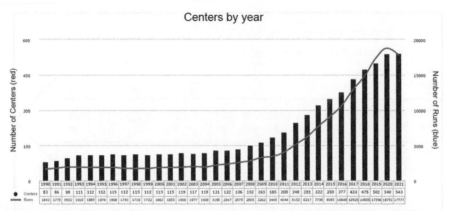

Fig. 3. ECLS Registry International Summary Report. ELSO. April 2022. Number of ECMO (all types) runs per year (*blue*) and centers (*red*) per year through December 2021. (Reprinted with permission of ELSO8 Organization ELS. ELSO Registry Report International Summary [Internet]. 2021 [cited 2022 Apr 3]. p. 1-40.)

Patient selection
The evaluation of adults with severe ARF for ECLS requires assessment for the cause of respiratory failure, the failure of conventional acute respiratory strategies, and the reversibility of the respiratory failure. In those patients with irreversible respiratory failure and eligible for lung transplant, ECLS is used as a bridge to transplant (BTT). Simply stated, VV ECLS is considered in patients with severe, refractory, acute, reversible respiratory failure. The decision to initiate ECLS should be balanced with the mortality of the patient despite conventional therapies without ECLS and the risks of ECLS. The RESP score and the Murray score, which are in-hospital survival/mortality prediction scores for ARF, are used to guide decision making around selection, but should not be used in isolation for patient selection[15,16] (**Table 1**). The RESP score provides predicted survival following initiation of ECLS. The Murray score provides predicted mortality without ECLS. The primary indications for VV ECLS are as a rescue for hypoxemic respiratory failure, for hypercarbic respiratory failure, and as a bridge to lung transplant or primary graft dysfunction after lung transplant. A full list of indications with proposed clinical scenarios are listed in **Table 2**.

Another clinical setting where ECLS has played an important role is in acute respiratory viral outbreaks, including H1N1, MERS-CoV, and COVID-19. Nonrandomized, retrospective small studies of patients with severe refractory ARDS related to acute respiratory viral outbreaks have demonstrated mortality benefits with early transfer to ECMO centers and, with strict patient selection, in-hospital mortality benefit.[17–21]

Recent evidence has provided some guidance on triggers for VV ECLS initiation in the setting of hypoxemia (Pao_2 < 80 mm Hg), Murray score > 3, and hypercarbia (pH < 7.25 and $Paco_2 \geq$ 60 mm Hg) only after conventional therapies (prone positioning) have been exhausted.[11,13,22] Early institution and optimization of the conventional medical therapies, coupled with early initiation of VV ECLS when those therapies are failing, should be a priority in the management of ARF to minimize morbidity and mortality.

The list of VV ECLS contraindications continue to decrease likely owing to the improved safety and ease of its use. Several relative contraindications for VV ECLS initiation persist, whereas the only absolute contraindication is irreversible disease without any chance for recovery despite VV ECLS[23] (**Table 3**). In the setting of

Table 1
Components to calculate a Murray score

Parameter, Score		Murray Score			
SCORE ≥ Predicted Mortality Related to ARDS at least 80%					
	0	1	2	3	4
Pao_2/Fio_2 (on 100%)	≥40 kPA	30–40 kPA	23–30 kPA	13–23 kPA	<13 kPA
	300 mm Hg	225–299 mm Hg	175–224 mm Hg	100–174 mm Hg	<100 mm Hg
CXR quadrants	Normal	1	2	3	4
PEEP (cm_{H_2O})	≤5	6–8	9–11	12–14	≥15
Compliance (mL/cm_{H_2O})	≥80	60–79	40–59	20–39	≤19

Averaged scores of all 4 parameters.[18]
Murray JF, Matthay MA, Luce JM, Flick MR. An expanded definition of the adult respiratory distress syndrome. *Am Rev Respir Dis.* Sep 1988;138(3):720-3. https://doi.org/10.1164/ajrccm/138.3.720

Table 2
Venovenous extracorporeal life support indications with examples of clinical conditions[14,16,24]

VV ECLS Indications	Clinical Scenarios
Hypoxemic respiratory failure: $Pao_2/$ $Fio_2 < 80$ mm Hg & Murray score >3; despite optimal medical management, including prone positioning	• Acute respiratory distress syndrome • Severe Inhalation Injury • Pulmonary hemorrhage/diffuse alveolar hemorrhage • Thoracic injury/pulmonary contusion • Eosinophilic pneumonia • Large bronchopleural fistula • Acute pulmonary embolism without shock
Hypercarbic respiratory failure: pH < 7.25 with a $Paco_2 \geq 60$ mm Hg despite optimal conventional mechanical ventilation including respiratory rate (RR) < 35 bpm & plateau pressure ≤ 30 cm$_{H_2O}$	• Status asthmaticus • COPD exacerbation
Bridge to lung transplant or primary graft dysfunction after lung transplant in the setting of requiring mechanical ventilation	• Peri-lung transplant requiring mechanical ventilation support

Peek GJ, Mugford M, Tiruvoipati R, et al. Efficacy and economic assessment of conventional ventilatory support versus extracorporeal membrane oxygenation for severe adult respiratory failure (CESAR): a multicentre randomised controlled trial. *Lancet.* Oct 17 2009;374(9698):1351-63. https://doi.org/10.1016/s0140-6736(0961069-2). Combes A, Hajage D, Capellier G, et al. Extracorporeal Membrane Oxygenation for Severe Acute Respiratory Distress Syndrome. *New England Journal of Medicine.* 2018/05/23/ 2018;378(21):1965-1975. Tonna JE, Abrams D, Brodie D, et al. Management of Adult Patients Supported with Venovenous Extracorporeal Membrane Oxygenation (VV ECMO): Guideline from the Extracorporeal Life Support Organization (ELSO). *ASAIO J.* 2021;67(6):601-610. https://doi.org/10.1097/mat.0000000000001432

---

multidisciplinary discussions, consideration of the relative contraindications should be evaluated based on individual risks and benefits to VV ECLS initiation.

Once a patient has been identified as an appropriate candidate for VV ECLS early initiation is favored. In centers where ECLS is not feasible, early transfer to established ECMO centers should be considered.[11]

Cannulation strategies

The basic principles of VV ECLS cannulation are to choose the strategy that provides the optimal flow rates, which match physiologic demands of the patient while balancing risks and benefits. Three different modalities of ECLS cannulation for ARF include single-lumen dual (SLDC) cannulation, bicaval dual-lumen single cannulation (DLSC), and the bifemoral venous cannulation. The SLDC consists of placement of the drainage cannula into the inferior vena cava (IVC)-atrial junction via percutaneous insertion into the femoral vein (FV) and the return cannula in the superior vena cava (SVC)-atrial junction via percutaneous insertion into the internal jugular vein (IJV). This strategy has the advantage of being placed by surface ultrasound and often permits higher ECMO flow rates. The disadvantages include the need for 2 cannulation sites and limited patient mobility. The bicaval DLSC consists of percutaneous placement of a dual-lumen cannula via the IJV under live fluoroscopic or echocardiographic imaging with the drainage locations being in the SVC and IVC in the same lumen of the cannula and the return location being in the right atrium (RA) with the jet directed toward the tricuspid valve. The advantages of the DLSC are only one cannulation site and increased liberation for mobility. The disadvantages include insertion difficulties,

Table 3
Venovenous extracorporeal life support contraindications[28]

	VV ECLS Contraindications
Absolute contraindications	• Irreversible disease with no chance for recovery despite ECMO
Relative contraindications	• Advanced age • Comorbidities: Immunosuppression, significant and irreversible central nervous system (CNS) injury/disease, terminal malignancy • Systemic or CNS bleeding • Contraindications to anticoagulation • High mechanical ventilation settings for >7 d (plateau pressures > 30 cm_{H_2O} and Fio_2 > 90%)

Tonna JE, Abrams D, Brodie D, et al. Management of Adult Patients Supported with Venovenous Extracorporeal Membrane Oxygenation (VV ECMO): Guideline from the Extracorporeal Life Support Organization (ELSO). *ASAIO Journal*. 2021;67(6):601-610. https://doi.org/10.1097/mat.0000000000001432

possible flow limitations, cannula movement resulting in recirculation, cerebral venous congestion, and some evidence for increased risk of intracerebral hemorrhage with larger-diameter cannulas.[24] Recently, the use of a DLSC inserted percutaneously into the IJV with RA as the drainage location and the pulmonary artery as the return location has been successfully used in ARF requiring VV ECLS.[25] This cannulation provides the advantage of bypassing the right ventricle (RV), which is often strained in patients with ARF. The bifemoral venous cannulation consists of percutaneous placement of the cannulas via the FVs with the drainage cannula located in the IVC and the return cannula located in the RA. The advantages of this strategy are like the SLDC. The disadvantages are similar to SLDC with mobility being more limited given cannulas are in both FVs.

MECHANICAL CIRCULATORY SUPPORT FOR CARDIOPULMONARY FAILURE
Intra-Aortic Balloon Pump

The intra-aortic balloon pump (IABP) is a device inserted into the femoral or axillary artery and positioned into the descending thoracic/aortic arch, which provides counterpulsation, inflating during diastole and collapsing during systole. This device augments coronary perfusion and increases cardiac output by 0.5 to 1.0 L per minute. The balloon size ranges in size from 22 to 27.5 cm long and 25 to 50 mL inflated, in order to accommodate a wide range of patient body sizes. Normally, the balloon is inserted into the femoral artery via an 8.5-French sheath and advanced under fluoroscopic guidance to within a few centimeters of the left subclavian artery in the aortic arch. The rationale for its use includes the augmentation of aortic pressure and coronary perfusion during inflation in and decrease in afterload and potential unloading of the left ventricle (LV) during systole (**Fig. 4**). The timing of the balloon inflation-deflation is synchronized to the cardiac cycle by either an electrocardiogram or an aortic pressure sensor.

The major advantages of this mode of MCS are the ease with which it can be implanted and its widespread availability.[6,26] There are several clinical circumstances leading to CS for which the IABP may be indicated for LV afterload reduction or improving coronary perfusion; these include the following:

1. Acute new-onset heart failure

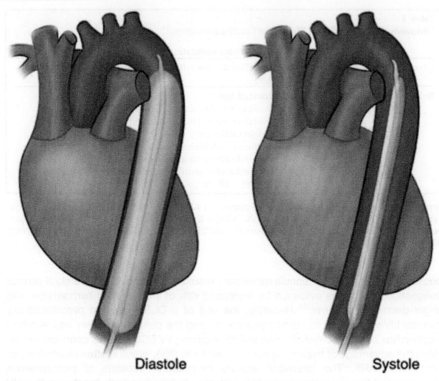

Diastole   Systole

Fig. 4. IABP: inflating during diastole and deflating during systole.

2. Cardiac arrest
3. Acute-on-chronic heart failure
4. Perioperative support for cardiac surgery
5. ST segment elevation myocardial infarction

In addition, when the IABP does not provide adequate support for a patient in CS, venoarterial (VA) ECLS may be added. The added benefit in this model is the afterload reduction that the IABP provides to a patient on VA ECLS, thus reducing the risk of LV distension.[27] Outcomes studies on the use of the IABP with VA ECLS versus VA ECLS alone are mixed.[28–30]

The IABP may be placed through the upper extremity as an open surgical technique with graft placement via the axillary artery.[31] Percutaneous placement using fluoroscopy or ultrasound via the radial, brachial, or axillary arterial approach avoids the risks of general anesthesia. The left side is preferred, as a right-sided approach is associated with a high incidence of displacement into the aortic arch, causing potential compromise of the anterior cerebral circulation (**Fig. 5**). Axillary placement of these devices facilitates a longer period of time for which the IABP may be left in place, allowing for medical optimization. Another advantage of axillary placement is the ability to ambulate should the patient's condition improve. Should rupture of the helium balloon occur, replacement of the IABP may be achieved using the same access site over a guide wire.

Impella

The Impella (Abiomed Impella, Danvers, MA, USA) is a microaxial flow pump that is catheter mounted. The traditional Impella is placed across the aortic valve. The inlet

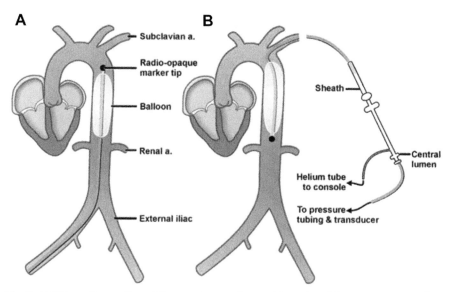

A

- Subclavian a.
- Radio-opaque marker tip
- Balloon
- Renal a.
- External iliac

B

- Sheath
- Central lumen
- Helium tube to console
- To pressure tubing & transducer

Fig. 5. IABP insertion options: (*A*) percutaneous femoral insertion; (*B*) percutaneous axillary insertion. a., aorta.

in the LV draws blood from the ventricle via the flow pump and accelerates blood flow to the outlet in the proximal aorta (**Fig. 6**). In this way, the Impella enhances systemic perfusion while simultaneously unloading the LV.[32] This displacement of blood from the LV to the proximal aorta occurs in a continuous, nonpulsatile manner.[33] The Impella may be inserted by either the axillary or the femoral artery. Because blood is withdrawn from the LV throughout the cardiac cycle, the Impella decreases end-diastolic volume and ameliorates chamber distension, which may decrease myocardial oxygen consumption.[34]

Four Impella devices are currently available for LV support, which provide different amounts of flow augmentation:

1. Impella 2.5 (2.5 L/min)
2. Impella CP (3.8 L/min)
3. Impella 5.0 (5 L/min)
4. Impella 5.5 (5.5 L/min)

The external controller gives the clinician feedback as to how the device is functioning, and which may signal malposition of either the LV inlet or the aortic outlet. The performance level (P level) with the corresponding flow, set and found on the controller, determines the amount of support that the patient receives from the device. Several waveforms are displayed on the console, including the motor current waveform for the microaxial pump, the aortic outlet waveform, the LV inlet waveform, the Impella flow, and the cardiac output. Because these devices provide continuous unloading of the LV throughout the cardiac cycle, they may reduce ventricular distension, left ventricular end-diastolic pressure (LVEDP), and thus may potentially improve native cardiac function.[35] Data exist detailing quantitative approaches to heart-Impella interactions, which can generate accurate measurements of LVEDP, cardiac output, and systemic vascular resistance.[36] Continuous and instantaneous monitoring of these parameters allow the clinician to titrate support from the Impella

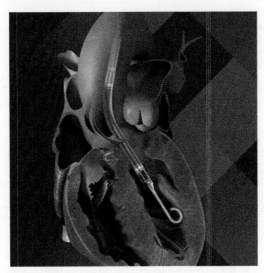

Fig. 6. Impella positioned across aortic valve into the LV.

accordingly. The Impella 2.5 and CP are smaller devices that can be inserted percutaneously into the femoral or axillary/subclavian arteries. Femoral artery insertion is most common, especially in emergency/urgent scenarios. The insertion of the Impella via the axillary arteries is favored when anticipated duration is long and alternative vessels are too calcified. The Impella 5.0 and 5.5 (larger) require a surgical cutdown and vascular graft.

Impella RP

The Impella RP, a right-sided support device that is inserted into the FV via a 23-French sheath and advanced until the outlet is in the main pulmonary artery and the inlet is resting in either the IVC or RA, is designed to support the failing right heart. The technology for this device is analogous to left-sided Impella support devices in that it uses a microaxial flow pump, which provides continuous, nonpulsatile forward motion of blood flow. The device bypasses the failing RV, sending blood from the IVC or RA directly to the pulmonary arterial circulation. Large randomized controlled trials for right-sided MCS devices are lacking. One prospective study (RECOVER RIGHT TRIAL) demonstrated patients with a failing RV to have an immediate increase in cardiac index (CI) and a decrease in central venous pressure (CVP). Although the trial was not powered to look at an effect on clinical outcomes, the 30-day mortality in the Impella RP patient was approximately 27%.[37–40] A more recent multicenter prospective study demonstrated an immediate improvement in hemodynamics with a marked increase in CI and a decrease in CVP. The overall survival at 30 days (or discharge) was 72%.[41]

Impella 5.5

The Impella 5.5 can generate flow rates of up to 6 L per minute and can be implanted via a surgical cutdown technique via the axillary artery or as an open chest procedure into the aortic root. One study at 3 medical centers enrolled 55 patients with CS of various causes (acute myocardial infarction, postpericardiotomy, and so forth) with 83% of these surviving to explant and 76% of these patients recovering native cardiac function.[42]

Venoarterial Extracorporeal Life Support

VA-ECLS is a form of MCS that provides both cardiac and pulmonary support to patients with hemodynamic instability. Blood is drained from the venous circulation (usually the IVC or the RA), pumped through the ECLS circuit, and returned to arterial circulation either peripherally (femoral artery, axillary artery cannula) or centrally via an aortic cannula. There are several indications for VA ECLS support. VA ECLS is indicated in the setting of refractory CS, which is usually defined as a CI of less than 2 L/min/m^2 and hypotension with systolic blood pressure less than 90 mm Hg. This can occur postmyocardial infarction despite maximal pharmacologic therapy,[43] with the recommendation that this should be performed early (60 minutes of appearance of refractory CS).[44,45]

Another common indication is refractory postcardiotomy shock in the operating room or postoperatively owing to profound shock or cardiac arrest.[46,47]

VA ECLS has been an invaluable tool with a favorable survival to discharge in the management of acute myocarditis, a condition that can be quite severe and deadly without MCS.[48–50] VA ECLS can be lifesaving in patients with massive pulmonary embolism by providing adequate perfusion to organs and unloading the right heart pending reduction of clot burdens by other interventions.[51]

Other indications include support of patients with acute-on-chronic decompensated heart failure and support during interventional cardiology procedures. VA ECLS is also used to rescue a failed return of spontaneous circulation (ROSC) despite adequate cardiopulmonary resuscitation, providing more optimal blood flow to vital organs pending treatment and recovery from underlying pathology. This method of rescue has shown promising results especially when used in younger patients after a witnessed arrest and early (within 10–15 minutes) in the resuscitation efforts[52,53] (**Boxes 1** and **2**).

Cannulation Techniques

There are 2 major techniques to cannulate for VA ECLS. The peripheral cannulation technique, which is faster and less invasive, can be performed at bedside and can support blood flow of 5 to 6 L/min with the right sized catheters. This ease of placement makes it ideal for emergency cannulation, especially for eCPR. Typically, blood is drained from the femoral or IJV and returned to the femoral artery to perfuse the body in a retrograde fashion[54] (**Fig. 7**).

Another option for peripheral arterial cannulation is to use the axillary artery. This provides anterograde arterial flow, and it is therefore more physiologic. It also has the added advantage of promoting ambulation, which is important for rehabilitation while on ECLS, either as part of the recovery efforts or as rehabilitation in preparation for transplantation.[55,56]

Central cannulation is more likely to be used in postcardiotomy patients. In these cases, venous blood is drained from the atrium and returned after gas exchange into the arterial cannulation and is placed directly into the ascending aorta (**Fig. 8**).

Hybrid Configurations

Venoarterial-veno extracorporeal life support

Venoarterial-veno (VAV) ECLS represents a hybrid of VA and VV ECLS. Blood is drained from the venous circulation, oxygenated, and pumped back into 2 return cannulas, one to the arterial side (VA) and the second, back to the venous side (VV). This configuration is considered when a patient with coexisting respiratory and circulatory failure requires ECLS..

> **Box 1**
> **Venoarterial extracorporeal life support indications**
>
> Indications for VA ECLS
> Cardiogenic shock
>   Postmyocardial infarction
>   Postcardiotomy shock
>   Acute myocarditis
>   Massive pulmonary embolism
>   Acute on chronic decompensated heart failure
>   eCPR
>
> Bridge to transplant
>
> Procedural support

Patients with circulatory failure supported with peripheral VA ECLS are at risk for North-South or Harlequin syndrome. This syndrome occurs when a contractile LV, be it marginal, ejects blood with poor oxygen tension into the circulation. This mixes with retrograde blood flow from the ECMO cannula, and depending on the mixing point or watershed area, the coronary and even cerebral circulations are at risk of hypoxemia. In VAV ECLS, a second return arterial delivers oxygenated blood via the venous to the right side of the heart in addition to the oxygenated blood delivered to the left circulation already. Flow though the 2 return cannulas can be controlled by a clamp based on measurement from a flow sensor.[57,58]

VAV can also be helpful as an adjunct to a VV ECLS configuration initially placed for isolated respiratory failure but subsequently developed cardiac dysfunction. An arterial cannula is added via a Y-connector to provide oxygenated blood to the arterial side, usually via a femoral artery cannula.

Venovenoarterial extracorporeal life support

This is VA ECLS with an extravenous drainage cannula. The function of the extravenous cannula is to enhance venous drainage, reduce LV distension, and improve arterial flow. This may be particularly useful in patients with large body habitus and small-size venous cannulas.[59]

Extracorporeal Life Support Complications

Despite advances in technology and knowledge, morbidity and mortality on ECLS remain high. ECLS can result in severe complications, which are potentially life-threatening. Complications from ECLS support are related to the placement of the cannulas or those related to maintenance (noncannulation related) on ECLS support. Bleeding, with rates as high as 50%, and thromboembolism represent the major non-cannula-related complications while on ECLS.[60] LV distension and North-South syndrome (previously described) are VA ECLS-specific complications. VA ECLS, especially peripheral ECLS, creates a

> **Box 2**
> **Venoarterial extracorporeal life support contraindications**
>
> Contraindications for VA ECLS
>   Unwitnessed cardiac arrest or prolonged resuscitation efforts
>   Advanced malignancy with poor prognosis
>   Severe brain injury incompatible with acceptable quality of life
>   Severe aortic regurgitation
>   Severe peripheral vascular disease for peripheral cannulation

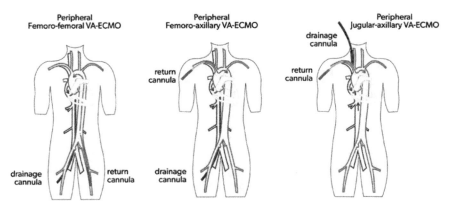

Fig. 7. Peripheral VA ECLS cannulation strategies. (Reprinted with permission from *ASAIO Journal 2022* Guidelines.63Gajkowski EF, Herrera G, Hatton L, Velia Antonini M, Vercaemst L, Cooley E. ELSO Guidelines for Adult and Pediatric Extracorporeal Membrane Oxygenation Circuits. *Asaio j.* Feb 1 2022;68(2):133-152. https://doi.org/10.1097/mat.0000000000001630)

state of increased afterload, which, in a failing heart, can lead to increased LVEDP, pulmonary edema, poor recovery of heart function as well as stasis of blood and thrombosis.[61–63] Measures to reduce LV distension include decreased ECMO flows, inotropes, vasodilation, diuretics, or invasive procedures, such as atrial septostomy, LV venting, Impella, and IABP, to name a few.[64]

Mechanical, cannula-related complications, albeit rare, lead to vessel injury with an associated increased morbidity (ie, limb ischemia, pseudoaneurysm) and mortality. A more complete list of ECLS complications are listed in **Table 4**. To minimize, and often avoid these complications, cannulation should be performed by a skilled, competent, and experienced cannulating physician.

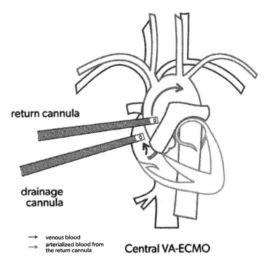

Fig. 8. Central VA ECLS cannulation strategies. Reprinted with permission from *ASAIO Journal 2022* Guidelines. Gajkowski EF, Herrera G, Hatton L, Velia Antonini M, Vercaemst L, Cooley E. ELSO Guidelines for Adult and Pediatric Extracorporeal Membrane Oxygenation Circuits. *Asaio j.* Feb 1 2022;68(2):133-152. doi:10.1097/mat.0000000000001630

Table 4	
More common extracorporeal life support complications	
Mechanical Cannula-Related Complications	**Noncannulation Related Complications**
Vessel perforation	Bleeding
Arterial dissection	Hemolysis
Distal limb ischemia	Thromboembolism
Malposition	LV distension
Incorrectly placed (ie, wrong vessel)	North-South syndrome (Harlequin syndrome)
Pseudoaneurysm	Acute kidney injury
	Infection

INTERMEDIATE- AND LONG-TERM (DURABLE) MECHANICAL CIRCULATORY SUPPORT

For patients with refractory heart failure, MCS may be considered for prolonged or permanent support. These devices can serve as a BTT; "bridge to recovery" for patients who require a temporary period of MCS for cardiac recovery from acute CS; "bridge to decision" in patients whose candidacy for transplantation or additional therapeutic options are being considered; or "destination therapy" (DT) for patients who require lifelong MCS as an alternative to heart transplantation.

Left Ventricular Assist Devices

LVADs pump blood from the LV into the ascending aorta, both increasing systemic blood flow and unloading the LV. Internal LVADs or "durable" devices use an LV apical inflow cannula, a pump, an ascending aortic outflow cannula, and a percutaneous driveline that attaches to a controller, powered by either wall power or batteries. First-generation devices used pulsatile flow and gave a survival benefit over maximal medical therapy,[65] but limitations included poor durability, large size, and noisiness. Second-generation devices were designed to have a smaller profile and greater durability, and they provide continuous rather than pulsatile flow. The HeartMate II (HMII; Abbott Labs, Chicago, IL, USA) LVAD (**Fig. 9**), a continuous-flow mechanical bearing axial pump, dramatically improved patient survival and quality of life[66] and was Food and Drug Administration (FDA) approved as BTT in 2008 and DT in 2010. Additional second-generation devices are listed in **Table 5**.

Third-generation LVADs, including HeartWare (HVAD, Medtronic, Minneapolis, MN, USA) and HeartMate 3 (HM3; Abbott Labs), also provide continuous flow but use a centrifugal pump with a smaller profile that fits inside the pericardium. Implantation can be performed either through traditional sternotomy or through a less-invasive approach involving a left anterolateral thoracotomy and either right miniature thoracotomy or hemisternotomy. The less-invasive approach aims to reduce surgical trauma and keep the pericardium closed, potentially reducing the incidence or severity RV failure.[67]

The HVAD pump is suspended by both magnetic and hydrodynamic forces with no mechanical bearings, minimizing friction, and it runs at a slower speed, giving it longer durability. The ADVANCE study compared HVAD with HMII as BTT and showed noninferiority, with 86% 1-year survival and marked improvement in quality of life.[68] The ENDURANCE trial compared HVAD with HMII in patients withDT and showed noninferiority in survival free from disabling stroke or the need for device replacement; however, there was a significantly higher risk of stroke, RV failure, and sepsis in the HVAD

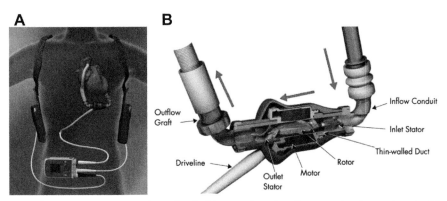

Fig. 9. (A) HeartMate II is trademark of Abbott or its related companies. Reproduced with permission of Abbott, © 2022. All rights reserved. (B) HeartMate II is trademark of Abbott or its related companies. Reproduced with permission of Abbott, © 2022. All rights reserved.

group compared with a higher risk of device malfunction in the HMII group.[69] HVAD was approved for BTT in 2012 and DT in 2017. In 2021, the FDA issued a class 1 recall of the HVAD, halting its sale and distribution because of an increased risk of neurologic adverse events and mortality as well as pump stoppages with failure to restart.[70]

The HM3 LVAD (**Fig. 10**) is a fully magnetically levitated centrifugal pump with an asynchronous "pulse" every 2 seconds that reduces stasis in the pump. It is currently the only FDA-approved durable LVAD.[7] The MOMENTUM 3 trial randomized patients with heart failure to HM3 versus HMII and found significantly improved survival free of disabling stroke or reoperation to replace or remove the device.[71] The primary outcome difference was driven by significantly more frequent reoperation for pump malfunction owing to pump thrombosis in the HMII group.[71] Two-year follow-up also revealed a significantly lower overall stroke risk in the HM3 group.[72] Follow-up in a continuous access protocol postpivotal trial study of 2200 HM3 patients showed 81.2% 2-year survival and 76.7% survival free of disabling stroke or reoperation to replace or remove the device.

The STS Interagency Registry for Mechanically Assisted Circulatory Support (INTERMACS) registry is a North American database of patients who receive FDA-approved MCS devices and their outcomes. Based on the most recent annual report, 1- and 2-year survival of patients undergoing isolated LVAD implant between 2015 and 2019 are 82.3% and 73.1%, respectively.[7]

COMPLICATIONS

Infection and major bleeding are the most common complications in the early and late periods after LVAD implantation, with only 59% and 67%, respectively, free from these complications at 1 year.[7] Bleeding can be multifactorial based on surgical factors, anticoagulation, and acquired von Willebrand factor deficiency (aVWFD). aVWFD is thought to occur because of shear stress leading to excessive cleavage of large multi-mers by the metalloproteinase ADAMTS.[73] Gastrointestinal bleeding is particularly common in patients with LVAD owing to the formation of arteriovenous malformations, thought to be caused by hypoxia of the intestinal mucosa from decreased pulse pressure during continuous flow physiology.[73] Device infections may occur within the pump, in the pump pocket, or most commonly, at the driveline site.[74] Additional

Table 5
Current durable Mechanical Circulatory Devices (MCDs)

Device Name	Manufacturer	Flow Profile	FDA Approved	Maximum Flow	Speed Range	Weight	Notes
HeartMate II	Abbott	Continuous (axial)	BTT 2008 DT 2010	10 L/min	6000–12,000 rpm	350 g	• Higher rate of pump thrombosis and stroke compared with HM3
Jarvik2000	JarvikHeart	Continuous (axial)	BTT 2005	8.5 L/min	8000–12,000 rpm	85 g	• Entire pump within LV cavity • Reduction in speed 8 s every 1 min • Option for retroauricular driveline
HeartMate 3	Abbott	Continuous (centrifugal)	BTT 2017 DT 2018	10 L/min	3000–9000 rpm	240 g	• Intrapericardial • Fully magnetically levitated • Artificial pulse every 2 s • Only commercially available LVAD currently
Heartware (HVAD)	Medtronic	Continuous (centrifugal)	BTT 2012 DT 2017	10 L/min	1800–4000 rpm	140 g	• Intrapericardial • Recalled in 2021 for pump stoppages and increased neurologic events
SynCardia Total Artificial Heart	SynCardia	Pulsatile	BTT 2004	9.5 L/min	Variable	160 g	• Replaces the heart • Restricted to larger chest size • 2 drivelines

A   **B**

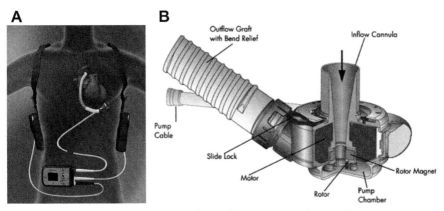

Fig. 10. (*A*) HeartMate 3 LVAD system during battery-powered operation. HeartMate 3 is trademark of Abbott or its related companies. Reproduced with permission of Abbott, © 2022. All rights reserved. (*B*) HeartMate 3 LVAD components. HeartMate 3 is trademark of Abbott or its related companies. Reproduced with permission of Abbott, © 2022. All rights reserved.

complications from LVAD include RV failure, cardiac arrhythmias, stroke, device malfunction, ARF, and renal dysfunction.

Right Ventricular Assist Devices after Left Ventricular Assist Device Placement

Decompression of the LV by an LVAD can lead to worsening RV function owing to septal shift to the left, distortion of RV geometry, and worsening tricuspid regurgitation. Titration of LVAD speed must consider maintaining septal position and optimizing RV function, as this is necessary to provide preload to the LVAD. The incidence of right ventricular failure (RVF) after LVAD placement is associated with higher mortality and longer length of stay.[41,75] Management of RVF includes the use of inotropes, pulmonary vasodilators, and echocardiogram-guided LVAD speed adjustment. In cases of RVF refractory to medical management, either a surgical or a percutaneous right ventricular assist device (RVAD) may be needed. A surgical RVAD uses an extracorporeal pump such as CentriMag (Abbott Labs, Chicago, IL, USA) with either FV or right atrial inflow and pulmonary artery outflow. ProtekDuo is a dual-lumen cannula that is placed percutaneously through an IJV with device inflow in the RA and outflow in the pulmonary artery. The Impella RP has also been used for mechanical RV support after LVAD placement. CentriMag is the only FDA-approved device for extended temporary support for up to 30 days, and there are no approved long-term devices.[76] Outcomes after biventricular assist devices (BiVAD) are significantly worse when compared with isolated LVADs.[75]

External Left Ventricular Assist Devices

For patients who are inadequately supported with or unable to be weaned from short-term left ventricular support and candidacy for a durable device is under consideration, an external LVAD can be placed as a bridge to recovery or durable device. Cannulation typically involves a left atrial or LV apical inflow to ascending aorta or axillary artery outflow with an external pump, such as a CentriMag; this device can be inserted without the use of cardiopulmonary bypass.[77] A variation with the addition of VA ECLS called "EC-VAD" gives biventricular support through the addition of a femoral venous drainage cannula to unload the RV.[77]

Table 6
Cardiac support device selection

Device	Maximum Flow	LV Unloading	RV Support	Duration of Support	Notes
IABP		Yes	No	Weeks	
Impella CP/5.5		Yes	No	Weeks	
Impella RP		N/A	Yes	Weeks	
VA ECMO		No	Yes	Weeks	
TandemHeart		Yes	No		Contraindications: Severe PVD
HM3 LVAD	10 L/min	Yes	No	Years	Durable device. Contraindications: severe liver or kidney dysfunction, RV failure
CentriMag LVAD	10 L/min	Yes	No	Up to 30 d	Variety of cannulation options
CentriMag RVAD	10 L/min	No	Yes	Up to 30 d	Oxygenator can be inserted
SynCardia TAH	9.5 L/min	N/A	Yes	Months to years	Consider patients with: biventricular failure, small, nondilated ventricles, postinfarction ventricular septal defect (VSD), end-stage congenital heart disease, intracardiac thrombus or tumor

Total Artificial Heart

Although LVADs are the preferred device for severe left ventricular dysfunction, the total artificial heart (TAH, SynCardia, Tucson, AZ, USA) remains an option for patients with profound biventricular failure or severe cardiac abnormalities that place them at risk for poor outcomes following LVAD implantation (eg, a small, nondilated LV, massive cardiac thrombus, or uncontrollable malignant arrhythmias).[78] The SynCardia TAH is the only commercially available TAH, and it was FDA-approved as BTT in 2004. The device consists of 2 pneumatically driven ventricles with mechanical valves to create unidirectional flow, replacing the native heart. Because of the device's size, there are significant chest size constraints on candidates for placement. A prospective nonrandomized study showed 1-year survival of 70%, with 1-year and 5-year survivals after bridge to heart transplant of 86% and 64%, respectively.[79] There have been no randomized studies comparing BIVAD with TAH, as most patients who receive TAH are deemed poor candidates for LVAD. Complications are similar to those of LVAD. Newer TAHs are currently being investigated.[80]

Selecting a Device

Selection of MCS involves first assessing the degree of relative cardiopulmonary dysfunction using cardiopulmonary imaging and pulmonary artery catheterization. Assessment of relative left, right, or biventricular dysfunction is necessary for selecting the appropriate type of support. Additional considerations include duration and degree of support needed, degree of ventricular unloading, percutaneous versus surgical approach, patient size and access constraints, and site capabilities in placement and management (**Table 6**).

CLINICS CARE POINTS

- Triggers for VV ECLS initiation include hypoxemia (PaO2 < 80 mm Hg), Murray score >3, and hypercarbia (pH <7.25 and PaCO2 60 mm Hg) after conventional therapies have been exhausted.

- The IABP improves coronary perfusion and unloads the LV with a small increase in LV output, but it is easily implanted and widely available. The Impella device provides greater cardiac output but is more complex to place since it crosses the aortic valve.

- VA ECLS can provide 5-6 L/min of flow to the systemic circulation as well as RV unloading, but it creates high LV afterload. An IABP or Impella device can be added to VA ECLS to prevent or treat LV distension.

- RV failure is a common complication after LVAD placement due to LV decompression, septal shift, and distortion of RV geometry. This can be managed with inotropic support, pulmonary vasodilators, echocardiogram-guided LVAD speed adjustment, and RV mechanical support in severe cases.

DISCLOSURE

The authors have nothing to disclose.

REFERENCES

1. Clowes GH Jr. Extracorporeal maintenance of circulation and respiration. Physiol Rev 1960;40:826–919.

2. Brogan TV, Lequier L, Lorusso R, et al. Extracorporeal life support: the ELSO red book. In: ELSO red book. 5th edition. Extracorporeal Life Support Organization; 2017.

3. Enciso JS. Mechanical circulatory support: current status and future directions. Prog Cardiovasc Dis 2016;58(4):444–54.

4. Terzi A. Mechanical circulatory support: 60 years of evolving knowledge. Int J Artif Organs 2019;42(5):215–25.

5. Munshi L, Walkey A, Goligher E, et al. Venovenous extracorporeal membrane oxygenation for acute respiratory distress syndrome: a systematic review and meta-analysi. Lancet Respir Med 2019;7(2):163–72.

6. Stretch R, Sauer CM, Yuh DD, et al. National Trends in the Utilization of Short-Term Mechanical Circulatory Support: Incidence, Outcomes, and Cost Analysis. J Am Coll Cardiol 2014;64(14):1407–15.

7. Molina EJ, Shah P, Kiernan MS, et al. The Society of Thoracic Surgeons Intermacs 2020 Annual Report. Ann Thorac Surg 2021;111(3):778–92.

8. Bellani G, Laffey JG, Pham T, et al. Epidemiology, Patterns of Care, and Mortality for Patients With Acute Respiratory Distress Syndrome in Intensive Care Units in 50 Countries. JAMA 2016;315(8):788–800.

9. Goligher EC, Tomlinson G, Hajage D, et al. Extracorporeal Membrane Oxygenation for Severe Acute Respiratory Distress Syndrome and Posterior Probability of Mortality Benefit in a Post Hoc Bayesian Analysis of a Randomized Clinical Trial. JAMA 2018;320(21):2251–9.

10. Combes A, Schmidt M, Hodgson CL, et al. Extracorporeal life support for adults with acute respiratory distress syndrome. Intensive Care Med 2020;46(12): 2464–76.

11. Peek GJ, Mugford M, Tiruvoipati R, et al. Efficacy and economic assessment of conventional ventilatory support versus extracorporeal membrane oxygenation for severe adult respiratory failure (CESAR): a multicentre randomised controlled trial. Lancet 2009;374(9698):1351–63.

12. Abrams D, Brodie D. Extracorporeal Membrane Oxygenation for Adult Respiratory Failure: 2017 Update. Chest 2017;152(3):639–49.

13. Combes A, Hajage D, Capellier G, et al. Extracorporeal Membrane Oxygenation for Severe Acute Respiratory Distress Syndrome. N Engl J Med 2018;378(21): 1965–75.

14. Organization ELS. ELSO Registry Report International Summary [Internet]. 2021 [cited 2022 Apr 3]. p. 1-40.

15. Joshi H, Flanagan M, Subramanian R, et al. Respiratory ECMO Survival Prediction (RESP) Score for COVID-19 Patients Treated with ECMO. ASAIO J 2022; 68(4):486–91.

16. Murray JF, Matthay MA, Luce JM, et al. An expanded definition of the adult respiratory distress syndrome. Am Rev Respir Dis 1988;138(3):720–3.

17. Noah MA, Peek GJ, Finney SJ, et al. Referral to an extracorporeal membrane oxygenation center and mortality among patients with severe 2009 influenza A (H1N1). JAMA 2011;306(15):1659–68.

18. Davies A, Jones D, Bailey M, et al. Extracorporeal Membrane Oxygenation for 2009 Influenza A (H1N1) Acute Respiratory Distress Syndrome. JAMA 2009; 302(17):1888–95.

19. Schmidt M, Bailey M, Sheldrake J, et al. Predicting survival after extracorporeal membrane oxygenation for severe acute respiratory failure. The Respiratory Extracorporeal Membrane Oxygenation Survival Prediction (RESP) score. Am J Respir Crit Care Med 2014;189(11):1374–82.

20. Barbaro RP, MacLaren G, Boonstra PS, et al. Extracorporeal membrane oxygenation support in COVID-19: an international cohort study of the Extracorporeal Life Support Organization registry. Lancet 2020;396(10257):1071–8.
21. Urner M, Barnett AG, Bassi GL, et al. Venovenous extracorporeal membrane oxygenation in patients with acute covid-19 associated respiratory failure: comparative effectiveness study. Bmj 2022;377:e068723.
22. Abrams D, Ferguson ND, Brochard L, et al. ECMO for ARDS: from salvage to standard of care? Lancet Respir Med 2019;7(2):108–10.
23. Tonna JE, Abrams D, Brodie D, et al. Management of Adult Patients Supported with Venovenous Extracorporeal Membrane Oxygenation (VV ECMO): Guideline from the Extracorporeal Life Support Organization (ELSO). ASAIO J 2021;67(6): 601–10.
24. Mazzeffi M, Kon Z, Menaker J, et al. Large Dual-Lumen Extracorporeal Membrane Oxygenation Cannulas Are Associated with More Intracranial Hemorrhage. ASAIO J 2019;65(7).
25. Mustafa AK, Alexander PJ, Joshi DJ, et al. Extracorporeal Membrane Oxygenation for Patients With COVID-19 in Severe Respiratory Failure. JAMA Surg 2020;155(10):990–2.
26. Ginsberg F, Parrillo JE. Cardiogenic shock: a historical perspective. Crit Care Clin 2009;25(1):103–14, viii.
27. Burkhoff D, Sayer G, Doshi D, et al. Hemodynamics of Mechanical Circulatory Support. J Am Coll Cardiol 2015;66(23):2663–74.
28. Ro SK, Kim JB, Jung SH, et al. Extracorporeal life support for cardiogenic shock: influence of concomitant intra-aortic balloon counterpulsation. Eur J Cardiothorac Surg 2014;46(2):186–92 ; discussion 192.
29. Park TK, Yang JH, Choi SH, et al. Clinical impact of intra-aortic balloon pump during extracorporeal life support in patients with acute myocardial infarction complicated by cardiogenic shock. BMC Anesthesiol 2014;14:27.
30. Li Y, Yan S, Gao S, et al. Effect of an intra-aortic balloon pump with venoarterial extracorporeal membrane oxygenation on mortality of patients with cardiogenic shock: a systematic review and meta-analysis. Eur J Cardiothorac Surg 2019; 55(3):395–404.
31. Bhimaraj A, Agrawal T, Duran A, et al. Percutaneous Left Axillary Artery Placement of Intra-Aortic Balloon Pump in Advanced Heart Failure Patients. JACC Heart Fail 2020;8(4):313–23.
32. Abiomed. Abiomed Impella CP. 2022. Available at: https://abiomed.com. Accessed May 1, 2022.
33. Stoliński J, Rosenbaum C, Flameng W, et al. The heart-pump interaction: effects of a microaxial blood pump. Int J Artif Organs 2002;25(11):1082–8.
34. Miyashita S, Kariya T, Yamada KP, et al. Left Ventricular Assist Devices for Acute Myocardial Infarct Size Reduction: Meta-analysis. J Cardiovasc Transl Res 2021; 14(3):467–75.
35. Esposito ML, Zhang Y, Qiao X, et al. Left Ventricular Unloading Before Reperfusion Promotes Functional Recovery After Acute Myocardial Infarction. J Am Coll Cardiol 2018;72(5):501–14.
36. Chang BY, Keller SP, Bhavsar SS, et al. Mechanical circulatory support device-heart hysteretic interaction can predict left ventricular end diastolic pressure. Sci Transl Med 2018;10:430.
37. Anderson MB, Goldstein J, Milano C, et al. Benefits of a novel percutaneous ventricular assist device for right heart failure: The prospective RECOVER RIGHT study of the Impella RP devic. J Heart Lung Transplant 2015;34(12):1549–60.

38. Maekawa K, Tanno K, Hase M, et al. Extracorporeal cardiopulmonary resuscitation for patients with out-of-hospital cardiac arrest of cardiac origin: a propensity-matched study and predictor analysis. Crit Care Med 2013;41(5):1186–96.
39. Holmberg MJ, Geri G, Wiberg S, et al. Extracorporeal cardiopulmonary resuscitation for cardiac arrest: A systematic review. Resuscitation 2018;131:91–100.
40. Ortega-Deballon I, Hornby L, Shemie SD, et al. Extracorporeal resuscitation for refractory out-of-hospital cardiac arrest in adults: A systematic review of international practices and outcomes. Resuscitation 2016;101:12–20.
41. Anderson M, Morris DL, Tang D, et al. Outcomes of patients with right ventricular failure requiring short-term hemodynamic support with the Impella RP device. J Heart Lung Transpl 2018;37(12):1448–58.
42. Ramzy D, Soltesz E, Anderson M. New Surgical Circulatory Support System Outcomes. ASAIO J 2020;66(7):746–52.
43. Rihal CS, Naidu SS, Givertz MM, et al. 2015 SCAI/ACC/HFSA/STS Clinical Expert Consensus Statement on the Use of Percutaneous Mechanical Circulatory Support Devices in Cardiovascular Care: Endorsed by the American Heart Association, the Cardiological Society of India, and Sociedad Latino Americana de Cardiologia Intervencion; Affirmation of Value by the Canadian Association of Interventional Cardiology-Association Canadienne de Cardiologie d'intervention. J Am Coll Cardiol 2015;65(19):e7–26.
44. Aoyama N, Imai H, Kurosawa T, et al. Therapeutic strategy using extracorporeal life support, including appropriate indication, management, limitation and timing of switch to ventricular assist device in patients with acute myocardial infarction. J Artif Organs 2014;17(1):33–41.
45. Smedira NG, Blackstone EH. Postcardiotomy mechanical support: risk factors and outcomes. Ann Thorac Surg 2001;71(3 Suppl):S60–6 ; discussion S82-5.
46. Ko WJ, Lin CY, Chen RJ, et al. Extracorporeal membrane oxygenation support for adult postcardiotomy cardiogenic shock. Ann Thorac Surg 2002;73(2):538–45.
47. Smedira NG, Moazami N, Golding CM, et al. Clinical experience with 202 adults receiving extracorporeal membrane oxygenation for cardiac failure: survival at five years. J Thorac Cardiovasc Surg 2001;122(1):92–102.
48. Diddle JW, Almodovar MC, Rajagopal SK, et al. Extracorporeal membrane oxygenation for the support of adults with acute myocarditis. Crit Care Med 2015;43(5):1016–25.
49. Hsu KH, Chi NH, Yu HY, et al. Extracorporeal membranous oxygenation support for acute fulminant myocarditis: analysis of a single center's experience. Eur J Cardiothorac Surg 2011;40(3):682–8.
50. Su TW, Tseng YH, Wu TI, et al. Extracorporeal life support in adults with hemodynamic collapse from fulminant cardiomyopathies: the chance of bridging to recovery. ASAIO J 2014;60(6):664–9.
51. Leacche M, Unic D, Goldhaber SZ, et al. Modern surgical treatment of massive pulmonary embolism: results in 47 consecutive patients after rapid diagnosis and aggressive surgical approach. J Thorac Cardiovasc Surg 2005;129(5):1018–23.
52. Reynolds JC, Frisch A, Rittenberger JC, et al. Duration of resuscitation efforts and functional outcome after out-of-hospital cardiac arrest: when should we change to novel therapies? Circulation 2013;128(23):2488–94.
53. Bossaert LL, Perkins GD, Askitopoulou H, et al. European Resuscitation Council Guidelines for Resuscitation 2015: Section 11. The ethics of resuscitation and end-of-life decisions. Resuscitation 2015;95:302–11.

54. Gajkowski EF, Herrera G, Hatton L, et al. ELSO Guidelines for Adult and Pediatric Extracorporeal Membrane Oxygenation Circuits. ASAIO J 2022;68(2):133–52.

55. Navia JL, Atik FA, Beyer EA, et al. Extracorporeal membrane oxygenation with right axillary artery perfusion. Ann Thorac Surg 2005;79(6):2163–5.

56. Moazami N, Moon MR, Lawton JS, et al. Axillary artery cannulation for extracorporeal membrane oxygenator support in adults: an approach to minimize complications. J Thorac Cardiovasc Surg 2003;126(6):2097–8.

57. Choi JH, Kim SW, Kim YU, et al. Application of veno-arterial-venous extracorporeal membrane oxygenation in differential hypoxia. Multidiscip Respir Med 2014; 9(1):55.

58. Hou X, Yang X, Du Z, et al. Superior vena cava drainage improves upper body oxygenation during veno-arterial extracorporeal membrane oxygenation in sheep. Crit Care 2015;19(1):68.

59. Takeda K, Garan AR, Topkara VK, et al. Novel minimally invasive surgical approach using an external ventricular assist device and extracorporeal membrane oxygenation in refractory cardiogenic shock. Eur J Cardiothorac Surg 2017;51(3):591–6.

60. Mazzeffi M, Greenwood J, Tanaka K, et al. Bleeding, Transfusion, and Mortality on Extracorporeal Life Support: ECLS Working Group on Thrombosis and Hemostasis. Ann Thorac Surg 2016;101(2):682–9.

61. Madershahian N, Weber C, Scherner M, et al. Thrombosis of the aortic root and ascending aorta during extracorporeal membrane oxygenation. Intensive Care Med 2014;40(3):432–3.

62. Rupprecht L, Flörchinger B, Schopka S, et al. Cardiac decompression on extracorporeal life support: a review and discussion of the literature. ASAIO J 2013; 59(6):547–53.

63. Weber C, Deppe AC, Sabashnikov A, et al. Left ventricular thrombus formation in patients undergoing femoral veno-arterial extracorporeal membrane oxygenation. Perfusion 2018;33(4):283–8.

64. Lorusso R, Shekar K, MacLaren G, et al. ELSO Interim Guidelines for Venoarterial Extracorporeal Membrane Oxygenation in Adult Cardiac Patients. ASAIO J 2021; 67(8):827–44.

65. Rose EA, Gelijns AC, Moskowitz AJ, et al. Long-term use of a left ventricular assist device for end-stage heart failure. N Engl J Med 2001;345(20):1435–43.

66. Kirklin JK, Naftel DC, Pagani FD, et al. Seventh INTERMACS annual report: 15,000 patients and counting. J Heart Lung Transpl 2015;34(12):1495–504.

67. Al-Naamani A, Fahr F, Khan A, et al. Minimally invasive ventricular assist device implantation. J Thorac Dis 2021;13(3):2010–7.

68. Aaronson KD, Slaughter MS, Miller LW, et al. Use of an intrapericardial, continuous-flow, centrifugal pump in patients awaiting heart transplantation. Circulation 2012;125(25):3191–200.

69. Rogers JG, Pagani FD, Tatooles AJ, et al. Intrapericardial Left Ventricular Assist Device for Advanced Heart Failure. N Engl J Med 2017;376(5):451–60.

70. Medtronic. Urgent Medical Device Communication. Available at: https://www.medtronic.com/content/dam/medtronic-com/global/HCP/Documents/hvad-urgent-medical-device-notice-june-2021.pdf. Accessed May 29, 2022, 2022.

71. Mehra MR, Uriel N, Naka Y, et al. A Fully Magnetically Levitated Left Ventricular Assist Device - Final Report. N Engl J Med 2019;380(17):1618–27.

72. Mehra MR, Goldstein DJ, Uriel N, et al. Two-Year Outcomes with a Magnetically Levitated Cardiac Pump in Heart Failure. N Engl J Med 2018;378(15):1386–95.

73. Patel SR, Vukelic S, Jorde UP. Bleeding in continuous flow left ventricular assist device recipients: an acquired vasculopathy? J Thorac Dis 2016;10:e1321–7.

74. O'Horo JC, Abu Saleh OM, Stulak JM, et al. Left Ventricular Assist Device Infections: A Systematic Review. ASAIO J 2018;64(3):287–94.

75. Cleveland JC Jr, Naftel DC, Reece TB, et al. Survival after biventricular assist device implantation: an analysis of the Interagency Registry for Mechanically Assisted Circulatory Support database. J Heart Lung Transpl 2011;30(8):862–9.

76. Turner KR. Right Ventricular Failure After Left Ventricular Assist Device Placement-The Beginning of the End or Just Another Challenge? J Cardiothorac Vasc Anesth 2019;33(4):1105–21.

77. Takeda K, Garan AR, Ando M, et al. Minimally invasive CentriMag ventricular assist device support integrated with extracorporeal membrane oxygenation in cardiogenic shock patients: a comparison with conventional CentriMag biventricular support configuration. Eur J Cardiothorac Surg 2017;52(6):1055–61.

78. Cook JA, Shah KB, Quader MA, et al. The total artificial heart. J Thorac Dis 2015; 7(12):2172–80.

79. Copeland JG, Smith RG, Arabia FA, et al. Cardiac replacement with a total artificial heart as a bridge to transplantation. N Engl J Med 2004;351(9):859–67.

80. Schroder JN, Milano CA. CARMAT Total Artificial Heart and the Quest to Improve Biventricular Mechanical Support. ASAIO J 2021;10:1109–10.

Management of Intraoperative Cardiac Arrest

Aalok K. Kacha, MD, PhD[a,b,]*, Megan Henley Hicks, MD[c],
Christopher Mahrous, MD[d], Allison Dalton, MD[a],
Talia K. Ben-Jacob, MD, MSc[e]

KEYWORDS

- Perioperative cardiac arrest • Advanced cardiac life support • Resuscitation
- Hemodynamic and respiratory compromise

KEY POINTS

- Intraoperative cardiopulmonary arrest is rare and management differs from cardiac arrest in other locations often due to knowledge of etiology and early initiation of treatment.
- Common intraoperative causes include arrhythmias, anaphylaxis, local anesthetic systemic toxicity, adverse effects of neuraxial agents, excessive dosing of intravenous or inhalation agents, malignant hyperthermia, traumatic cardiac arrest, tension pneumothorax or hemothorax, pericardial tamponade, and pulmonary embolism.
- Metabolic abnormalities (eg, hyperkalemia, hypokalemia, hypomagnesemia, hypoglycemia, and hyperglycemia) should be corrected.
- Patients are at high risk for hemodynamic and/or respiratory compromise during transport from the operating room to another interventional location or to the intensive care unit after cardiac arrest.

INTRODUCTION

Advanced cardiac life support (ACLS), is a set of clinical guidelines for the urgent and emergent treatment of life-threatening cardiovascular conditions that will cause or have caused cardiopulmonary arrest. Originally created for community-based emergency

[a] Department of Anesthesia and Critical Care, Section of Critical Care Medicine, University of Chicago, 5841 South Maryland Avenue, MC 4028, Chicago, IL 60637, USA; [b] Department of Surgery, Section of Transplant Surgery, University of Chicago, 5841 South Maryland Avenue, MC 4028, Chicago, IL 60637, USA; [c] Department of Anesthesiology, Wake Forest University School of Medicine, Atrium Health Wake Forest Baptist Medical Center, 1 Medical Center Boulevard, Winston-Salem, NC 27157, USA; [d] Department of Anesthesiology, Cooper Medical School of Rowan University, One Cooper Plaza, Dorrance 2nd Floor, Camden, NJ 08103, USA; [e] Department of Anesthesiology, Division of Critical Care, Cooper Medical School of Rowan University, One Cooper Plaza, Dorrance 2nd Floor, Camden, NJ 08103, USA
* Corresponding author. Department of Anesthesia and Critical Care, Section of Critical Care Medicine, University of Chicago, 5841 South Maryland Avenue, MC 4028, Chicago, IL 60637.
E-mail address: akacha@bsd.uchicago.edu

Anesthesiology Clin 41 (2023) 103–119
https://doi.org/10.1016/j.anclin.2022.10.002
anesthesiology.theclinics.com

services and subsequently translated for application in the emergency department and other hospital locations, ACLS has become the mainstay of cardiac arrest management.[1]

Cardiac arrest during anesthesia is distinct from other settings because it is usually witnessed and frequently anticipated. Consequently, aggressive measures can be taken to support the patient's physiology and avoid or delay the need for ACLS. These key differences are associated with better outcomes compared with out-of-hospital or unwitnessed in-hospital cardiac arrests.[2,3]

This article reviews specific ACLS recommendations and approaches for management of intraoperative cardiac arrest.

Incidence and Outcomes of Intraoperative Cardiac Arrest

Intraoperative cardiopulmonary arrest (ICA) in the United States is rare, occurring in approximately five to six per 10,000 anesthetic cases.[4–6] One study noted that only 0.74 per 10,000 ICAs were thought to be associated with anesthesia-related causes.[6] However, hypoxemia, acidosis, and hypovolemia due to fluid shifts or blood loss are often contributory factors.

The etiology of ICA is often readily apparent during a surgical procedure because arrest is almost always witnessed by clinician(s) familiar with the patient's medical history, and the precipitating cause may be known and rapidly reversible. Thus, the initiation of treatment is usually timely and focused, resulting in better outcomes in terms of survival or residual neurologic deficits compared with arrest in other settings.[2,7] In one retrospective registry study of patients suffering ICA, one-third survived to hospital discharge, with good neurologic outcomes seen in two-thirds of the survivors.[8]

Considerations for Patients at Risk for Cardiac Arrest

ICA occurs most frequently in patients undergoing cardiac, thoracic, or vascular surgery.[4] Comorbidities including congestive heart failure, pulmonary circulation disorders, peripheral vascular disease, end-stage renal disease, or fluid and electrolyte abnormalities are often present. Patients in shock and those who have suffered major trauma are also at risk. In one study, intraoperative calls for help in the intraoperative setting were most frequently for airway, cardiac, or hemorrhagic emergencies.[9]

Standard intraoperative monitoring should include electrocardiography (ECG) for immediate recognition and treatment of arrhythmias. A five-lead ECG with computerized ST-segment trending may also be useful for diagnosis of abnormalities suggestive of ischemia or pericarditis (ST segment changes), pericardial effusion (low voltage of the QRS complex or electrical alternans), or pulmonary embolism (S1Q3T3 pattern, new right bundle branch block, or anterior T-wave inversion).

For patients at risk for arrhythmias leading to cardiac arrest, transcutaneous defibrillator adhesive patches with pacing capability should be placed before induction of anesthesia as defibrillation, cardioversion, or transcutaneous pacing may become necessary.[2,3] During cardiac arrest, delay in defibrillation for longer than 2 minutes is associated with decreased survival in the perioperative setting.[10]

Intra-arterial catheters allow for continuous monitoring of blood pressure (BP) in critical illness states (low cardiac output state, preoperative infusion of vasoactive agents), for evaluation of respirophasic variations in the arterial pressure waveform to predict fluid responsiveness and for frequent blood sampling. Of all the nonstandard monitoring techniques, arterial catheterization for continuous monitoring of BP is probably the most important additional monitoring method and should be frequently used. Central venous catheters (CVCs) may be inserted for patients who need central access for infusion of vasoactive drugs, fluid or blood administration, measurement of central venous pressure, or measurement of central-mixed venous oxygen saturation.

Pulmonary artery catheters are used less frequently but are appropriate if the patient would benefit from measurement of cardiac output, systemic vascular resistance, pulmonary artery pressure, pulmonary vascular resistance, and mixed venous oxygen saturation.

Transesophageal echocardiography (TEE) monitoring or point-of-care ultrasonography (POCUS) may be useful for continuous monitoring of cardiac function and intravascular volume status in high-risk patients. Even if a TEE probe is not inserted initially, "rescue" TEE can be performed urgently to diagnose the cause of cardiac arrest or refractory hypotension. POCUS is an alternative modality for diagnosis or confirmation of the cause of shock or cardiac arrest. Although invasive cardiovascular monitors may be helpful for recognition and management of the cause of cardiopulmonary arrest and may also provide useful information as subsequent interventions are performed, attempts to insert an intra-arterial catheter, CVC, or TEE probe should not delay treatment.

Recognition of impending or actual cardiopulmonary arrest may be challenging in the operating room compared with other settings as patients are typically sedated or under general anesthesia with controlled ventilation. Thus, the loss of consciousness, physical collapse, and sudden apnea cannot be observed. Patients with pacemakers will continue to demonstrate electrical activity on ECG. In addition, patient positioning for the surgical procedure and the presence of sterile drapes covering most of the body typically make assessment difficult.[2,3] For example, it may not be possible to access and check a central pulse.

Of note, the pulse oximeter may be unreliable or nonfunctioning in a patient with shock. In some patients, body habitus (eg, obesity) or pathology (eg, burns, hypothermia, anasarca, and vasculopathy) impede noninvasive monitor function. The overall positive predictive value for alarms built into anesthesia machines and clinical monitors is very poor, and the vast majority of these alarms are false.[11]

Recognition and Management of Cardiac Arrest

In the intraoperative setting, the most commonly recognized indicators of cardiopulmonary arrest are:

a. A nonperfusing rhythm evident on the ECG (eg, pulseless rhythms including ventricular fibrillation, ventricular tachycardia, severe bradycardia, or asystole). It is critically important to check for a carotid (or other accessible) pulse as soon as an abnormal rhythm is detected. Loss of pulse for greater than 10 seconds is an indicator of cardiopulmonary arrest.[2]

b. "Loss" of the intra-arterial pressure waveform tracing.

c. Loss of pulse oximetry plethysmography.

d. Loss of the end-tidal carbon dioxide ($EtCO_2$) tracing or low $EtCO_2$ values.

As in any other setting, cardiopulmonary resuscitation (CPR) and ACLS should be initiated as soon as cardiac arrest is recognized[2,3] This includes the performance of excellent chest compressions, ensuring ventilation, and defibrillation as rapidly as possible if ventricular fibrillation or pulseless ventricular tachycardia is present. Once pulselessness has been detected, delays greater than 2 minutes in initiation of CPR with chest compressions, defibrillation if warranted, and administration of epinephrine have each been associated with lower survival after witnessed in-hospital cardiac arrest.[12] There is limited evidence to specifically guide the management of cardiac arrest in the perioperative setting, but some literature-supported recommendations are available.[13]

The effectiveness of chest compressions can also be gauged by measuring $EtCO_2$ levels; a sudden increase in $EtCO_2$ to 35 to 40 mm Hg indicates return of spontaneous circulation (ROSC). However, this must be confirmed by noting the presence of an arterial waveform, palpable carotid or femoral pulse, and/or by obtaining a noninvasive BP cuff measurement. $EtCO_2$ readings greater than 20 mm Hg during CPR are associated with better outcome and survival, whereas $EtCO_2$ readings less than 10 mm Hg for 20 minutes are associated with failure of ROSC.[14]

The nadir pressure occurring during the release of each chest compression (ie, diastolic relaxation pressure) can be measured if an intra-arterial catheter is in place during CPR. Compressions that result in a diastolic BP between 30 and 40 mm Hg have a higher chance of successful ROSC.[14]

SPECIAL TOPICS
Non-Supine Positioning

Starting chest compressions without delay in the operating room is challenging if the patient is positioned in prone, lateral, steep Trendelenburg, beach chair, or other non-supine positions to facilitate the surgical procedure. Ideally, the patient should be rapidly repositioned to be supine. Also, the patient's back must be against a hard surface to provide uniform force and sternal counterpressure during chest compressions. However, CPR and defibrillation in the prone position are a reasonable alternative when the airway is already secured.[15]

Case reports, simulation-based studies, and cadaver feasibility studies have described ROSC or other successful outcomes after CPR performed in unusual positions.[16–20] For example, during CPR in the prone position, attempts are made to deliver effective compressions on the thoracic spine by using the same rate and force that would be delivered in a supine position.[17–19] Also, case reports have described successful intraoperative CPR with apparently adequate chest compressions performed on patients in the lateral position by placing a hard surface positioned behind the patient during CPR or having a second rescuer provide back support.[16,17,20,21]

For cardiopulmonary arrest in the pregnant patient, left lateral uterine displacement is necessary, if fundal height is at or above the umbilicus to minimize aortocaval compression, optimize venous return (preload), and generate adequate stroke volume during CPR. Manual uterine displacement is preferred so that supine positioning of the upper torso is preserved to facilitate optimal chest compression vector forces. A hand is used to apply maximal leftward push to the right upper border of the uterus to achieve uterine displacement of approximately 1.5 inches from the midline.[22] Other aspects of management are similar to cardiac arrests in nonpregnant adults,[23] as discussed separately.

Anaphylaxis

Hypersensitivity reactions including anaphylaxis have been reported to have an incidence of 1 in 6825 procedures.[24] Drug-induced reactions comprise the majority of cases, with antibiotics, analgesics, and non-depolarizing muscle relaxants being the usual culprits. Intraoperative identification of anaphylaxis may be challenging, as common findings in an awake patient, including subjective dyspnea, nausea, vomiting, dizziness, and altered mental status, are usually not reportable by anesthetized patients. Further, wheezing and mucosal and skin changes including angioedema and urticaria may not be recognized due to surgical draping and limited access to the patient.

The profound systemic vasodilation and increased capillary permeability of anaphylaxis cause a decrease in preload and relative hypotension, as well as potentially malignant arrhythmias, which can cause cardiovascular collapse. When suspected as a potential etiology of intraoperative arrest, all presumable offending agents should be immediately ceased and avoided. The mainstay of therapy is cessation of mast cell degranulation with epinephrine; recommended doses start at 100 μg intravenously (IV) in patients with a pulsatile cardiac rhythm and escalating as needed.[25] In the absence of IV access, 500 μg intramuscular (IM) can be given in the lateral thigh and repeated every 5 minutes until IV access is established. IV infusions of epinephrine, vasopressin, and norepinephrine may be required to maintain hemodynamics.

In patients without a definitive airway, it is critical that emergent endotracheal intubation be performed, given the potential for rapidly progressive oropharyngeal and laryngeal edema; surgical airway access should be considered early.[3] Monitoring for auto-PEEP and its resultant hemodynamic compromise are important given the likelihood of bronchospasm. Inhaled anesthetic agents may be used to treat refractory bronchospasm if hemodynamics allow. IV fluid boluses with crystalloid may be beneficial by offsetting the vasodilatory decrease in preload. Adjuvant agents to consider in severe anaphylaxis include IV corticosteroids, inhaled B2 adrenergic agents, and H1 and H2 antihistamines for severe anaphylaxis.[3] If available, extracorporeal life support can be considered and has been successfully deployed in rare instances.[26] As anaphylactic reactions are bimodal in nature with a high rate of recurrence, monitoring in an intensive care setting for at least 24 hours postoperatively is recommended.[3]

Obstructive Physiology

Obstructive or tension physiology from pneumothorax, hemothorax, or combination hemopneumothorax results in increased intrathoracic pressure from the accumulation and trapping of air, fluid, or blood in the chest. This elevated pressure is then transmitted to the mediastinum and potentially contralateral hemithorax, when these pressures rise sufficiently to impair venous return to the heart or impaired gas exchange, cardiorespiratory collapse with pulseless electrical activity (PEA) can occur.[3]

Potential causes of tension physiology include spontaneous pneumothorax, ruptured emphysematous blebs, trauma, and iatrogenic causes including lung puncture with central line placement, intercostal injury from thoracentesis or tube thoracostomy, and mediastinal or thoracic surgical bleeding, particularly in the patient who is status post recent cardiothoracic surgery.[27]

Symptoms of this syndrome in the awake patient include dyspnea, tachypnea, hypoxemia, and decreased breath sounds on the effected side.[3] In the sedated and ventilated patient, subjective symptoms are absent, but hypoxia, hypotension—particularly in the setting of pneumoperitoneum for laparoscopic cases, decreased or absent breath sounds, tracheal deviation, increased airway pressures, and in the case of pneumothorax, subcutaneous emphysema may be present.[27] Subcutaneous emphysema is characterized by crepitus on palpation of affected skin, and if air is not evacuated, often spreads to the neck and face. In patients with increasing subcutaneous emphysema, the chest should be emergently decompressed and the airway rapidly secured to avoid distortion of airway landmarks, which may result in difficult intubation.

The diagnosis of tension physiology is largely clinical, and although chest x-ray is used for diagnosis, it is less useful in the OR due to limited availability. Thoracic POCUS has emerged as a useful tool for intraoperative diagnosis.[3] A low threshold for empiric intervention without confirmatory diagnosis by imaging is reasonable, particularly in the trauma population.

Management of these patients hinges on the emergent decompression of the affected chest via needle, finger, or tube thoracostomy. Recent evidence suggests higher rates of successful decompression when performed in the fourth or fifth intercostal space at the anterior axillary line.[28] Any underlying etiology for the parenchymal injury or bleeding should then be investigated and controlled.[3]

Local Anesthetic Systemic Toxicity

Local anesthetic systemic toxicity (LAST) is a potentially devastating iatrogenic complication of surgical and anesthetic use of local anesthetics. With a published incidence of 1 to 10 per 10,000 cases, it is rare. Symptoms range from mild neurologic symptoms including tinnitus, metallic taste, and drowsiness to more severe including agitation, obtundation, and seizures. Cardiac symptoms, due to the inhibition of cardiac sodium channels by the anesthetics, also progress with the degree of toxicity, ranging from cardiac irritability to lethal arrhythmias and myocardial depression and ultimately, cardiovascular collapse.

As neurologic symptoms usually precede cardiovascular symptoms, albeit to varying degrees based on the specific medication, dose, and route used, early recognition and prompt intervention at the first signs of neurologic decline are key. Priorities include halting further local anesthetic dosing, airway management, administration of lipid emulsion, and administration of benzodiazepines for seizures. In the event of cardiac arrest due to LAST, standard ACLS doses of epinephrine as well as other inotropes and vasopressors are contraindicated, and small doses of approximately 1 µg/ kg should be used instead.[29] Prolonged arrest is common, and thus resuscitation in severe cases may be expected to last hours before return of circulation. In these cases, extracorporeal membranous oxygenation (ECMO) has been successfully deployed and early consideration should be given to its use when feasible.[30]

Malignant Hyperthermia

Malignant hyperthermia is a rare autosomal dominant hereditary myopathy resulting from a mutation in the calcium release channel ryanodine receptor 1 of skeletal muscle, which when unrecognized or left untreated, is often fatal.[31] When triggered by administration of succinylcholine or volatile anesthetic agents in susceptible individuals, a hypermetabolic state results in profound hypercarbia, respiratory acidosis, hyperthermia, and rhabdomyolysis, potentially leading to severe electrolyte abnormalities.

Early recognition and cessation of triggering anesthetic agents are key, so as to allow prompt administration of dantrolene, which blocks further calcium release from the skeletal muscle. Other priorities include rapid cooling, aggressive ventilation for CO_2 elimination, and fluid administration for management of rhabdomyolysis and to account for accelerated losses from hyperpyrexia. Unrecognized, electrolyte abnormalities including hyperkalemia and the profound acidosis of malignant hyperthermia (MH) may precipitate cardiac arrest.

Given the extremely low incidence of between 1 in 62,000 and 500,000 anesthetics, most anesthesiologists may never see the syndrome. As such, the Malignant Hyperthermia Association of the United States is an outstanding resource that should be used for guidance during an intraoperative event.[3] Given the risk of recrudescence and weakness resulting from the calcium inhibition by dantrolene, patients who have suffered an MH crisis should be monitored closely for at least 24 hours.[31]

Hyperkalemia

Hyperkalemia in the perioperative setting is largely related to acute and chronic renal dysfunction and medication effects and can have devastating cardiac consequences. Rarely, other circumstances, including succinylcholine administration in immobilized patients, malignant hyperthermia, trauma and burns with evolving rhabdomyolysis, and reperfusion after limb or organ ischemia may occur intraoperatively, leading to symptomatic hyperkalemia. The threshold for severe hyperkalemia is difficult to define, but intervention is largely recommended when serum potassium exceeds 6 mmol/L.

Diagnosis for the anesthetized patient largely depends on electrocardiographic ECG findings, which are variable and potentially subtle, particularly in patients who have chronically elevated potassium. Classically, peaked T waves are seen, but other conduction abnormalities including widened QRS, flattened P waves, ventricular ectopy, bradycardia, varying degrees of atrioventricular (AV) nodal block, and malignant ventricular arrhythmias may be noted.

Treatment hinges on membrane stabilization with calcium and temporizing measures to shift potassium intracellularly while working to ultimately decrease serum potassium through renal or bowel excretion or in the event of cardiac arrest, hemodialysis. Treating any underlying pathologies leading to the hyperkalemia is also key.

Embolism

Cardiac arrest due to acute venous or arterial thromboembolism, venous gas embolism, fat embolism, or amniotic fluid embolism is relatively rare but devastating complications of the perioperative period. Venous thromboembolism comprises the majority of acute pulmonary embolism cases leading to intraoperative cardiac arrest.

Symptoms of acute embolism include rapidly developed hypotension, desaturation, low end-tidal CO_2, arrhythmia, and rapid degradation to PEA and cardiac arrest. The pathophysiology and management of acute embolic disease hinges largely on V/Q mismatch and right ventricular (RV) dysfunction resulting from acutely elevated RV afterload. Intraoperative echocardiography, usually via TEE, but alternatively with TTE when the precordium is accessible, is the mainstay in diagnosis and relies on the diagnosis of RV dysfunction.

In cases where risk exists for acute venous air embolism, including laparoscopic cases, hysteroscopy, endoscopic retrograde cholangiopancreatography, and prone or sitting-position neurosurgical or orthopedic cases with the operative field above the heart, a high index of suspicion is key. Cessation of air entrainment by flooding the surgical field with saline and rapid patient repositioning to prevent ventricular air lock are critical components of resuscitation of this syndrome.

Management hinges on both elimination of the embolism and supportive care, particularly for the right heart. Anticoagulation with systemic or catheter-directed thrombolytic therapy and heparin are most commonly deployed, but surgical and percutaneous thrombectomy are also potential options. Aside from minimizing hypoxia and hypercarbia, inotropic infusions and RV afterload reduction by way of pulmonary vasodilators, including epoprostenol and nitric oxide, are key to supporting the RV through acute obstructive physiology. Vasopressin is the preferred vasopressor in this situation due to its sparing of the pulmonary vasculature. Prolonged resuscitation is frequent in these cases, and ECMO may be a useful adjunct.

SPECIAL POPULATIONS
Cardiac Transplant

As longevity of patients status post-cardiac transplantation has improved, the likelihood of encountering such a patient in the perioperative setting for both cardiac and noncardiac surgery has increased.[32] In many ways, these patients can be approached as if they have a healthy heart; however, some physiology, particularly cardiac automaticity and thus heart rate management is innately different due to the sympathetic and parasympathetic denervation which occurs with transplantation. In recent years, evidence has demonstrated that delayed reinnervation may occur in up to 70% of transplant patients.[33]

The resting heart rate of the denervated heart is usually relatively high, usually between 90 and 110 beats per minute, with absent compensatory reflexes and minimal reaction to increased physiologic demand and stress states including exercise, pain, and hypotension.[33] Indirect sympathomimetics, including ephedrine, and medications which induce tachycardia via a reflexive vagal response, including atropine and glycopyrrolate, will be ineffective in this population.

In the event of lethal arrhythmia and fulminant cardiovascular collapse, standard ACLS pathways should be followed. Management of bradycardia in the immediate postoperative setting from transplant usually hinges on pacing. In the absence of pacing capabilities, Epinephrine is often the most easily accessible medications in the acute phase, but if available, the beta agonist isoproterenol is a very effective alternative.[31] Norepinephrine and glucagon are other suitable medications.[31]

Left Ventricular Assist Device

With the increasing utilization of long-term mechanical circulatory support with implantable left ventricular assist devices (LVADs), so too has the incidence of cardiac arrest in these patients.[34]

Cardiac arrest in this population is largely secondary to pump failure, which is most likely a result of power failure or disconnection or driveline malfunction. RV dysfunction due to acute embolism, arrhythmia, or acute ischemia leading to LVAD underfilling or "suckdown events" due to hypovolemia, which can themselves incite ventricular arrhythmias are rarer etiologies for arrest overall in this population, but more frequently encountered with ICA in LVAD patients. Certainly, this population may also suffer from non-cardiogenic causes of cardiac arrest, including hypoglycemia, respiratory arrest, and neurologic complications including intracranial hemorrhage given chronic anticoagulation. Individuals with an LVAD present a unique clinical challenge in that their physiology usually precludes palpation of a pulse. Functionally, these patients live in hemodynamically stable PEA.[34] As such, conventional monitoring via physical examination, pulse oximetry, and sphygmomanometry with palpation or a stethoscope are often impossible in these patients, even at baseline. Frequently, the only available monitoring is $EtCO_2$ sampling as a measure of ROSC and adequate cardiac output. Furthermore, manual BP measurement with Doppler ultrasound or intra-arterial monitoring is important tools in the intraoperative setting. Classically, it has been taught that chest compressions are contraindicated in these patients, however, evidence now supports compressions as a key component of ACLS in this population.[35]

Electrophysiologic and Catheterization Laboratory Complications

Electrophysiologic procedures ranging from transcatheter cardiac ablations to transvenous cardiac lead extractions carry the risk of major complications. Although the bulk of these complications are considered *extra*-procedural, about 19% are *intra*-procedural complications which include large vessel tears, cardiac wall perforations, leading to acute cardiac tamponade or development of aberrant rhythms.[36]

Acute cardiac tamponade is life-threatening and demands swift relief of the cardiac compression as well as correction of the underlying insult. Vigilance and coordination between the surgical team and anesthetic team during cases with increased chances of transmural insult are paramount and echocardiographic imaging, in addition to anesthetic monitors. Initial management includes drainage of the pericardial accumulation with either pericardiocentesis or surgical evacuation in addition to appropriate resuscitation aimed at maintaining euvolemia.[37] It should be noted that inotropic support in these patients is controversial, as it is presumed that endogenous inotropic stimulation of a heart experiencing tamponade physiology is already maximized.[37]

If possible, mechanical ventilation with positive airway pressures should be avoided, or at least limited to the lowest tolerable pressures and minute ventilation, as increased intrathoracic pressures further decrease cardiac output. Should a patient experience cardiac arrest secondary to acute cardiac tamponade, CPR without evacuation of the effusion is of little to no value as the cardiac chambers have little room for filling and external pressures applied to the chest will have minimal benefits to circulation.[37]

Extracorporeal Support

Mechanical circulatory support in the form of ECMO has emerged as a useful adjunct to prolonged resuscitative efforts in refractory cardiac arrest.[26,30,38] When deployed during cardiopulmonary arrest, support is referred to as extracorporeal CPR (ECPR).[39] Since the first reported successes of ECPR in the literature in the 1950s, its utilization has increased to over 1500 cases per year, with a notable surge in its use after the 2009 influenza pandemic, which expanded the number of ECMO-capable facilities.[39]

In cases of refractory arrest, femoral arterial and venous cannulation and initiation of venoarterial ECMO during ongoing ACLS allows for restoration of systemic perfusion to vital end-organs, whereas reversible underlying causes are treated.

Observational studies indicate improved in-hospital survival and neurologic outcomes in patients who have successful resuscitation with ECPR, particularly for in-hospital arrests, when compared with conventional CPR; however, the relative paucity of cases is consistent with the lack of a national standard for ECPR protocols as well as the cost and resource limitations with which EPCR is fraught.

Automated Cardiopulmonary Resuscitation Devices

Originally created for the out-of-hospital setting, automated, electronic CPR devices are increasingly available in hospitals as a means of standardizing the delivery of adequate, appropriate chest compressions for a sustained period of time. Some of these devices, notably the Lund University Cardiac Assist System, are also designed to assist in the adequate recoiling of the chest wall, thereby optimizing negative intrathoracic pressure and preload in a patient receiving compressions. In addition, the integration of an impedance threshold device—which prevents positive ventilation during chest recoiling—with automated CPR provides another layer of complexity when examining the outcomes of automated CPR. However, the adoption of these devices is controversial, as there is concern regarding the rates of thoracic and abdominal injuries with automated CPR devices.[40] Until further studies are conducted, the best method of CPR delivery is likely the one with which the resuscitation team is most comfortable and allows sustained, good quality CPR.

Liver transplantation

Although ICA is overall rare, the incidence during orthotopic liver transplant (OLT) is higher, with a reported rate of 3.7% in OLT with an associated intraoperative mortality of 31.6%.[41] Approximately 90% of these events occur in the neohepatic phase of OLT, with 65% of ICA occurring within 5 minutes of graft reperfusion.[42] Risk factors for ICA during OLT include higher Model for End-Stage Liver Disease (MELD) score, extremes of body mass index, greater cold ischemic times, hemorrhage, longer surgical duration and clamping, post-reperfusion syndrome (PRS), non-living donor case, and re-transplant.

PRS was originally described as cardiac collapse after graft reperfusion and is now defined as a greater than 1 minute decrease in mean arterial pressure (MAP) of greater than 30% within 5 minutes of reperfusion.[43] PRS is the major cause of ICA during OLT, accounting for 38.2% of arrests.[42] In addition to hemodynamic instability due to an acute decrease in systemic vascular resistance (SVR), increased pulmonary vascular resistance, left or right ventricular dysfunction, bradycardia, asystole, and supraventricular arrhythmias may be observed. The anticipatory use of norepinephrine, epinephrine, and ephedrine before hepatic reperfusion can improve post-reperfusion hemodynamics and may avoid ICA.

Risk factors for PRS include age greater than 60 years, higher MELD score, more severe hyponatremia, and increased cold ischemic time.[44] Certain donor characteristics are also associated with the development of PRS. PRS was observed in 37.5% of patients receiving a graft with steatosis of $\geq$ 30%, whereas grafts with less fat had a lower rate of PRS of 18.8%.[45] Cardiac arrest rates in matched patients receiving grafts with $\geq$ 30%, 10% to 29% steatosis, and no steatosis were 8.3%, 1.0%, and 0%, respectively. The use of grafts from donation after cardiac death (DCD) donors has been associated with greater hyperkalemia and increased rate of PRS.[46] Hypothermic machine perfusion will likely result in a lower rate of PRS when using grafts from DCD donors.[47]

Pulmonary embolus is the second most common cause of ICA during OLT, accounting for 35.3% of cases.[42] With more widespread use of TEE, intracardiac thrombus is sometimes an incidental finding or associated with hemodynamic instability without ICA. In the event of significant hemodynamic instability or cardiac arrest, IV low-dose recombinant tissue plasminogen activator (0.5–4 mg) can be used.[48] Multiple rescue options exist, including the use of VA ECMO for stabilization and surgical management with either evacuation of thrombus via the inferior vena cava (IVC) or sternotomy and cardiac embolectomy.

Traumatic cardiac arrest
Traumatic cardiac arrest (TCA) is a lethal pathology, with less than 4% of patients surviving regardless of mechanism and largely due to hemorrhagic shock, tension physiology, asphyxia, or pericardial tamponade.[49,50] Initial rhythm in TCA is usually PEA or asystole. Survival depends on prompt intervention, aggressive resuscitation and blood transfusion, and synchronous management of reversible causes.[3]

Well-coordinated, communicative, resourced, multidisciplinary teams, working in parallel, are best poised to achieve swift management of the situation. Patients presenting with TCA should undergo immediate bedside imaging with POCUS to diagnose reversible pathologies including hemorrhage, tension pneumothorax, and cardiac tamponade, whereas ACLS and securing the airway are ongoing. Hemorrhage control via compression, tourniquet, or topical hemostatic agents should be performed to all visible and compressible injuries. Restoration of adequate circulating volumes is paramount, and many institutions rely on coordinated massive transfusion protocols during damage control resuscitation (DCR). Resuscitation with whole blood or equal ratios of packed red blood cells, fresh frozen plasma, and platelets should continue until the patient is hemodynamically stable.

In patients with TCA due to hemorrhage, placement of a resuscitative endovascular balloon occlusion of the aorta device, emergent damage control surgery, and tranexamic acid administration can be considered.[3,51] In cases of chest or epigastric penetrating trauma or suspicion for cardiac tamponade, resuscitative thoracotomy should be performed.[3]

Avoidance of hyperventilation until volume status is restored is beneficial. Small tidal volumes with infrequent delivery of breaths reduce the total overall positive pressure in the chest cavity, thereby optimizing venous return to the heart.

Cardiac arrest in coronavirus disease 2019

Emerging as a devastating global pandemic in 2019, coronavirus disease 2019 (COVID-19), caused by severe acute respiratory syndrome coronavirus 2 (SARS-CoV-2) infection, often presents as a severe respiratory illness.

Cardiac complications are common in patients with COVID with a range of etiologies including acute uni- or biventricular dysfunction due to viral myocarditis, right heart dysfunction due to severe hypoxemia and hypercarbia, tension physiology due to barotraumic pneumothorax, saddle pulmonary embolism due to hypercoagulability, and QT prolongation as a medication effect.[52,53]

COVID-19 is marked by a high incidence of cardiac arrhythmia and sudden cardiac death.[53] Cardiac arrest in these patients, which composed up to 13% of intensive care unit patients in some studies, correlates with the severity of illness and is thus thought to be largely due to systemic illness rather than the virus itself.[53] Of note, most cardiac arrests have a first noted rhythm of PEA or asystole rather than a preceding lethal arrhythmia, further confirming that the arrests were unlikely to be primarily cardiac in nature.[53]

Overall, resuscitation of COVID-19 patients should be guided by the standard ACLS protocols. However, specific attention should be paid to the etiologies above when attempting to treat underlying causes.

Literature has recently suggested much worse outcomes in patients with COVID-19 suffering an in-hospital cardiac arrest compared with those without COVID-19, prompting international debate regarding the ethics of resuscitation in these patients.[53]

POST-ARREST MANAGEMENT

Post-cardiac arrest syndrome occurs as the result of total body ischemia followed by reperfusion. This physiologic process results in organ dysfunction characterized by post-anoxic brain injury, cardiovascular impairment and systemic inflammation.[54] In addition to identification of the underlying cause of arrest, post-resuscitation care should focus on airway protection, ensuring adequate oxygenation and ventilation, hemodynamic monitoring and management and preventing further neurologic injury.

ECG may be useful in guiding diagnosis and treatment of perioperative cardiac arrest. In patients with ST elevation following ROSC, emergent cardiac catheterization with possible percutaneous coronary intervention is recommended. There may also be utility of cardiac catheterization for patients without ST elevations who do not have another clear noncardiac etiology for cardiac arrest, especially if they remain hemodynamically unstable post-ROSC.[55] TEE may provide utility in diagnosis and management peri-arrest. For patients without an obvious cardiac etiology, early consideration for computed tomography (CT) for diagnosis of neurologic and pulmonary conditions may be beneficial and may guide further treatment.

Airway, Oxygenation, and Ventilation

Optimizing oxygenation and ventilation may improve survival following cardiac arrest. Patients not already intubated for their surgical procedure should have an endotracheal tube placed to provide the improved control of ventilation and oxygenation.

During resuscitation efforts, ventilation should be limited to avoid hypotension related to decreased venous return from elevated intrathoracic pressure and auto-

PEEP. Post-ROSC patients should receive oxygen to achieve a saturation of 94% to 98%.[56] Prolonged hyperoxia should be avoided. Goal PCO_2 post-ROSC is 35 to 45 mm Hg. Hyperventilation and PCO_2 less than 35 mm Hg are associated with cerebral vasoconstriction, lower cerebral blood flow, and potential exacerbation of cerebral injury, and PCO_2 greater than 45 is associated with cerebral vasodilation, hyperemia, and cerebral edema.

Hemodynamic Management

Arterial cannulation is recommended to ensure mean MAP of at least 65 mm Hg. Patients with chronic hypertension or altered autoregulation may benefit from higher patient-specific MAP targets based on their preoperative baseline pressures. BP should be maintained with IV fluids, vasoconstrictors, and/or inotropes as appropriate. Patients with hypotension despite fluid, inotropic, and vasopressor support may require mechanical circulatory support (ie, Impella, ECMO) post-arrest.

Electrolyte Correction

Frequent monitoring of electrolytes and acid-base status is imperative in the immediate post-arrest state. Cardiac arrest is frequently associated with metabolic acidosis that should improve assuming no regional perfusion concerns still exist. Bicarbonate therapy is usually avoided in arrest-associated metabolic acidosis as its administration is associated with hypernatremia, continued or worsening acidosis, poor neurologic outcomes and increases in mortality.[57]

Hyperkalemia is common during cardiac arrest. Hyperkalemia should be treated with standard measures including calcium. While not standard therapy, one may consider therapy with bicarbonate in the setting of severe hyperkalemia with coinciding metabolic acidosis. Following ROSC, endogenous catecholamine release and correction of metabolic and respiratory acidosis lead to intracellular shifts of potassium and resultant hypokalemia. Hypomagnesemia is common post-ROSC and may require supplementation to decrease likelihood of arrhythmia.

Glucose should be maintained between 140 and 180 mg/dL, with avoidance of both hypoglycemia and hyperglycemia.

Post-Arrest Neurologic Function

Neurologic injury is a common cause of death and disability following cardiac arrest.[58] Post-resuscitation care should focus on attenuating progression of neurologic injury related to anoxia and preventing the occurrence of secondary post-arrest brain injury from inflammation, tissue hypoxia, endothelial damage, and excitotoxicity.

Temperature management is effective in minimizing neurologic damage related to anoxic brain injury following cardiac arrest. Decreases in temperature are associated with decreased cerebral metabolic rate, decreased release of excitatory amino acids and decreased production of free radicals.[59,60] Targeted temperature management (TTM) is indicated in patients who remain unresponsive following ROSC post-arrest. The goal of TTM is to lower core body temperature to 32°C to 36°C for at least 24 hours and avoid fever for at least 72 hours post-arrest.

The TTM trial randomized patients to TTM goals of 33°C versus 36°C and found no statistical difference in mortality or neurologic outcome at 6 months, which initially led to a change in practice to target higher temperatures during TTM.[61] Although the optimal duration of TTM is largely unknown, many centers target 24 hours. A trial randomizing patients to TTM at 33°C for 24 hours compared with 48 hours found no difference in neurologic outcome or mortality at 6 months post-arrest.[62] In the TTM-2 trial, compared with normothermia (avoidance of temperature $\geq$37.8°C), there is no mortality benefit to TTM at 33°C.[63] TTM at lower temperatures or prolonged cooling may be associated with increased adverse effects including decreased heart rate, hypotension, need for vasopressor support, elevated lactate, and bleeding.[54,64]

TTM can be accomplished via conventional cooling methods such as the placement of ice to highly vascularized areas of the body or IV infusion of cold fluids. Alternatively, cooling blankets or pads can be applied to the patient and are equipped with the ability to set a target temperature. Cooling catheter systems provide more precise control of temperature but are not associated with improved outcomes as compared with surface cooling techniques.[65]

Neurologic Prognostication

Given the high morbidity and mortality related to neurologic injury following cardiac arrest, early neurologic prognostication is a priority. Unfortunately, at this time, there are no modalities or combination of studies to predict poor neurologic outcome with absolute certainty. Findings with high reliability in predicting negative outcomes include bilateral absence of pupillary responses or corneal reflexes, high serum levels of neuron-specific enolase, absent N20 waves of somatosensory evoked potentials, diffuse cerebral edema on brain CT at 24 hours, and reduced diffusion on MRI at 2 to 5 days post-arrest.[66] Electroencephalogram (EEG) may also be used for both diagnosis of seizures and for prognostication.

SUMMARY

In conclusion, ICA is rare and the etiology is usually more readily apparent than in other settings because the arrest is witnessed by clinicians familiar with the patient's medical history, and the precipitating cause may be known and rapidly reversible. Initiation of treatment is usually timely and focused, resulting in better outcomes compared with other settings.

CLINICS CARE POINTS

- Prompt initiation of CPR followed by etiology-specific treatment for intraoperative cardiac arrest requires early recognition of non-perfusing rhythm, decreased end-tidal carbon dioxide, loss of pulse oximetry signal, and/or loss of arterial pressure waveform.

- Intraoperative cases of cardiac arrest should be evaluated with an expanded differential diagnosis that includes etiologies specific to the perioperative setting and informed by the patient's known comorbidities and special circumstances related to the surgical procedure and anesthetic technique.

- Post-arrest management should maintain adequate MAP, correct electrolyte abnormalities, and avoid hyperoxia, hyperthermia, and hyperventilation.

DISCLOSURE

None of the authors has any conflicts of interest related to the material in this article.

REFERENCES

1. Berg RA, Hemphill R, Abella BS, et al. Part 5: adult basic life support: 2010 American Heart Association Guidelines for Cardiopulmonary Resuscitation and Emergency Cardiovascular Care. Circulation 2010;122(18 Suppl 3):S685–705.

2. Moitra VK, Einav S, Thies KC, et al. Cardiac arrest in the operating room: resuscitation and management for the anesthesiologist: part 1. Anesth Analg 2018; 126(3):876–88.

3. McEvoy MD, Thies KC, Einav S, et al. Cardiac arrest in the Operating Room: Part 2-Special Situations in the Perioperative Period. Anesth Analg 2018;126(3): 889–903.

4. Fielding-Singh V, Willingham MD, Fischer MA, et al. A Population-Based Analysis of Intraoperative Cardiac Arrest in the United States. Anesth Analg 2020;130(3): 627–34.

5. Nunnally ME, O'Connor MF, Kordylewski H, et al. The incidence and risk factors for perioperative cardiac arrest observed in the national anesthesia clinical outcomes registry. Anesth Analg 2015;120(2):364–70.

6. Sobreira-Fernandes D, Teixeira L, Lemos TS, et al. Perioperative cardiac arrests - A subanalysis of the anesthesia -related cardiac arrests and associated mortality. J Clin Anesth 2018;50:78–90.

7. Sprung J, Warner ME, Contreras MG, et al. Predictors of survival following cardiac arrest in patients undergoing noncardiac surgery: a study of 518,294 patients at a tertiary referral center. Anesthesiology 2003;99(2):259–69.

8. Ramachandran SK, Mhyre J, Kheterpal S, et al. Predictors of survival from perioperative cardiopulmonary arrests: a retrospective analysis of 2,524 events from the Get With The Guidelines-Resuscitation registry. Anesthesiology 2013; 119(6):1322–39.

9. Ricks CJ, Ma MW, Gastelum JR, et al. A Prospective Observational Cohort Study of Calls for Help in a Tertiary Care Academic Operating Room Suite. Anesth Analg 2019;129(3):e83–5.

10. Mhyre JM, Ramachandran SK, Kheterpal S, et al. American Heart Association National Registry for Cardiopulmonary Resuscitation I. Delayed time to defibrillation after intraoperative and periprocedural cardiac arrest. Anesthesiology 2010; 113(4):782–93.

11. Schmid F, Goepfert MS, Kuhnt D, et al. The wolf is crying in the operating room: patient monitor and anesthesia workstation alarming patterns during cardiac surgery. Anesth Analg 2011;112(1):78–83.

12. Bircher NG, Chan PS, Xu Y. American Heart Association's Get With The Guidelines-Resuscitation I. Delays in Cardiopulmonary Resuscitation, Defibrillation, and Epinephrine Administration All Decrease Survival in In-hospital Cardiac Arrest. Anesthesiology 2019;130(3):414–22.

13. Chalkias A, Mongardon N, Boboshko V, et al. Clinical practice recommendations on the management of perioperative cardiac arrest: A report from the PERIOPCA Consortium. Crit Care 2021;25(1):265.

14. Sandroni C, De Santis P, D'Arrigo S. Capnography during cardiac arrest. Resuscitation 2018;132:73–7.

15. Anez C, Becerra-Bolanos A, Vives-Lopez A, et al. Cardiopulmonary Resuscitation in the Prone Position in the Operating Room or in the Intensive Care Unit: A Systematic Review. Anesth Analg 2021;132(2):285–92.

16. Bengali R, Janik LS, Kurtz M, et al. Successful cardiopulmonary resuscitation in the lateral position during intraoperative cardiac arrest. Anesthesiology 2014; 120(4):1046–9.

17. Bhatnagar V, Jinjil K, Dwivedi D, et al. Cardiopulmonary Resuscitation: Unusual Techniques for Unusual Situations. J Emerg Trauma Shock 2018;11(1):31–7.

18. Mazer SP, Weisfeldt M, Bai D, et al. Reverse CPR: a pilot study of CPR in the prone position. Resuscitation 2003;57(3):279–85.

19. Wei J, Tung D, Sue SH, et al. Cardiopulmonary resuscitation in prone position: a simplified method for outpatients. J Chin Med Assoc 2006;69(5):202–6.
20. Yunoki K, Sasaki R, Taguchi A, et al. Successful recovery without any neurological complication after intraoperative cardiopulmonary resuscitation for an extended period of time in the lateral position: a case report. JA Clin Rep 2016;2(1):7.
21. Song Y, Oh J, Chee Y, et al. Effectiveness of chest compression feedback during cardiopulmonary resuscitation in lateral tilted and semirecumbent positions: a randomised controlled simulation study. Anaesthesia 2015;70(11):1235–41.
22. Kundra P, Khanna S, Habeebullah S, et al. Manual displacement of the uterus during Caesarean section. Anaesthesia 2007;62(5):460–5.
23. Helviz Y, Einav S. Maternal cardiac arrest. Curr Opin Anaesthesiol 2019;32(3): 298–306.
24. Gonzalez-Estrada A, Campbell RL, Carrillo-Martin I, et al. Incidence and risk factors for near-fatal and fatal outcomes after perioperative and periprocedural anaphylaxis in the USA, 2005-2014. Br J Anaesth 2021;127(6):890–6.
25. Houseman BT, Bloomstone JA, Maccioli G. Intraoperative cardiac arrest. Anesthesiology Clin 2020;38(4):859–73.
26. Carelli M, Seco M, Forrest P, et al. Extracorporeal membrane oxygenation support in refractory perioperative anaphylactic shock to rocuronium: a report of two cases. Perfusion 2019;34(8):717–20.
27. Roberts DJ, Leigh-Smith S, Faris PD, et al. Clinical presentation of patients with tension pneumothorax: a systematic review. Ann Surg 2015;261(6):1068–78.
28. Inaba K, Branco BC, Eckstein M, et al. Optimal positioning for emergent needle thoracostomy: a cadaver-based study. J Trauma 2011;71(5):1099–103, discussion 1103.
29. Neal JM, Bernards CM, Butterworth JFt, et al. ASRA practice advisory on local anesthetic systemic toxicity. Reg Anesth And Pain Med 2010;35(2):152–61.
30. Bacon B, Silverton N, Katz M, et al. Local Anesthetic Systemic Toxicity Induced Cardiac Arrest After Topicalization for Transesophageal Echocardiography and Subsequent Treatment With Extracorporeal Cardiopulmonary Resuscitation. J Cardiothorac Vasc Anesth 2019;33(1):162–5.
31. Ellinas H, Albrecht MA. Malignant Hyperthermia Update. Anesthesiology Clin 2020;38(1):165–81.
32. Joglar JA, Wan EY, Chung MK, et al. Management of Arrhythmias After Heart Transplant: Current State and Considerations for Future Research. Circ Arrhythm Electrophysiol 2021;14(3):e007954.
33. Awad M, Czer LS, Hou M, et al. Early Denervation and Later Reinnervation of the Heart Following Cardiac Transplantation: A Review. J Am Heart Assoc 2016; 5(11). https://doi.org/10.1161/JAHA.116.004070.
34. Peberdy MA, Gluck JA, Ornato JP, et al. Cardiopulmonary Resuscitation in Adults and Children With Mechanical Circulatory Support: A Scientific Statement From the American Heart Association. Circulation 2017;135(24):e1115–34.
35. Mabvuure NT, Rodrigues JN. External cardiac compression during cardiopulmonary resuscitation of patients with left ventricular assist devices. Interact Cardiovasc Thorac Surg 2014;19(2):286–9.
36. Hussain SK, Eddy MM, Moorman L, et al. Major complications and mortality within 30 days of an electrophysiological procedure at an academic medical center: implications for developing national standards. J Cardiovasc Electrophysiol 2015;26(5):527–31.
37. Spodick DH. Acute cardiac tamponade. N Engl J Med 2003;349(7):684–90.

38. Karami M, Mandigers L, Miranda DDR, et al. Survival of patients with acute pulmonary embolism treated with venoarterial extracorporeal membrane oxygenation: A systematic review and meta-analysis. J Crit Care 2021;64:245–54.

39. Abrams D, MacLaren G, Lorusso R, et al. Extracorporeal cardiopulmonary resuscitation in adults: evidence and implications. Intensive Care Med 2022; 48(1):1–15.

40. Frascone RJ. The risk versus benefit of LUCAS: is it worth it? Anesthesiology 2014;120(4):797–8.

41. Smith NK, Zerillo J, Kim SJ, et al. Intraoperative cardiac arrest during adult liver transplantation: incidence and risk factor analysis from 7 academic centers in the United States. Anesth Analg 2021;132(1):130–9.

42. Matsusaki T, Hilmi IA, Planinsic RM, et al. Cardiac arrest during adult liver transplantation: a single institution's experience with 1238 deceased donor transplants. Liver Transpl 2013;19(11):1262–71.

43. Manning MW, Kumar PA, Maheshwari K, et al. Post-reperfusion syndrome in liver transplantation-an overview. J Cardiothorac Vasc Anesth 2020;34(2):501–11.

44. Sahmeddini MA, Tehran SG, Khosravi MB, et al. Risk factors of the post-reperfusion syndrome during orthotopic liver transplantation: a clinical observational study. BMC Anesthesiol 2022;22(1):89.

45. Croome KP, Lee DD, Croome S, et al. The impact of postreperfusion syndrome during liver transplantation using livers with significant macrosteatosis. Am J Transpl 2019;19(9):2550–9.

46. Pan X, Apinyachon W, Xia W, et al. Perioperative complications in liver transplantation using donation after cardiac death grafts: a propensity-matched study. Liver Transpl 2014;20(7):823–30.

47. van Rijn R, Schurink IJ, de Vries Y, et al. Hypothermic machine perfusion in liver transplantation - a randomized trial. N Engl J Med 2021;384(15):1391–401.

48. Verbeek TA, Stine JG, Saner FH, et al. Hypercoagulability in end-stage liver disease: review of epidemiology, etiology, and management. Transpl Direct 2018; 4(11):e403.

49. Zwingmann J, Mehlhorn AT, Hammer T, et al. Survival and neurologic outcome after traumatic out-of-hospital cardiopulmonary arrest in a pediatric and adult population: a systematic review. Crit Care 2012;16(4):R117.

50. Kleber C, Giesecke MT, Lindner T, et al. Requirement for a structured algorithm in cardiac arrest following major trauma: epidemiology, management errors, and preventability of traumatic deaths in Berlin. Resuscitation 2014;85(3):405–10.

51. Castellini G, Gianola S, Biffi A, et al. Resuscitative endovascular balloon occlusion of the aorta (REBOA) in patients with major trauma and uncontrolled haemorrhagic shock: a systematic review with meta-analysis. World J Emerg Surg 2021; 16(1):41.

52. Ippolito M, Catalisano G, Marino C, et al. Mortality after in-hospital cardiac arrest in patients with COVID-19: A systematic review and meta-analysis. Resuscitation 2021;164:122–9.

53. Bhatla A, Mayer MM, Adusumalli S, et al. COVID-19 and cardiac arrhythmias. Heart Rhythm 2020;17(9):1439–44.

54. Kirkegaard H, Taccone FS, Skrifvars M, et al. Postresuscitation care after out-of-hospital cardiac arrest: clinical update and focus on targeted temperature management. Anesthesiology 2019;131(1):186–208.

55. Neumann FJ, Sousa-Uva M, Ahlsson A, et al. 2018 ESC/EACTS Guidelines on myocardial revascularization. Eur Heart J 2019;40(2):87–165.

56. Nolan JP, Sandroni C, Bottiger BW, et al. European resuscitation council and european society of intensive care medicine guidelines 2021: post-resuscitation care. Resuscitation 2021;161:220–69.
57. Kawano T, Grunau B, Scheuermeyer FX, et al. Prehospital sodium bicarbonate use could worsen long term survival with favorable neurological recovery among patients with out-of-hospital cardiac arrest. Resuscitation 2017;119:63–9.
58. Laver S, Farrow C, Turner D, et al. Mode of death after admission to an intensive care unit following cardiac arrest. Intensive Care Med 2004;30(11):2126–8.
59. McCullough JN, Zhang N, Reich DL, et al. Cerebral metabolic suppression during hypothermic circulatory arrest in humans. Ann Thorac Surg 1999;67(6): 1895–9, discussion 1919-21.
60. Gunn AJ, Thoresen M. Hypothermic neuroprotection. NeuroRx 2006;3(2):154–69.
61. Nielsen N, Wetterslev J, Cronberg T, et al. Targeted temperature management at 33 degrees C versus 36 degrees C after cardiac arrest. N Engl J Med 2013; 369(23):2197–206.
62. Kirkegaard H, Soreide E, de Haas I, et al. Targeted temperature management for 48 vs 24 hours and neurologic outcome after out-of-hospital cardiac arrest: a randomized clinical trial. JAMA 2017;318(4):341–50.
63. Dankiewicz J, Cronberg T, Lilja G, et al. Hypothermia versus normothermia after out-of-hospital cardiac arrest. N Engl J Med 2021;384(24):2283–94.
64. Annborn M, Bro-Jeppesen J, Nielsen N, et al. The association of targeted temperature management at 33 and 36 degrees C with outcome in patients with moderate shock on admission after out-of-hospital cardiac arrest: a post hoc analysis of the target temperature management trial. Intensive Care Med 2014;40(9):1210–9.
65. Gillies MA, Pratt R, Whiteley C, et al. Therapeutic hypothermia after cardiac arrest: a retrospective comparison of surface and endovascular cooling techniques. Resuscitation 2010;81(9):1117–22.
66. Sandroni C, D'Arrigo S, Cacciola S, et al. Prediction of poor neurological outcome in comatose survivors of cardiac arrest: a systematic review. Intensive Care Med 2020;46(10):1803–51.

Intraoperative Ventilator Management of the Critically Ill Patient

Erin Hennessey, MD, MEHP[a],*, Edward Bittner, MD, PhD, MSEd, FCCM[b], Peggy White, MD[c], Alan Kovar, MD[d], Lucas Meuchel, MD[e]

KEYWORDS

- Intraoperative lung-protective ventilation • Ventilator-induced lung injury
- Respiratory mechanics • Postoperative pulmonary complications
- Critically ill patients • Operating room

KEY POINTS

- Although low tidal volume and reduced airway pressures are standard components of lung-protective ventilation, further individualization of ventilation may be necessary based on patient characteristics and surgical conditions.
- Noninvasive tools that provide real-time, continuous, dynamic lung imaging (lung ultrasound, electrical impedance tomography) or pressure measurements (esophageal manometry) may help to better identify different lung morphology including lung overdistension and atelectatic components as well as response to specific interventions.
- Using predictive risk scores to identify patients at risk for postoperative pulmonary complications in addition to recognition of specific patient populations (those with obesity, sepsis, or acute respiratory distress syndrome) or surgical procedures (laparoscopic, abdominal, or one-lung ventilation needs) that are at risk can help physicians implement ventilator management plans in the operating room to those that may benefit from lung-protective strategies.

INTRODUCTION

More than 2 decades ago, we learned that low tidal volumes (TVs; 6 mL/kg predicted body weight [PBW]) and lower plateau pressures ($\leq$30 cmH$_2$O) resulted in reduced patient mortality for patients suffering from acute respiratory distress syndrome (ARDS).[1]

[a] Stanford University - School of Medicine Department of Anesthesiology, Perioperative and Pain Medicine, 300 Pasteur Drive, Room H3580, Stanford, CA 94305, USA; [b] Department of Anesthesia, Critical Care and Pain Medicine, Harvard Medical School, Massachusetts General Hospital, Boston, MA 02114, USA; [c] University of Florida College of Medicine, Department of Anesthesiology, 1500 SW Archer Road, PO Box 100254, Gainesville, FL 32610, USA; [d] Oregon Health and Science University, 3161 SW Pavilion Loop, Portland, OR 97239, USA; [e] Oregon Health and Science University, 3181 SW Sam Jackson Park Road, Portland, OR 97239, USA
* Corresponding author.
E-mail address: erinkh@stanford.edu

Anesthesiology Clin 41 (2023) 121–140
https://doi.org/10.1016/j.anclin.2022.11.004
1932-2275/23/© 2022 Elsevier Inc. All rights reserved.

These strategies are now frequently referred to as lung-protective ventilation (LPV) and are distinctively different from the historical large TVs of 10 to 12 mL/kg used intraoperatively to promote lung recruitment and provide optimal oxygenation. With the growing evidence to support LPV in the management of ARDS in critically ill patients, anesthesiologists and intensivists have translated these strategies for the operating room (OR) in efforts to minimize postoperative pulmonary complications (PPCs) and prevent ventilator-induced lung injury (VILI). However, despite a solid trend in intraoperative ventilator strategies suggesting practice has changed, such as decreased TV[2] and the increased use of positive-end-expiratory pressure (PEEP)[3] during the past decade, the evidence for specific intraoperative lung-protective ventilation (IOLPV) strategies that parallel those in the intensive care unit (ICU) remains incomplete.

As clinicians are faced with decisions regarding which strategies are beneficial in the OR versus the ICU, there are a growing number of critically ill patients that require surgical and procedural interventions during their hospital course. For simplicity of intraoperative management, there is an understandable desire to standardize mechanical ventilation for all patients undergoing surgery, yet there is evidence that this standardized approach may not be optimal or may even be detrimental depending on patient characteristics and surgical conditions.[4] Furthermore, selective targeting of a fixed TV, airway pressure, or gas exchange value may conflict with other protective ventilation goals.[5] Importantly, the stress and strain applied to the lung are not directly measured with standard LPV settings but are inferred from respiratory mechanics. Limitations of intraoperative mechanical ventilators, decreased access to ancillary staff and equipment, dynamic physiologic and positional changes occurring during surgery, in addition to the heterogeneity of the critically ill patient population, are all frequent barriers to implementing a single IOLPV framework for all ICU patients in the OR. Based on these challenges, an individualized approach to intraoperative mechanical ventilation that combines advanced monitoring tools and targets is increasingly becoming a point of focus for reducing PPCs.[6–9]

BACKGROUND

Deleterious outcomes of positive pressure ventilation (PPV) are not new concepts. Well before and directly contributing to the motivation for the landmark ARDSnet study,[1] Ventilator-induced lung injury (VILI) is described in reports of human disease following PPV as well as being studied in animal models preceding this and the term "respirator lung" was coined for patients exhibiting evidence of lung tissue disruption following mechanical ventilation.[10] Evidence of lung tissue damage, pulmonary edema, and development of hyaline membranes as precursors of pending severe and potentially life-threatening lung disease is present in the literature from the 1960s

---

Box 1
Definitions for the underlying pathophysiology of ventilator-induced lung injury

Barotrauma: Elevated pressure applied to the airways and alveoli affecting the microvasculature of the lung.

Volutrauma: Due to the overdistension of the respiratory apparatus, even in the absence of elevated pressure.

Atelectrauma: Repetitive opening and closing of small airways and alveoli or frequent atelectasis.

Biotrauma: The presence of a panoply of inflammatory substances that results in alveolar damage.

and 1970s.[11,12] Currently, 4 classical concepts for the underlying cause of VILI persist and are further defined in **Box 1**.

Studies focusing on barotrauma revealed that the amount of distension[12] and the transpulmonary pressure (airway pressure–pleural pressure) are both of importance.[13] For example, subjects with low airway but high transpulmonary pressure due to air hunger or significant spontaneous respiratory effort can generate significant gradients associated with lung injury.[14] Similar to barotrauma, but more specifically related to damage resulting from overdistension of alveoli, high volumes during mechanical ventilation lead to alveolar rupture and potentially large air leak.[13,15,16] Just as overdistension of alveoli causes epithelial barrier disruption, repetitive opening and closing of the distal alveoli similarly results in the development of injury from pulmonary edema, epithelial cell dislodgement, and ultimately development of hyaline membranes.[12] PEEP has been shown to reduce this cyclic opening and closing and helps to minimize atelectrauma.[17,18] Indeed, utilization of PEEP to maintain respiratory airway recruitment is now nearly ubiquitous following multiple publications and has been suggested as yet another basis for increased survival in patients with ARDS requiring mechanical ventilation.[19] In a fourth mechanism, stimulation of the inflammatory cytokines leads to an upregulation of hypertrophy and/or hyperplasia of airway epithelium and eventual pulmonary remodeling.[20,21] Notable substances include TNF-alpha, IL-8, and IL-6, and patients prescribed lung-protective ventilation seem to show reduced levels of these cytokines.[22]

In terms of mitigation of VILI, current therapy includes application of reduced lung volumes,[1] reducing airway pressure to the minimum required to provide adequate gas exchange, titration of ventilator settings to transpulmonary pressure as assessed through esophageal pressure monitoring,[23] prone positioning,[24,25] and finally neuromuscular blockade in critically ill patients requiring mechanical ventilation.[26] With studies providing evidence of lung injury through altered structure and ultimately function, the clinician is left without doubt that mechanical ventilation, although lifesaving and often necessary in the OR and the ICU, must be tailored to the individual patient just as any other therapy.

DISCUSSION

The goal of intraoperative mechanical ventilation management is to optimize lung recruitment without overdistending compliant alveoli. In the critically ill patient, the low TV strategy has proven beneficial in preventing mechanisms of VILI that result in improved outcomes. Similarly, low TV ventilation (<8 mL/kg) versus high (>8 mL/kg) with general anesthesia (GA) has been associated with a decrease in PPCs.[27–30] Going beyond low TV as the solo physiologic target for LPV and instead focusing on individualized targets for mechanical ventilation based on physiologic principles and dynamic monitoring may provide more effective intraoperative ventilation and reduce the occurrence of VILI.

ADVANCED PHYSIOLOGIC TARGETS
Alveolar Recruitment

Most patients develop atelectasis during anesthesia and surgery, the extent of which is determined by the type and duration of surgery, surgical technique, positioning, and underlying medical conditions.[31] PEEP can be used to prevent atelectrauma by alveolar recruitment. However, too much PEEP can have a hemodynamic effect, cause overdistention of aerated alveoli leading to increased dead space and shunt, and increased risk of cor pulmonale.[32] PEEP must be carefully titrated to balance the risk/benefit ratio. This approach has been described using P:F tables,[32] stepwise recruitment maneuvers,[33] and the use of advanced monitoring techniques described below.[32,34,35]

The use of PEEP alone cannot reopen all collapsed alveoli, so it is essential to use a recruitment maneuver (RM) to enable a complete reopening. Several methods for performing RMs have been described in the literature.[36] Most commonly, RMs are performed manually using the "bag squeezing" method of applying and holding a set inflation pressure for a specific duration of time using the airway pressure-limiting valve of the anesthesia machine.[37] However, ventilator-driven RMs are preferred to minimize the loss of PPV when switching back to the ventilator. Provided there are no contraindications, an inspiratory pressure of 40 cmH$_2$O for 7 to 8 seconds is likely to result in full recruitment in most nonobese patients with healthy lungs.[38,39] Higher pressures and longer times may be needed for certain patients. For anesthesia ventilators that allow pressure-controlled ventilation, RMs can be performed by increasing PEEP up to 20 cmH$_2$O in steps of 5 cmH$_2$O (30–60 seconds per step) while maintaining a constant driving pressure of 15 to 20 cmH$_2$O.[37] Although RMs have the potential to improve respiratory mechanics and gas exchange, they also have the potential to increase lung injury depending on the clinical circumstances.[40] Consequently, it is important to assess the extent of atelectasis and monitor the response when performing RMs. The recruitment-to-inflation ratio is a recently proposed approach to estimate recruitability at the bedside.[41]

Driving Pressure

Driving pressure (DP) is defined as the difference between plateau pressure and PEEP and is linearly related to lung strain.[42] Retrospective studies have shown that DP is related to mortality in patients with ARDS even among those who received traditional protective ventilation.[43,44] The threshold value of DP for higher mortality in patients with ARDS is approximately 15 cmH$_2$O, and each 1-cmH$_2$O increase of DP was associated with a 5% increment in mortality. Higher DP values have also been associated with increased mortality in patients receiving pressure support ventilation.[45] In surgical patients, a meta-analysis of 17 randomized controlled trials found that intraoperative high driving pressure was associated with the development of PPCs, whereas no association was found with TV and PEEP.[46] The deleterious effect of DP is believed to result from the concept of "functional lung size"—the volume of aerated lung available for ventilation. "Functional lung size" is reduced in patients with lung pathologic conditions such as atelectasis, consolidation, effusion, or fibrosis. Therefore, if lungs are either overdistended or underventilated in relation to their "functional lung size," DP will increase. It has been suggested that DP may be used to set PEEP because the best compromise between overinflation and recruitment is determined at the lowest DP.[47] However, although studies clearly show that elevated DP is associated with increased complications, they do not confirm that active control of DP improves outcomes. Although a causal effect has not been demonstrated, it has been recommended that at least for patients with ARDS, DP should be targeted less than 13 cmH$_2$O.[48]

Stress Index

Analysis of the pressure–time curve during volume control ventilation can provide useful information to help set the ventilation parameters.[49] During inspiration in volume control ventilation with constant airflow, the airway pressure–time relationship can be described by the power equation[5]:

$$P_{P-T} = a \times t^{SI} + c,$$

where the coefficient *a* represents the slope of the pressure time (P_{P-T}) curve at a given time of measurement *t*, and *c* is the pressure at the initiation of inspiration. The constant SI, referred to as the "stress index," is a number that describes the shape of P_{P-T} curve.

Linearity of the P_{P-T} curve (SI = 1) denotes compliance during TV insufflation, which is minimally injurious. Nonlinearity of the pressure–time curve denotes a nonconstant compliance during TV insufflation. If compliance increases during inspiration, as occurs with intratidal lung recruitment, the slope of the pressure–time curve decreases over time, resulting in a downward concavity (SI < 1). Implementation of increased PEEP to avoid the cyclic opening and closing of respiratory units, a mechanism of VILI, is beneficial in this instance. In contrast, if compliance decreases during inspiration, as suggested by an upward concavity of the pressure–time curve (SI > 1), this suggests that the lung is cyclically overdistended during inspiration. In this case, a reduction of PEEP and/or TV might be warranted. Use of the SI allows adjustment of the ventilatory settings to respiratory system characteristics of the patient, modifying VT and PEEP. Although measuring the SI requires complex calculations that are clinically onerous, it can be easily estimated by visualizing the P_{P-T} curve and is demonstrated in **Fig. 1**.[50,51]

Mechanical Power

Mechanical power (MP) is a summary construct that attempts to relate the different ventilatory parameters set by the clinician at the bedside to the amount of energy transferred from the mechanical ventilator to the respiratory system.[52] MP can be estimated using a simplified equation of motion:

$$MP = RR \times \Delta V^2 \times \{(0.5 \times Ers + RR \times (1 + I:E)/60 \times I:E \times Raw) + \Delta V \times PEEP),$$

where ΔV is tidal change in lung volume, RR is respiratory rate, Ers is respiratory system elastance, and Raw is airway resistance, and I:E is the inspiratory–expiratory ratio.

The MP equation illustrates the relative importance of each respiratory variable on the energy delivered to the lungs during mechanical ventilation. For example, the

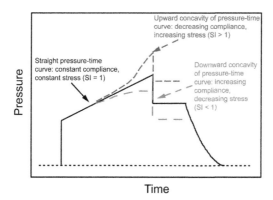

Fig. 1. A dynamic airway pressure during volume control ventilation with a constant inspiratory flow. The stress index (SI) is derived from changes in the slope of the pressure time during inspiration. Upward concavity of the pressure–time curve reflects decreasing compliance (overdistension, SI > 1) while downward concavity of the pressure–time curve indicates increasing compliance (atelectasis, SI < 1). (*From* [Kallet RH. Should PEEP Titration Be Based on Chest Mechanics in Patients with ARDS? *Respir Care*. Jun 2016;61(6):876-90]; with permission.)

effect of TV, which is squared in the MP calculation, is predominant. The effect of PEEP is dichotomous: PEEP directly increases the MP but can also indirectly reduce it through a reduction in Ers. The MP equation also illustrates that the respiratory rate is linearly related to the amount of the energy delivered to the lungs. Studies have reported that increasing values of MP are associated with an increased risk of lung injury.[53,54]

The MP calculation is too cumbersome for clinical use and simpler formulas are being evaluated.[55] It is also important to recognize that despite low MP values, lung damage is still possible with inhomogeneous ventilation where atelectasis and hyperinflation simultaneously coexist.[6]

Dead Space

An important determinant of the appropriate size of the delivered TV during mechanical ventilation is the size of the dead space—the volume of inhaled gas that does not take part in gas exchange.[56] Dead space is divided into the anatomic dead space—which exists in the large and small airways that do not normally participate in gas exchange—and the alveolar dead space, which results when there is absence of blood flow to an area of lung that is still receiving ventilation. Physiologic dead space, the sum of anatomical and alveolar dead space, is a global measure of the efficiency of the lung function. It has been associated with outcome in patients with respiratory failure and may be helpful for selecting optimal PEEP.[9,57] However dead space is not routinely measured in anesthetic practice, due to difficulties in interpreting capnograms and in calculation methods. Use of minute ventilation is unable to adequately describe ventilation efficiency because it does not distinguish between alveolar and anatomic dead space ventilation. Volumetric capnography (VCap), which measures the volume of expired CO_2 in one single breath, is a reliable real-time method for measuring dead space. In addition, VCap provides information about pulmonary perfusion, end-expiratory lung volume, and pulmonary ventilation inhomogeneities, which can be used for optimization of ventilation at the bedside.[58–60] Although further investigation is needed to establish the optimal use of VCap in the intraoperative setting, it is a potentially useful noninvasive tool to measure dead space and optimize intraoperative ventilation.

ADVANCED MONITORING TOOLS
Electrical Impedance Tomography

Electrical impedance tomography (EIT) is a noninvasive, radiation-free portable monitoring technique that provides images based on the electrical conductivity of tissue in the chest. Electrodes are placed on the chest wall, which record the surface voltage after the repeated application of a small amount of electrical current. The changes of electrical impedance over time are displayed dynamically in color-code images. By imaging breath-by-breath changes in ventilation distribution, EIT can be used intraoperatively to dynamically optimize ventilator settings.[61] EIT measurements of TV and ventilation distribution have been validated as accurate surrogates in comparison to CT scan and nitrogen washout, respectively.[62] EIT monitoring can identify regional ventilation heterogeneity, overdistention, and atelectasis, that are otherwise not identifiable by traditional protective ventilator-based metrics.

EIT helps inform the mechanical compromise between ventilation of nondependent and dependent lung regions, minimizing both overdistension and collapse. These beneficial effects are more pronounced in obese patients and those undergoing interventions that impair normal respiratory mechanics (eg, laparoscopy procedures or

Trendelenburg positioning).[63] A variety of EIT-derived indices have been proposed to quantify temporal and spatial ventilation heterogeneity including the "global inhomogeneity index," "regional ventilation delay," and "dynamic relative regional strain." Lung perfusion monitoring is another important feature of EIT that can be evaluated during general anesthesia. An IV injection of hypertonic saline during an expiratory breath-hold allows the calculation of pulmonary perfusion through impedance time-curves. Comparisons of impedance data for both ventilation and perfusion can then be analyzed and ventilator strategies can be altered based on knowledge of ventilation/perfusion mismatch.[64] Although the usefulness of EIT has been highlighted by a growing body of literature; limitations to its use include lower spatial resolution; lack of intrapatient and interpatient reproducibility secondary to variations in electrode placement; and deterrence due to setup time, equipment costs, and training of personnel.

Esophageal Manometry

Esophageal manometry is a clinical method used to separate the pressure applied to the respiratory system (P_{aw}) into the component distending the chest wall (ie, pleural pressure, P_{pl}), and that distending the lung transpulmonary pressure (P_L).[65,66] Transpulmonary pressure is defined as the difference between the airway pressure and the pleural pressure.

$$P_L = P_{aw} - P_{pl}$$

Esophageal manometry estimates the P_{pl} through an air-filled balloon catheter inserted in the esophagus. Although esophageal manometry is best known for its role in guiding mechanical ventilation in patients with ARDS,[34] it has also been used in the OR to optimize PEEP instead of relying on standard protective parameters that target P_{aw} alone. To prevent atelectasis, it has been proposed to adjust PEEP such that expiratory transpulmonary pressure is slightly positive, so as to ensure that the lung (if recruitable) is maintained open.[66] To prevent injury from overdistension, attempts are also made to limit the inspiratory transpulmonary pressure.

Esophageal manometry can be used not only to monitor respiratory system mechanics during controlled ventilation but also to monitor patient's respiratory muscle activity during spontaneous breathing. Although evidence-based guidelines recommend limiting inspiratory plateau pressure (P_{plat}) to 30 cmH$_2$O especially in ARDS; however, P_{aw} cannot be measured during normal spontaneous breathing. In contrast, P_L can be measured during spontaneous breathing because it is calculated based on both P_{aw} and P_{pl}. Studies in healthy individuals indicate that a P_L of 25 cmH$_2$O is the upper limit encountered by the lungs in normal life but it is unclear whether this limit is safe in injured lungs, and, a lower threshold than that experienced in healthy breathing may be required.[67]

Despite these potential benefits of esophageal manometry, only limited studies have demonstrated a positive influence of esophageal manometry on patient outcomes.[68] In the OR setting, esophageal manometry may be especially helpful for selecting PEEP in patients with chest-wall abnormalities, such as those with obesity, or with surgical conditions such as increased intra-abdominal pressure due to laparoscopy or Trendelenburg positioning. Setting a desired target for transpulmonary pressures is another proposed method for determining appropriate TVs based on patient's respiratory mechanics.[69] **Fig. 2** demonstrates an example of using esophageal manometry and EIT together to optimize mechanical ventilation during pneumoperitoneum and Trendelenburg positioning in an obese patient.

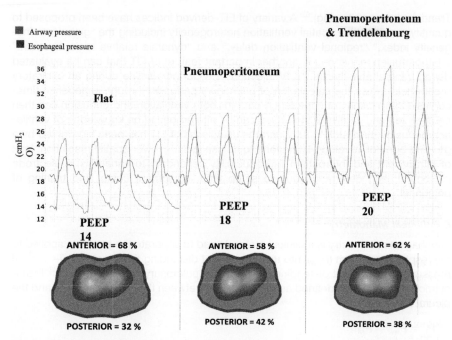

Fig. 2. The use of esophageal manometry and electrical impedance for intraoperative mechanical ventilation optimization in an obese patient.

Lung Ultrasound

Lung ultrasonography (LUS) is a noninvasive bedside tool that can quantify aerated lung mass and provide real-time information during mechanical ventilation.[70] In the perioperative setting, LUS has been used to dynamically detect the development of intraoperative atelectasis, alveolar consolidation, as well as diaphragmatic dysfunction and weakness.[71–73] LUS can be used to assess PEEP-induced lung recruitment, enabling optimization of the ventilatory settings. It can also help discriminate between a cardiac, lung parenchymal, or diaphragmatic cause of loss of lung aeration and, as a consequence, help to determine the most appropriate approach to management.[74] Although lung aeration reaeration can be evaluated using LUS, the ability to predict lung overinflation has been more challenging and the source of ongoing investigation.[75,76]

METHODS TO INCREASE ADHERENCE TO INTRAOPERATIVE LUNG-PROTECTIVE VENTILATION

With multiple physiologic targets, equations, and studies to recall, creating an individualized approach to mechanical ventilation in the OR can be cumbersome and can be limited by the individual's education and comfortability of IOLPV. IOLPV strategies that institute physiologic TVs (6–8 mL/kg cmH_2O) and avoid zero PEEP settings can be facilitated by institutional quality improvement measures. Interventions that have shown improvement in the adherence to IOLPV include the removal of older anesthesia machines,[77] modification of default anesthesia ventilator settings,[78] and near real-time feedback with individualized performance data regarding personal adherence with a peer comparison.[79] For the critically ill patient requiring mechanical ventilation in the OR, the use of a standardized hand-off tool to incorporate mechanical ventilation goals and targets between the ICU and OR team can be instrumental in continuing LPV in the OR setting.

CLINICAL RELEVANCE
Risk Evaluation and Prediction Scores

Selection of an individualized intraoperative ventilation strategy begins with an awareness of the factors that pose the greatest risk for PPCs. Acknowledging known risk factors and using risk prediction models can be useful, particularly in patients that seem to have healthy lungs despite being at risk for PPC or critical illness.[80,81] Recent studies show that patients with a higher risk of PPCs are not routinely receiving IOLPV in the OR.[82] **Table 1** demonstrates the use of 3 different prediction/risk scores available: risk of PPC in patients undergoing surgical procedures (ARISCAT),[83] risk of ALI in-patients with predisposing conditions (lung injury prediction score [LIPS]),[84] and hospitalized patients at risk for progression to PPV due to worsening pulmonary dynamics (early acute lung injury [EALI]).[85] Incorporating these models into your intraoperative mechanical ventilation plan can help minimize "second-hit" exposures in conjunction with a LPV strategy.[84]

Induction

Although 20% to 40% of ICU patients require mechanical ventilation, it is not uncommon to encounter spontaneously breathing critically ill patients that need a life-sustaining intervention in the operating suite to advance care. In these cases, it is vital to remember that protective ventilation begins with induction. Atelectasis occurs in 90% of patients undergoing GA, and it can persist for weeks postoperatively.[27] This is usually tolerated well by young, otherwise healthy patients. However, patients who are aged older than 50 years or who have a body mass index (BMI) greater than 40 kg/m^2, an American Society of Anesthesiologists physical status greater than II, or obstructive sleep apnea may have less tolerance for the decreased functional residual capacity (FRC), shortening the time allowable for intubation. Supine positioning during anesthetic induction results in cephalad displacement of abdominal contents and compression of dependent lung regions. The 30-degree head-up and reverse Trendelenburg positions are associated with less reduction in FRC and should be used during anesthetic induction especially in obese individuals.[27] Critically ill patients are at a high risk for airway complications due to pathophysiologic alterations recently defined as the "physiologically difficult airway," which can hinder optimal intubation times.[86] There is some literature to support the use of noninvasive positive pressure ventilation during induction to reduce atelectasis, minimize desaturations, and allow more time for intubation.[27,86]

Sepsis

Sepsis remains one of the leading causes of ICU admission. Timely source control remains vital to standard treatment. Adequate source control within 6 hours of sepsis onset is associated with reduced risk-adjusted odds of 90-day mortality.[87] One-third of hospitalized patients with sepsis will undergo source-control procedures,[88] and although the use of minimally invasive procedures has increased, anesthetic consideration and ventilation strategies are necessary for many of these procedures. Sepsis and septic shock are known risk factors for ARDS.[84] The requirement for mechanical ventilation in the setting of sepsis can range from airway protection for procedures or altered mental status, to acute respiratory failure secondary to pneumonia,

Table 1
Risk and prediction models for postoperative pulmonary complications and acute lung injury

Assess Respiratory Risk in Surgical Patients in Catalonia (ARISCAT) Risk Score		LIPS		EALI Score	
Parameters	Score	Predisposing Conditions	LIPS Points	Component	Points
Age (y)		Shock	2	O_2 requirement	
≤50	0	Aspiration	2	>2–6 L/min	1
51–80	3	Sepsis	1	>6 L/min	2
>80	16	Pneumonia	1.5	Tachypnea (RR > 30)	1
Preop S_pO_2[a]		High-risk surgery[b]		Immune suppression	1
≥96%	0	Orthopedic spine	1		
91%–95%	8	Acute abdomen	2		
≤50%	24	Cardiac	2.5		
Respiratory infection last 30d		Aortic vascular	3.5		
No	0	High-risk trauma			
Yes	17	Traumatic brain injury	2		
Surgical incision		Smoke inhalation	2		
Peripheral	0	Near drowning	2		
Upper abdominal	15	Lung contusion	1.5		
Intrathoracic	24	Multiple fractures	1.5		
Duration of surgery		Modifiable risk factors			
<2	0	Alcohol abuse	1		

EALI score greater than or equal to 2 identified patients who progressed to ALI and the need for PPV (median time of progression 20 h)

LIPS >4 was associated with an increased frequency of ALI/ARDS with a positive likelihood ration of 3.10

2–3	16	Obesity (body mass index >30)	1
>3	23	Hypoalbuminemia	1
Emergency procedure		Chemotherapy	1
No	0	$F_IO.35$ (4 L/min)	2
Yes	8	Tachypnea (RR > 30)	1.5
ARISCAT has three levels of risk for PPC: <26 points, low (1.6%); 26–44 points, moderate (13.3%); and > 45 points, high risk (42.1%)		SpO_2 < 95%[a]	1
		Acidosis (pH<7.35)	1.5
		Diabetes mellitus[c]	-1

[a] Arterial oxyhemoglobin saturation by pulse oximetry.
[b] Add 1.5 points if emergency surgery.
[c] Only if sepsis.

or to sepsis-induced ARDS. A multidisciplinary team coordination for induction and intubation is important given the possibility of hypoxemia, hypotension, and cardiac collapse that can result in the setting of a physiologically difficult airway. Given the high possibility of a metabolic acidemia at the time of induction and intubation, one must take caution of allowing permissive hypercapnia in the setting of low TVs in at risk patients, resulting in a worsening acidosis.[89] The Surviving Sepsis Campaign Guidelines outline mechanical ventilation strategies for septic patients, which are summarized in **Box 2**.[90] Many of the recommendations parallel to those already discussed, with the exception of a suggestion to use low TV compared with high TV ventilation for adults with sepsis-induced respiratory failure (without ARDS). While stating that the evidence is low and the recommendation is weak, given that sepsis is an independent risk factor for the development of ARDS, they recommend utilizing low TV strategies to avoid the underuse of or the delayed implementation of LPV in an at-risk population.[90]

Acute Respiratory Distress Syndrome

ARDS affects approximately 200,000 patients each year in the United States and results in nearly 75,000 deaths annually.[91] The clinical trials during the past 50 years exploring ways to prevent, mitigate, and treat ARDS are extensive and beyond the scope of this article. However, as this article does focus on the intraoperative strategies for critically ill patients, many of the parameters that were already explored are relevant to IOLPV in patients meeting criteria for the definition of ARDS. Institution of low TVs, high PEEP, and prone positioning for more than 12 hours have shown beneficial results in the outcomes of patients with ARDS and should be incorporated into IOLPV protocols to minimize VILI.[91,92] Although proning patients in the OR may not be practical, considerations of performing bedside interventions in the ICU to limit interruptions in proning protocols could be considered. Anesthesiologists frequently use intraoperative neuromuscular blocking agents (NMBA) to facilitate intraoperative

---

Box 2
Surviving sepsis campaign guidelines for ventilator strategies in adults with sepsis

In sepsis-induced respiratory failure (without ARDS):
- Suggest using low TV as compared with high TV ventilation
  - Low quality evidence, weak recommendation

In sepsis-induced ARDS:
- Recommend using a low TV ventilation strategy (6 mL/kg) over a high TV strategy (>10 mL/kg)
  - High quality evidence, strong recommendation

In sepsis-induced severe ARDs:
- Recommend using an upper limit goal for plateau pressures of 30 cmH$_2$O
  - Moderate quality evidence, strong recommendation

In sepsis-induced moderate–severe ARDS:
- Suggest using higher PEEP over lower PEEP
  - Moderate quality weak recommendation
- Suggest using traditional recruitment maneuvers
  - Moderate quality weak recommendation
- Suggest using intermittent neuromuscular blocking agents (NMBA) over NMBA continuous infusion
  - Moderate quality weak recommendation
- Suggest using veno-venous extracorporeal membrane oxygenation when conventional mechanical ventilation fails
  - Low quality of evidence weak recommendation

ventilator synchrony and optimize surgical conditions. However, the most recent studies suggest that prolonged NMBA are no longer beneficial for ARDS and new recommendations regard limiting their use or implementing intermittent boluses over continuous infusions.[93] The OR and ICU team should coordinate goals for NMBA before transport and incorporate these new guidelines in the OR when feasible.

Special Surgical Cases and Patient Populations

Patient positioning and surgical conditions are important to consider in determining an LPV strategy. Laparoscopic surgery can have negative effects on respiratory mechanics resulting from the pneumoperitoneum, which reduces FRC and promotes atelectasis formation. Pneumoperitoneum also results in reduced compliance of the respiratory system such that a greater amount of pressure will be required to expand the chest wall to achieve a given TV. Many laparoscopic procedures also use the Trendelenburg position that further increases the transmission of intra-abdominal pressure to the chest. Other unique considerations include lateral positioning and single lung ventilation, which also result in changes in lung compliance, resistance, and in TV distribution. The PROTHOR study found a decrease in PPCs in one-lung ventilation with the use of low TV ventilation (6 mL/kg PBW), RMs, and high PEEP.[94] In addition, compliance of the ventilated lung was improved and as a result, driving pressure was decreased. Other trials, such as the iPROVE-OLV are ongoing.[95]

Patients with a BMI greater than 35 can develop rapid atelectasis, a decrease in FRC, and are susceptible to positioning changes in the OR. A recent study in JAMA compared the use of high PEEP (12 cmH_2O) with RMs with low PEEP (4 cmH_2O) with no RMs. Both groups received low TV ventilation of 7 mL/kg PBW in obese (BMI >35) patients undergoing noncardiac surgery. No differences in PPCs were found. The higher PEEP group had lower driving pressures but they were limited by hemodynamic instability.[96] A secondary analysis of this same cohort compared the fixed PEEP strategy to an individualized PEEP strategy using EIT.[97] The individualized PEEP was superior to either fixed low levels or hither level PEEP with regards to oxygenation, driving pressures, and indices of regional ventilation but did not show a difference in PPCs. Ventilator settings often need to be readjusted in response to surgical conditions, adding complexity to the ventilatory management of patients in the OR, and further studies may be needed to elucidate optimization of intraoperative mechanical ventilation in special patient populations.

RECOMMENDATIONS FOR INTRAOPERATIVE LUNG PROTECTIVE VENTILATION

Recent guidelines and several reviews focusing on intraoperative ventilation for patients with and without ARDS have recently been published.[7,27] Based on these publications and the prior discussion in this article, some recommendations for an individualized approach to IOLPV are provided.

Ventilatory parameters should be selected and titrated based on close monitoring of targeted physiologic variables and individualized goals. Although low TV and reduced airway pressures are standard components of LPV, further individualization of ventilation may be necessary based on patient characteristics and surgical conditions. Lung recruitability is essential to identify to determine the potential benefit of RMs and PEEP titration. DPs provide a target to adjust TV and possibly to optimize PEEP. For most patients, DP should be maintained less than 13 cmH_2O. Advanced monitoring tools including EIT, esophageal manometry, and LUS require additional effort and skill for interpretation but should be considered for patients and during surgical procedures that compromise respiratory mechanics and make standard interpretation difficult. Measures including mechanical power, stress index, and dead space provide additional insight into physiology of mechanical ventilation and may provide targets for further optimization.

SUMMARY

Based on the past 20 years of evidence for LPV in ARDS, anesthesiologists have an opportunity to advance intraoperative ventilatory management of critically ill patients in the OR. Delineating which parameters and strategies are best used in the OR versus the ICU will still require more investigation; however, the trend for low TVs, adequate PEEP, and driving pressure targets have gained traction as strategies to prevent PPCs and ARDS. Implementing educational strategies using the EMR and feedback dashboards and resetting default ventilator settings are 2 methods that can be used to change practice. Incorporating more advanced monitoring tools and assessments of respiratory mechanics may help anesthesiologists improve respiratory care provided at the individual level.

CLINICS CARE POINTS

- When implementing a LPV strategy in the OR include both low TVs and the use of PEEP in ventilator settings and avoid the use of low TVs without PEEP given the risk of atelectrauma.

- When monitoring driving pressure in the OR, target driving pressures that increase compliance or to a goal of less than 13.

- When performing a recruitment maneuver in the OR, look for evidence of atelectasis and recruitability by using the stress index and avoid using recruitment maneuvers in patients with overdistension.

- When performing recruitment maneuvers in the OR, consider setting the peak inspirator pressure at 40 cmH$_2$O for 7 to 8 seconds or an upward titration of PEEP up to 20 cmH$_2$O in a pressure-controlled mode but avoid the "bag squeezing" technique to minimize the loss of positive pressure ventilation.

- When inducing anesthesia and providing mechanical ventilation for patients with obesity, limiting atelectasis starts with induction and patients should be intubated in the 30-degree head-up and reverse Trendelenburg position.

- When intubating critically ill patients in the OR at risk for a physiological difficult airway, use noninvasive mechanical ventilation during induction.

- If your patient presents in sepsis or with septic shock, use low TV strategies in the OR given the high risk of ARDS in patients with sepsis.

- When caring for patients with sepsis or septic shock who require mechanical ventilation in the OR, avoid worsening acidemia with permissive hypercapnia.

- If a patient undergoing laparoscopic surgery develops worsening gas exchange with insufflation, increase PEEP and try recruitment maneuvers and consider a change in position or surgical technique if unsuccessful.

REFERENCES

1. Brower RG, Matthay MA, Morris A, et al. Ventilation with lower tidal volumes as compared with traditional tidal volumes for acute lung injury and the acute respiratory distress syndrome. N Engl J Med 2000;342(18):1301–8.
2. Schaefer MS, Serpa Neto A, Pelosi P, et al. Temporal changes in ventilator settings in patients with uninjured lungs: a systematic review. Anesth Analg 2019; 129(1):129–40.

3. Bender SP, Paganelli WC, Gerety LP, et al. Intraoperative Lung-Protective Ventilation Trends and Practice Patterns: A Report from the Multicenter Perioperative Outcomes Group. Anesth Analg 2015;121(5):1231–9.
4. Kirov MY, Kuzkov VV. Protective ventilation from ICU to operating room: state of art and new horizons. Korean J Anesthesiol 2020;73(3):179–93.
5. Ball L, Costantino F, Fiorito M, et al. Respiratory mechanics during general anaesthesia. Ann Transl Med 2018;6(19):379.
6. Fogagnolo A, Montanaro F, Al-Husinat Li, et al. Management of Intraoperative Mechanical Ventilation to Prevent Postoperative Complications after General Anesthesia: A Narrative Review.
7. Meier A, Hylton D, Schmidt UH. Intraoperative Ventilation in the High-Risk Surgical Patient. Respir Care 2021;66(8):1337–40.
8. Eikermann M, Kurth T. Apply Protective Mechanical Ventilation in the Operating Room in an Individualized Approach to Perioperative Respiratory Care. Anesthesiology 2015;123(1):12–4.
9. Nieman GF, Satalin J, Andrews P, et al. Personalizing mechanical ventilation according to physiologic parameters to stabilize alveoli and minimize ventilator induced lung injury (VILI). Intensive Care Med Exp 2017;5(1):8.
10. Respirator lung syndrome. Minn Med 1967;50(11):1693–705.
11. Ashbaugh DG, Bigelow DB, Petty TL, et al. Acute respiratory distress in adults. Lancet 1967;2(7511):319–23.
12. Webb HH, Tierney DF. Experimental pulmonary edema due to intermittent positive pressure ventilation with high inflation pressures. Protection by positive end-expiratory pressure. Am Rev Respir Dis 1974;110(5):556–65.
13. Slutsky AS, Ranieri VM. Ventilator-induced lung injury. N Engl J Med 2013; 369(22):2126–36.
14. Yoshida T, Uchiyama A, Matsuura N, et al. Spontaneous breathing during lung-protective ventilation in an experimental acute lung injury model: high transpulmonary pressure associated with strong spontaneous breathing effort may worsen lung injury. Crit Care Med 2012;40(5):1578–85.
15. Beitler JR, Malhotra A, Thompson BT. Ventilator-induced Lung Injury. Clin Chest Med 2016;37(4):633–46.
16. Albert RK. The role of ventilation-induced surfactant dysfunction and atelectasis in causing acute respiratory distress syndrome. Am J Respir Crit Care Med 2012; 185(7):702–8.
17. Caironi P, Cressoni M, Chiumello D, et al. Lung opening and closing during ventilation of acute respiratory distress syndrome. Am J Respir Crit Care Med 2010; 181(6):578–86.
18. Amato MB, Barbas CS, Medeiros DM, et al. Effect of a protective-ventilation strategy on mortality in the acute respiratory distress syndrome. N Engl J Med 1998; 338(6):347–54.
19. de Durante G, del Turco M, Rustichini L, et al. ARDSNet lower tidal volume ventilatory strategy may generate intrinsic positive end-expiratory pressure in patients with acute respiratory distress syndrome. Am J Respir Crit Care Med 2002; 165(9):1271–4.
20. Tremblay L, Valenza F, Ribeiro SP, et al. Injurious ventilatory strategies increase cytokines and c-fos m-RNA expression in an isolated rat lung model. J Clin Invest 1997;99(5):944–52.
21. Curley GF, Laffey JG, Zhang H, et al. Biotrauma and Ventilator-Induced Lung Injury: Clinical Implications. Chest 2016;150(5):1109–17.

22. Ranieri VM, Suter PM, Tortorella C, et al. Effect of mechanical ventilation on inflammatory mediators in patients with acute respiratory distress syndrome: a randomized controlled trial. JAMA 1999;282(1):54–61.
23. Baedorf Kassis E, Schaefer MS, Maley JH, et al. Transpulmonary pressure measurements and lung mechanics in patients with early ARDS and SARS-CoV-2. J Crit Care 2021;63:106–12.
24. Sud S, Friedrich JO, Taccone P, et al. Prone ventilation reduces mortality in patients with acute respiratory failure and severe hypoxemia: systematic review and meta-analysis. Intensive Care Med 2010;36(4):585–99.
25. Piedalue F, Albert RK. Prone positioning in acute respiratory distress syndrome. Respir Care Clin N Am 2003;9(4):495–509.
26. Sottile PD, Albers D, Moss MM. Neuromuscular blockade is associated with the attenuation of biomarkers of epithelial and endothelial injury in patients with moderate-to-severe acute respiratory distress syndrome. Crit Care 2018; 22(1):63.
27. Young CC, Harris EM, Vacchiano C, et al. Lung-protective ventilation for the surgical patient: international expert panel-based consensus recommendations. Br J Anaesth 2019;123(6):898–913.
28. Wolthuis EK, Choi G, Dessing MC, et al. Mechanical ventilation with lower tidal volumes and positive end-expiratory pressure prevents pulmonary inflammation in patients without preexisting lung injury. Anesthesiology 2008;108(1):46–54.
29. Yang D, Grant MC, Stone A, et al. A Meta-analysis of Intraoperative Ventilation Strategies to Prevent Pulmonary Complications: Is Low Tidal Volume Alone Sufficient to Protect Healthy Lungs? Ann Surg 2016;263(5):881–7.
30. Serpa Neto A, Hemmes SN, Barbas CS, et al. Protective versus conventional ventilation for surgery: a systematic review and individual patient data meta-analysis. Anesthesiology 2015;123(1):66–78.
31. Hedenstierna G, Edmark L. Mechanisms of atelectasis in the perioperative period. Best Pract Res Clin Anaesthesiol 2010;24(2):157–69.
32. Dianti J, Tisminetzky M, Ferreyro BL, et al. Association of positive end-expiratory pressure and lung recruitment selection strategies with mortality in acute respiratory distress syndrome: a systematic review and network meta-analysis. Am J Respir Crit Care Med 2022;205(11):1300–10.
33. Meade MO, Cook DJ, Guyatt GH, et al. Ventilation strategy using low tidal volumes, recruitment maneuvers, and high positive end-expiratory pressure for acute lung injury and acute respiratory distress syndrome: a randomized controlled trial. JAMA 2008;299(6):637–45.
34. Talmor D, Sarge T, Malhotra A, et al. Mechanical ventilation guided by esophageal pressure in acute lung injury. N Engl J Med 2008;359(20):2095–104.
35. Beitler JR, Sarge T, Banner-Goodspeed VM, et al. Effect of Titrating Positive End-Expiratory Pressure (PEEP) With an Esophageal Pressure-Guided Strategy vs an Empirical High PEEP-Fio2 Strategy on Death and Days Free From Mechanical Ventilation Among Patients With Acute Respiratory Distress Syndrome: A Randomized Clinical Trial. JAMA 2019;321(9):846–57.
36. Hess DR. Recruitment Maneuvers and PEEP Titration. Respir Care 2015;60(11): 1688–704.
37. Güldner A, Kiss T, Serpa Neto A, et al. Intraoperative protective mechanical ventilation for prevention of postoperative pulmonary complications: a comprehensive review of the role of tidal volume, positive end-expiratory pressure, and lung recruitment maneuvers. Anesthesiology 2015;123(3):692–713.

38. Rothen HU, Neumann P, Berglund JE, et al. Dynamics of re-expansion of atelectasis during general anaesthesia. Br J Anaesth 1999;82(4):551–6.
39. Tusman G, Groisman I, Fiolo FE, et al. Noninvasive monitoring of lung recruitment maneuvers in morbidly obese patients: the role of pulse oximetry and volumetric capnography. Anesth Analg 2014;118(1):137–44.
40. Fan E, Checkley W, Stewart TE, et al. Complications from recruitment maneuvers in patients with acute lung injury: secondary analysis from the lung open ventilation study. Respir Care 2012;57(11):1842–9.
41. Chen L, Del Sorbo L, Grieco DL, et al. Potential for Lung Recruitment Estimated by the Recruitment-to-Inflation Ratio in Acute Respiratory Distress Syndrome. A Clinical Trial. Am J Respir Crit Care Med 2020;201(2):178–87.
42. Aoyama H, Yamada Y, Fan E. The future of driving pressure: a primary goal for mechanical ventilation? J Intensive Care 2018;6:64.
43. Amato MB, Meade MO, Slutsky AS, et al. Driving pressure and survival in the acute respiratory distress syndrome. N Engl J Med 2015;372(8):747–55.
44. Guérin C, Papazian L, Reignier J, et al. Effect of driving pressure on mortality in ARDS patients during lung protective mechanical ventilation in two randomized controlled trials. Crit Care 2016;20(1):384.
45. Bellani G, Grassi A, Sosio S, et al. Driving Pressure Is Associated with Outcome during Assisted Ventilation in Acute Respiratory Distress Syndrome. Anesthesiology 2019;131(3):594–604.
46. Neto AS, Hemmes SN, Barbas CS, et al. Association between driving pressure and development of postoperative pulmonary complications in patients undergoing mechanical ventilation for general anaesthesia: a meta-analysis of individual patient data. Lancet Respir Med 2016;4(4):272–80.
47. Meier A, Sell RE, Malhotra A. Driving pressure for ventilation of patients with acute respiratory distress syndrome. Anesthesiology 2020;132(6):1569–76.
48. Pelosi P, Ball L, Barbas CSV, et al. Personalized mechanical ventilation in acute respiratory distress syndrome. Crit Care 2021;25(1):250.
49. Grasso S, Terragni P, Mascia L, et al. Airway pressure-time curve profile (stress index) detects tidal recruitment/hyperinflation in experimental acute lung injury. Crit Care Med 2004;32(4):1018–27, ad.
50. Sun XM, Chen GQ, Chen K, et al. Stress index can be accurately and reliably assessed by visually inspecting ventilator waveforms. Respir Care 2018;63(9):1094–101.
51. Kallet RH. Should PEEP Titration Be Based on Chest Mechanics in Patients With ARDS? Respir Care 2016;61(6):876–90.
52. Gattinoni L, Tonetti T, Cressoni M, et al. Ventilator-related causes of lung injury: the mechanical power. Intensive Care Med 2016;42(10):1567–75.
53. Giosa L, Busana M, Pasticci I, et al. Mechanical power at a glance: a simple surrogate for volume-controlled ventilation. Intensive Care Med Exp 2019;7(1):61.
54. Karalapillai D, Weinberg L, Neto AS, et al. Intra-operative ventilator mechanical power as a predictor of postoperative pulmonary complications in surgical patients: A secondary analysis of a randomised clinical trial. Eur J Anaesthesiol 2022;39(1):67–74.
55. Silva PL, Ball L, Rocco PRM, et al. Power to mechanical power to minimize ventilator-induced lung injury? Intensive Care Med Exp 2019;7(Suppl 1):38.
56. Robertson HT. Dead space: the physiology of wasted ventilation. Eur Respir J 2015;45(6):1704–16.

57. Morales-Quinteros L, Schultz MJ, Bringué J, et al. Estimated dead space fraction and the ventilatory ratio are associated with mortality in early ARDS. Ann Intensive Care 2019;9(1):128.

58. Suárez-Sipmann F, Villar J, Ferrando C, et al. Monitoring Expired CO. Front Physiol 2021;12:785014.

59. Verscheure S, Massion PB, Verschuren F, et al. Volumetric capnography: lessons from the past and current clinical applications. Crit Care 2016;20(1):184.

60. Suarez-Sipmann F, Bohm SH, Tusman G. Volumetric capnography: the time has come. Curr Opin Crit Care Jun 2014;20(3):333–9.

61. Spinelli E, Mauri T, Fogagnolo A, et al. Electrical impedance tomography in perioperative medicine: careful respiratory monitoring for tailored interventions. BMC Anesthesiol 2019;19(1):140.

62. Rubin J, Berra L. Electrical impedance tomography in the adult intensive care unit: clinical applications and future directions. Curr Opin Crit Care 2022;28(3): 292–301.

63. Ukere A, März A, Wodack KH, et al. Perioperative assessment of regional ventilation during changing body positions and ventilation conditions by electrical impedance tomography. Br J Anaesth 2016;117(2):228–35.

64. Xu M, He H, Long Y. Lung Perfusion Assessment by Bedside Electrical Impedance Tomography in Critically Ill Patients. Front Physiol 2021;12:748724.

65. Akoumianaki E, Maggiore SM, Valenza F, et al. The application of esophageal pressure measurement in patients with respiratory failure. Am J Respir Crit Care Med 2014;189(5):520–31.

66. Yoshida T, Amato MBP, Grieco DL, et al. Esophageal manometry and regional transpulmonary pressure in lung injury. Am J Respir Crit Care Med 2018; 197(8):1018–26.

67. Pham T, Telias I, Beitler JR. Esophageal manometry. Respir Care 2020;65(6): 772–92.

68. Cammarota G, Lauro G, Sguazzotti I, et al. Esophageal pressure versus gas exchange to set PEEP during intraoperative ventilation. Respir Care 2020;65(5): 625–35.

69. Grieco DL, Chen L, Brochard L. Transpulmonary pressure: importance and limits. Ann Transl Med 2017;5(14):285.

70. Mojoli F, Bouhemad B, Mongodi S, et al. Lung Ultrasound for Critically Ill Patients. Am J Respir Crit Care Med 2019;199(6):701–14.

71. Cylwik J, Buda N. The impact of ultrasound-guided recruitment maneuvers on the risk of postoperative pulmonary complications in patients undergoing general anesthesia. J Ultrason 2022;22(88):e6–11.

72. Umbrello M, Formenti P. Ultrasonographic assessment of diaphragm function in critically ill subjects. Respir Care 2016;61(4):542–55.

73. Moury PH, Cuisinier A, Durand M, et al. Diaphragm thickening in cardiac surgery: a perioperative prospective ultrasound study. Ann Intensive Care 2019;9(1):50.

74. Vetrugno L, Brussa A, Guadagnin GM, et al. Mechanical ventilation weaning issues can be counted on the fingers of just one hand: part 2. Ultrasound J 2020;12(1):15.

75. Tang KQ, Yang SL, Zhang B, et al. Ultrasonic monitoring in the assessment of pulmonary recruitment and the best positive end-expiratory pressure. Medicine (Baltimore) 2017;96(39):e8168.

76. Tonelotto B, Pereira SM, Tucci MR, et al. Intraoperative pulmonary hyperdistention estimated by transthoracic lung ultrasound: A pilot study. Anaesth Crit Care Pain Med 2020;39(6):825–31.

77. Blum JM, Davila V, Stentz MJ, et al. Replacement of anesthesia machines improves intraoperative ventilation parameters associated with the development of acute respiratory distress syndrome. BMC Anesthesiol 2014;14:44.
78. Chiao SS, Colquhoun DA, Naik BI, et al. Changing default ventilator settings on anesthesia machines improves adherence to lung-protective ventilation measures. Anesth Analg 2018;126(4):1219–22.
79. Parks DA, Short RT, McArdle PJ, et al. Improving adherence to intraoperative lung-protective ventilation strategies using near real-time feedback and individualized electronic reporting. Anesth Analg 2021;132(5):1438–49.
80. Miskovic A, Lumb AB. Postoperative pulmonary complications. Br J Anaesth 2017;118(3):317–34.
81. O'Gara B, Talmor D. Perioperative lung protective ventilation. BMJ 2018;362: k3030.
82. investigators LV. Epidemiology, practice of ventilation and outcome for patients at increased risk of postoperative pulmonary complications: LAS VEGAS - an observational study in 29 countries. Eur J Anaesthesiol 2017;34(8):492–507.
83. Canet J, Gallart L, Gomar C, et al. Prediction of postoperative pulmonary complications in a population-based surgical cohort. Anesthesiology 2010;113(6): 1338–50.
84. Gajic O, Dabbagh O, Park PK, et al. Early identification of patients at risk of acute lung injury: evaluation of lung injury prediction score in a multicenter cohort study. Am J Respir Crit Care Med 2011;183(4):462–70.
85. Levitt JE, Calfee CS, Goldstein BA, et al. Early acute lung injury: criteria for identifying lung injury prior to the need for positive pressure ventilation. Crit Care Med 2013;41(8):1929–37.
86. Kornas RL, Owyang CG, Sakles JC, et al, Committee SfAMsSP. Evaluation and Management of the Physiologically Difficult Airway: Consensus Recommendations From Society for Airway Management. Anesth Analg 2021;132(2):395–405.
87. Reitz KM, Kennedy J, Li SR, et al. Association Between Time to Source Control in Sepsis and 90-Day Mortality. JAMA Surg 2022. https://doi.org/10.1001/jamasurg. 2022.2761.
88. Jimenez MF, Marshall JC, Forum IS. Source control in the management of sepsis. Intensive Care Med 2001;27(Suppl 1):S49–62.
89. Maccagnan Pinheiro Besen BA, Tomazini BM, Pontes Azevedo LC. Mechanical ventilation in septic shock. Curr Opin Anaesthesiol 2021;34(2):107–12.
90. Evans L, Rhodes A, Alhazzani W, et al. Surviving sepsis campaign: international guidelines for management of sepsis and septic shock 2021. Crit Care Med 2021;49(11):e1063–143.
91. Fan E, Brodie D, Slutsky AS. Acute respiratory distress syndrome: advances in diagnosis and treatment. JAMA 2018;319(7):698–710.
92. Munshi L, Del Sorbo L, Adhikari NKJ, et al. Prone position for acute respiratory distress syndrome. a systematic review and meta-analysis. Ann Am Thorac Soc 2017;14(Supplement_4):S280–8.
93. Alhazzani W, Belley-Cote E, Møller MH, et al. Neuromuscular blockade in patients with ARDS: a rapid practice guideline. Intensive Care Med 2020;46(11):1977–86.
94. Kiss T, Wittenstein J, Becker C, et al. Protective ventilation with high versus low positive end-expiratory pressure during one-lung ventilation for thoracic surgery (PROTHOR): study protocol for a randomized controlled trial. Trials 2019; 20(1):213.
95. Carramiñana A, Ferrando C, Unzueta MC, et al. Rationale and Study Design for an Individualized Perioperative Open Lung Ventilatory Strategy in Patients on

One-Lung Ventilation (iPROVE-OLV). J Cardiothorac Vasc Anesth 2019;33(9): 2492–502.

96. Bluth T, Serpa Neto A, Schultz MJ, et al. Effect of intraoperative high positive end-expiratory pressure (PEEP) with recruitment maneuvers vs low PEEP on postoperative pulmonary complications in obese patients: a randomized clinical trial. JAMA 2019;321(23):2292–305.

97. Simon P, Girrbach F, Petroff D, et al. Individualized versus fixed positive end-expiratory pressure for intraoperative mechanical ventilation in obese patients: a secondary analysis. Anesthesiology 2021;134(6):887–900.

Postoperative Respiratory Failure and Advanced Ventilator Settings

Christopher Choi, MD[a],*, Gretchen Lemmink, MD[b],
Jose Humanez, MD[c]

KEYWORDS

- Postoperative respiratory failure • Postoperative pulmonary complications
- Pneumonia • ARDS

KEY POINTS

- Postoperative respiratory failure is the most common postoperative pulmonary complication and is associated with high mortality.
- The multiple-hit theory of postoperative respiratory failure calls for both preoperative and intraoperative risk stratification and prevention.
- Chest physiotherapy, pain control, and early treatment of postoperative hypoxemia are critical.

INTRODUCTION

Postoperative pulmonary complications (PPCs) are associated with increased mortality and higher health care costs for both cardiac and noncardiac surgery patients.[1–3] Specifically, postoperative pneumonia in abdominal surgery patients has been correlated with an increased length of stay of 11 days and an increased cost of $31,000.[4] Readmissions are also affected, with pneumonia and respiratory failure contributing to 2.8% and 1.4% of rehospitalizations.[3] Although much effort has been dedicated to identifying and reducing cardiac complications after surgery, PPCs are twice as common as well as underappreciated.[3,5] PPCs have varying definitions in the literature but can be generally described as any condition affecting the respiratory tract that can negatively impact a patient's postoperative course. The incidence of pulmonary

The authors have nothing to disclose.
[a] Department of Anesthesiology and Pain Management, University of Texas Southwestern Medical Center, 5323 Harry Hines Boulevard, Dallas, TX 75390-9068, USA; [b] Department of Anesthesiology, University of Cincinnati College of Medicine, 231 Albert Sabin Way, Cincinnati, OH 45267-0531, USA; [c] Department of Anesthesiology, University of Florida College of Medicine - Jacksonville, 655 West 8th Street, C72, Jacksonville, FL 32209, USA
* Corresponding author.
E-mail address: christopher.choi@utsouthwestern.edu

complications following major surgery has a wide range in the literature from less than 1% to 23%.[1] Thoracic surgery traditionally has been associated with the highest prevalence of PPCs, although one meta-analysis found a similar rate of postoperative lung injury in abdominal surgery.[6] Out of the aforementioned PPCs, postoperative respiratory failure (PORF) is the most common,[7] with an incidence between 2.7% and 3.4%.[8] When present, mortality can exceed 25%.[9]

DEFINITION

Respiratory failure by itself is well-defined as inadequate exchange of oxygen and carbon dioxide. Measurement of arterial partial pressure of oxygen (PaO_2) and carbon dioxide ($PaCO_2$) are the grounds for diagnosis: PaO_2 less than 60 mm Hg and/or $PaCO_2$ more than 50 mm Hg breathing air at sea level (inspiratory oxygen fraction [FIO_2], 0.21). In the clinical setting, the severity of hypoxemia is defined by calculating the ratio of PaO_2 to FiO_2 (P/F ratio). Therefore, a P/F ratio of less than 300 mm Hg is considered respiratory failure, keeping in mind that respiratory failure secondary to cardiac dysfunction is excluded from this definition.

PORF can be defined as pulmonary gas exchange impairment that presents after a surgical procedure and as a result of the changes induced by anesthesia and surgery. The Agency for Healthcare Research and Quality (AHRQ) defines PORF as the failure to wean from mechanical ventilation within 48 hours of surgery or unplanned intubation/reintubation postoperatively,[10] whereas the European Perioperative Clinical Outcomes define PORF as a partial pressure of oxygen less than 60 mm Hg on room air, a peripheral oxygen saturation less than 90%, and a PaO_2/FiO_2 ratio less than 300 mm Hg while using oxygen therapy,[11] a definition that does not consider intubation or reintubation. Severity of PORF can range from transient hypoxemia in the early postoperative period to acute respiratory disease syndrome (ARDS), its most life-threatening form. Although AHRQ sets a timeframe of 48 hours, the time in which PORF can be attributed to surgery or anesthesia is not clear. Some authors consider 7 days as the appropriate timeframe,[12,13] but others have broadened this timeframe up to 30 days.[10,14]

Mechanism of Postoperative Respiratory Failure

The pathological anatomy of respiratory complications can be categorized as respiratory muscle dysfunction or as disease of the airway itself. Acute upper airway collapse or laryngo/bronchospasm can cause negative pressure pulmonary edema secondary to high negative pulmonary pressures generated against a closed airway. Atelectasis is the most frequent mechanism of perioperative desaturation and occurs minutes after induction of general anesthesia due to reduction of regional transpulmonary pressure and reduction of muscle tone. This can lead to subsequent reduction in thorax diameters, lung volumes, and airway dimensions. These changes are followed by the development of airway closure and atelectasis, especially in the dependent parts of the lungs. Said changes lead to ventilation–perfusion mismatch and shunt followed by abnormal gas exchange.

Intraoperatively, perfusion mismatch and shunt can be accentuated by inflammation triggered by surgical incision and bacterial translocation, chest wall restriction, cephalad displacement of the diaphragm by surgical retractors, and supine position.[15] The injurious effects of perioperative atelectasis are magnified by pain, high driving pressure, and inflammation. Accordingly, the anesthetic and surgical perioperative insults can create conditions of "multiple-hit" lung injury, which can be further augmented by the tissue stress induced by intraoperative mechanical ventilation.[16]

Postoperatively, a restrictive lung pattern secondary to diaphragmatic dysfunction is observed, compromising respiratory mechanics and gas exchange. Respiratory muscle function in this period is a determinant of whether a patient develops PORF or not.[17] Normal physiology of the respiratory system relies on balance between respiratory pump muscles—which create a negative pressure leading to an urge to ventilate and the upper airway dilator muscles—which counterbalance the collapsing forces of the negative pressure and ensure upper airway patency.

During emergence from anesthesia and over the postoperative period, respiratory muscle function is affected to different degrees. Early after surgery, residual effects of sedatives and opiates reduce central stimulation of both the upper airway (hypoglossal nerve) and pump muscles (phrenic nerve).[18] At the same time, residual curarization is often present, affecting the upper airway dilator muscles to a greater extent than the diaphragm.[19] Taken together, these events increase upper airway collapsibility and predispose patients to PORF, particularly in the presence of comorbid conditions such as obesity, obstructive sleep apnea, chronic obstructive pulmonary disease, or smoking addiction. Later, the effects of surgery or trauma can further favor the development of PORF, mainly due to functional disruption of the respiratory muscles, postoperative pain, or direct diaphragmatic dysfunction from phrenic nerve injury.

Postoperative Respiratory Failure and Acute Respiratory Disease Syndrome

As mentioned, the worst presentation of PORF is the development of ARDS, in which lung damage occurs, leading to hypoxemia. **Box 1** shows the definition criteria for ARDS per the Berlin consensus.[20] One of the criteria is a respiratory failure that seems within a week of a recognized insult (such as surgery and anesthesia). ARDS starts with an exudative phase which is triggered by a variety of mechanical, chemical, and biological insults. This phase is characterized by diffuse alveolocapillary membrane damage occurring heterogeneously across the lung regions.[21] **Table 1** shows a different level of respiratory impairment found in ARDS. Mortality associated to ARDS is very high, ranging from 17% in the mild form to more than 58% in the severe form.[22] Incidence of ARDS ranges from 0.2% in the general surgical population[13] to 7.8% for high-risk procedures to 10.2% for cardiac surgery.[23]

Multiples factors are involved in the pathogenesis of postoperative ARDS. According to the multiple-hit theory mentioned before, there is a first hit that comes from factors related to a patient's initial status and the scheduled procedure, including the

---

Box 1
Berlin criteria for acute respiratory disease syndrome

1. Symptom onset within 1 week of known insult or new or worsening symptoms in the past 1 week

2. Bilateral opacities on chest imaging not fully explained by effusions, lung collapse, or nodules

3. $PaO_2/FiO_2 \leq 300$ while on PEEP ≥ 5 cm H_2O^a

4. Cannot be fully attributed to cardiac failure and/or volume overload

[a]Can be delivered noninvasively for mild ARDS group.*Abbreviations:* ARDS, acute respiratory distress syndrome; PEEP, positive-end expiratory pressure.

Ranieri VM, Rubenfeld GD, Thompson BT, et al. Acute respiratory distress syndrome: the Berlin Definition. JAMA 2012; 307:2526–2533.

Table 1	
Acute respiratory disease syndrome severity	
Severity	P/F Ratio
Mild	200–300
Moderate	100–200
Severe	<100

Abbreviations: ARDS, acute respiratory distress syndrome; P/F ratio, PaO_2/FiO_2.

anesthetic technique. These factors would not by themselves lead directly to alveolar damage, but the addition of second hits further increases the likelihood of ARDS.[24] Possible second hits in the surgical setting include aspects of intraoperative ventilatory management, aspiration, fluid therapy, transfusion, and inadequate control of infection. Postoperative atelectasis, which can trigger an inflammatory reaction, postoperative lung inflammation, and later pulmonary infection, can be considered second hits that favor ARDS.[25]

Prevention of Postoperative Respiratory Failure

Determining which patients are at increased risk for PORF helps clinicians anticipate adverse events postoperatively and improves allocation of resources after surgery. **Box 2** shows the main risk factors associated with PORF.[26] Following the idea of multiple-hit theory of ARDS in PORF, risk stratification and prevention can be divided into preoperative and intraoperative preventative measures. The first stage considers threats associated with the patient's condition and the planned procedure (preoperative information). The second stage considers intraoperative events, which would modulate first-hit risk and indicate the patient's definitive risk. Preoperatively screening patients is important to identify those at high risk for PORF in order to optimize them before surgery and anesthesia. PORF has a strong association with comorbid conditions; thus, it is important to use available data on demographics and comorbidities to make predictions regarding respiratory complication risk. There are several risk calculators, but one useful and easy to apply tool is the score for prediction of postoperative respiratory complications.[26] In addition to the presence of comorbid conditions, the clinical presentation of wheezing and clinical signs and symptoms of fluid overload favor the development of PORF. Active smokers have increased mortality risk following major surgery.[26] Smoking cessation at least 1 year before surgery decreases postoperative mortality risk and the respiratory event rate.[27]

Intraoperative and postoperative measures to prevent PORF can be divided into ventilator and non-ventilatory techniques. Ventilatory measures are listed in **Box 3**. Non-ventilatory measures are listed in **Box 4**. The main objective with these measures is to avoid the second hit in the multiple-hit theory. Therefore, it is reasonable to use intraoperative lung-protective management of ventilation to avoid ventilator-induced lung injury in all patients, not just those at high risk.[16,28] The goal is avoiding damage from atelectrauma by applying positive end-expiratory pressure (PEEP) and avoidance of volutrauma or overdistension by holding airway pressure and tidal volumes within limits. Fractional inspired oxygen should be adjusted throughout the anesthetic procedure as administration of high oxygen concentration may promote atelectasis,[29] although this is controversial.[30] Also, application of recruitment maneuvers during emergence has been shown to improve oxygenation and to reduce the development of atelectasis.[31] Intraoperative non-ventilatory measures include infection prevention, judicious fluid therapy, limiting transfusions, and using appropriately chosen and

---

Box 2
Risk factors for postoperative respiratory failure

- Age
- History of chronic obstructive pulmonary disease and/or congestive heart failure
- Smoking
- Functional dependence
- Serum albumin <3 g/dL
- ASA score 3 or greater
- Emergency surgery
- If referred from a high-risk service

Abbreviation: ASA, American Society of Anesthesiologists.

---

accurately dosed anesthetics. Choosing less invasive surgical approaches reduces the risk of PORF. Postoperatively, the use of multimodal pain control and/or regional anesthetic techniques, physiotherapy, and early treatment of postoperative hypoxemia has been shown to prevent PORF.

COVID-19 and Postoperative Respiratory Failure

Postoperative respiratory outcomes of patients infected with SARS-CoV-2, the virus responsible for COVID-19 disease, require special discussion. Literature suggests that postoperative respiratory complications occur in half of the patients diagnosed with SARS-CoV-2 in the perioperative period.[32] Patients with symptomatic COVID-19 disease presenting for high-risk surgery understandably have increased morbidity and mortality. However, it is becoming increasingly apparent that even patients with occult infection presenting for low or intermediate risk surgical procedures are predisposed to higher rates of PORF and have increased risk of progression to ARDS in the postoperative period.[33–36] Faced with this knowledge, nonurgent procedures in infected patients should be postponed, and nonoperative treatments should be promoted when possible. Perioperative guidelines for the management of these high-risk patients presenting for elective surgery exist and should be adhered to when feasible. Current recommendations suggest delaying elective surgery for 7 weeks after SARS-CoV-2 infection is diagnosed in unvaccinated patients.[37–41]

Box 3
Intraoperative ventilatory measures

Titration of FiO_2

Avoid atelectrauma
- Apply PEEP
- Recruitment maneuvers after intubation, after circuit disconnections, during hypoxemia and before extubation

Avoid volutrauma
- Limit plateau pressure <30 cm H_2O
- Tidal volume < 8 mL/Kg in non-risk patients
- Tidal volume <6 mL/Kg in high-risk patients

Abbreviations: FiO_2, inspired fraction of oxygen; PEEP, positive-end expiratory pressure.

Box 4
Intraoperative non-ventilatory measures

Anesthetic technique
• Choose neuroaxial or regional technique if feasible
• Use inhaled anesthetics to decrease pulmonary inflammatory response
• Accurate administration and monitoring of neuromuscular blockade

Emergence
• Complete reversal of the neuromuscular blockade
• Minimize atelectasis
• Adequate postoperative analgesia
• Avoid overuse of opiates and excessive sedation

Restrict fluids and minimize transfusions
• Optimize preoperative anemia
• Consider cell salvage

Decrease risk of pulmonary infection
• Antibiotic prophylaxis
• Tooth brushing and oral decontamination
• Endotracheal tube management
   ○ Check cuff pressure
   ○ Use appropriate cuff shape and material
• Avoid unnecessary nasogastric tube placement

Surgical technique
• Choose thoracoscopic or laparoscopic approach if feasible
• Decrease surgical duration

Regardless of risk of perioperative complications, patients with active SARS-CoV-2 infection often require urgent/emergent surgery, especially in times of increased community spread. These patients should be considered high risk from a respiratory standpoint and optimized preoperatively in a similar fashion to other patients with noninfectious pulmonary comorbidities. Postoperatively the patient's severity of disease should be assessed, and pharmacologic management specific to COVID-19 pneumonia should be considered and/or continued on an individualized basis based on the most current treatment guidelines.[42]

Noninvasive Versus Invasive Ventilation

As already mentioned, general anesthesia causes reduction of muscle tone and eventually, atelectasis. This, combined with typical intraoperative supine positioning, has a detrimental effect on lung mechanics. Noninvasive ventilation (NIV) has become a popular tool for patients in respiratory failure from chronic obstructive pulmonary disease (COPD) or cardiogenic pulmonary edema.[43,44] It also has a role in PORF, as hypoxemia and atelectasis are thought to be the major cause of postoperative pneumonia, a severe PPC that can lead to ARDS.[45,46] A continuous positive air pressure (CPAP) or bilevel positive airway pressure (BiPAP) device is used for respiratory support; BiPAP is typically used when hypoxemia and hypercarbia are present. The positive pressure supplied helps with lung re-expansion as well as weak respiratory effort. When applied, NIV reduces the risk of tracheal re-intubation[47,48]; however, the routine use of prophylactic NIV postoperatively is not currently indicated.[49]

High-flow nasal cannula (HFNC) is another option for delivering supplemental oxygen in the perioperative setting. It works by administering air through short and larger nasal prongs, which allows for high flows. The high flow rate reduces entrainment of room air, allowing for up to 100% oxygen administration. It also provides positive airway pressure ($\sim$1 cm water pressure for 10 L flow).[50] HFNC is not inferior to NIV in preventing post-extubation respiratory failure.[51] In the postoperative setting, HFNC may be preferred due to patient comfort and ability to access the oropharynx for pulmonary physiotherapy. Importantly, NIV is not recommended if a patient progresses to postoperative ARDS as NIV can do more harm than good.[52] NIV can create a false sense of security and delay life-saving tracheal intubation. It is also more difficult to control a patient's minute ventilation and provide high levels of PEEP with this modality, likely leading to further lung damage. In fact, patients with ARDS that were treated with NIV had increased mortality in a recent international study.[53]

Fluid Management in Postoperative Respiratory Failure /Acute Respiratory Disease Syndrome

The pathophysiology of postoperative ARDS includes increased pulmonary endothelial permeability and neutrophil infiltration mediated by systemic pro-inflammatory cytokines resulting in part from surgical trauma.[54] Increased vascular permeability results in the hallmark noncardiogenic pulmonary edema associated with early ARDS. This may be exacerbated in patients who were over-resuscitated intraoperatively or who may concurrently be suffering from other pulmonary pathologies such as aspiration pneumonia, transfusion-associated circulatory overload, or transfusion-associated acute lung injury. In such instances, a conservative fluid management strategy may increase ventilator-free days and decrease intensive care unit (ICU) length of stay and mortality.[55,56] In patients who no longer require ongoing volume resuscitation to manage a shock state and in who hypotension and organ hypoperfusion can be avoided, it is reasonable to target either euvolemia or even a negative fluid balance. This is especially true for those patients who exhibit signs of volume overload in the postoperative period. Such "de-resuscitation" can be achieved pharmacologically with a variety of diuretic mediations including loop diuretics (eg, furosemide) or medications from the thiazide family (eg, metolazone). Every effort should be made for all patients at risk for PORF to initiate early oral fluid therapy with discontinuation of postoperative IV fluid therapy as soon as it can be tolerated.[57]

Adjunctive Pharmacological Therapies for Acute Respiratory Disease Syndrome

Systemic glucocorticoid therapy in postoperative ARDS should be individualized according to severity and duration of ARDS as well as risk of steroid administration in the setting of surgical wound healing. Generally, systemic glucocorticoid therapy is recommended for patients with moderate to severe ARDS ([PaO_2/FiO_2] ratio <200) who are early in the disease course (within 14 days of onset).[58] This recommendation can be extrapolated to the perioperative period, provided the risk of steroids from a surgical standpoint is not determined to outweigh their anticipated respiratory benefit. The exact pharmacologic regimen remains controversial as specific agents and dosing regimens vary widely in available clinical trials.[59,60]

Inhaled pulmonary vasodilators (eg, nitric oxide and epoprostenol) have long been used in the ICU to improve oxygenation in patients with severe ARDS, especially those with hypoxemia refractory to other therapies.[61] These mediations act locally to improve ventilation/perfusion (V/Q) mismatch by dilating only the pulmonary vasculature associated with well-ventilated lung units. Despite their long-standing clinical use and established ability to improve oxygenation in the short term, none have been shown to improve morbidity or mortality in ARDS patients.[62,63] The choice of agent is often institution-specific and based on health system economics given their similar safety and efficacy profiles.[62,64] Systemic side effects are minimal due to selective action on local pulmonary vasculature, though it has been suggested that nitric oxide may increase risk for renal impairment in ARDS patients.[64,65] Further studies are needed to elucidate the true risk versus benefit profile of these agents in severe ARDS. Given their lack of impact on meaningful clinical outcomes, use in patients with PORF should be limited to those with severe ARDS and ongoing hypoxemia refractory to other medical therapies.

Neuromuscular-blocking agents (NMBAs) are perhaps the most used pharmacologic therapy for ARDS, and their use has increased in the postoperative period over the past two decades. These agents are used to facilitate mechanical ventilation and improve ventilator synchrony in the moderate/severe ARDS patient. Continuous cisatracurium infusion is the most well-studied agent in this patient population, and early literature had suggested its use in moderate to severe ARDS improves oxygenation, increases ventilator-free days, and decreases mortality without an increased incidence of ICU-acquired weakness.[66,67] Unfortunately, newer data do not support these findings, instead showing no difference in outcomes for patients receiving NMBAs versus controls.[68] In the setting of conflicting data, it is reasonable to avoid the use of NMBAs unless the patient is experiencing severe ventilator desynchrony refractory to ventilator adjustments and sedation optimization.

Physiotherapy and Mobility

Chest physiotherapy is often started in the postoperative period in hopes of preventing PPCs. This usually involves a combination of lung expansion maneuvers and airway clearance techniques. At the most basic level, deep breathing exercises, huffing, and coughing are used. The forced expiration technique is 1 to 2 forced expirations (huffs) followed by breathing control.[69] This may be the most effective component of chest clearance, as it loosens and moves secretions toward larger airways. Early mobilization is also critical, as it improves peripheral and arterial oxygenation when started within 2 hours.[70] It decreases atelectasis, lessens opiate medication use, and shortens recovery time.[71] Incentive spirometry is the most widespread lung expansion device in use today; however, its benefits are controversial,[72,73] especially when not paired with other physiotherapy actions.

Overall, a multifactorial program is recommended. The centers for disease control and prevention (CDC) encourages deep breathing exercises and ambulation to prevent PPCs as well as incentive spirometry use in patients that are high-risk for pneumonia.[74] When implemented, chest physiotherapy programs decrease rates of postoperative pneumonia.[71,75,76] Of note, patient education is an underappreciated component of physiotherapy. In one study, including patient education in the preoperative assessment clinic and preoperative holding area in a multidisciplinary patient care program reduced the rates of pneumonia as well as unplanned intubation.[75] When patients are unable to participate in physiotherapy, CPAP may be a viable alternative.[77] Importantly, patient positioning is the single most important factor. All these maneuvers in the sitting or upright position help increase lung volumes, strength of coughing, and secretion clearance.[78]

Proning

Another established therapy for patients suffering from moderate/severe ARDS is mechanical ventilation in the prone position. It has been recognized for years that this technique improves oxygenation over traditional supine positioning. Proning is typically used in settings of hypoxemia refractory to classic lung-protective ventilation strategies. There is evidence suggesting a substantial mortality benefit when prone therapy is initiated early in the course of moderate/severe ARDS.[79,80] The benefits of prone therapy are multifactorial. Its favorable effect on the transpulmonary pressure differences between the ventral and dorsal alveoli has been shown to homogenize ventilation between these two areas. Prone therapy also decreases lung compression and improves V/Q matching.[81–85] The methods and support needed to initiate prone therapy are not standardized, and risks related to positioning do exist. These include pressure ulcers, nerve damage, retinal damage, and accidental dislodgement of medical devices while turning. Contraindications to prone therapy exist and include unstable fractures (eg, spine, pelvis, and face), elevated intracranial pressure refractory to treatment, and recent sternotomy.[80] It is viewed as a safe and effective therapy when done in experienced centers, and it should be used early in the course of disease in patients with moderate/severe ARDS. It is advisable to consider transferring these patients to a facility with the resources to initiate prone therapy if it cannot be safely achieved in their current hospital setting.

Airway Pressure Release Ventilation

Airway pressure release ventilation (APRV) was introduced into clinical practice over 20 years ago. This mode of ventilation has been called different names depending on the manufacturer of the ventilator, such as BiLevel (Covidien), APRV (Drager), Bi-Vent (Maquet), BiPhasic (CareFusion), and DuoPAP (Hamilton). It involves a mix of inverse ratio, pressure controlled, and intermittent mandatory ventilation with unrestricted spontaneous breathing. It has several advantages over conventional ventilation, including alveolar recruitment, improved oxygenation, preservation of spontaneous breathing, improved hemodynamics, and potential lung-protective effects.[86] Disadvantages are related to risk of volutrauma, increased work of breathing, and increased energy expenditure compared with spontaneous breathing. APRV is used mainly as a rescue therapy for refractory hypoxemia in the setting of ARDS. APRV settings include "P high," "T high," "P low," and "T low," in addition to fractional inspired oxygen (FiO_2) and pressure support (**Fig. 1**). The mandatory breaths applied by APRV are time-triggered, pressure-targeted, time-cycled breaths, whereas the spontaneous breaths can occur both during and between mandatory breaths. The amplitude of the time-triggered mandatory breath (inspiratory pressure) and the duration of it (inspiratory time) are known as "P high" and "T high," respectively. The expiratory pressure is called "P low," and the expiratory time (release time) is called "T low."[87]

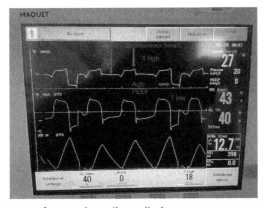

Fig. 1. Sample APRV waveform and ventilator display.

Studies comparing APRV and conventional mechanical ventilation are limited by small sample size, but they tend to show a faster improvement in oxygenation with APRV, albeit without a mortality benefit.[88] APRV shares some similar features with other non-conventional modes of ventilation (eg, inverse ratio ventilation [IRV] and high-frequency oscillatory ventilation [HFOV]), but these modes cause more patient discomfort, thereby requiring sedation and sometimes the use of paralytic agents.[89] Most authors recommend setting P high according to the plateau pressure of the volume-controlled mode or the peak Paw of the pressure-controlled mode.[90] The recommendation is to limit the P high to 30–35 cm H_2O while setting the P low at zero cm H_2O and setting a very short T low. The short T low creates auto-PEEP to maintain end-expiratory lung volume. This method takes into consideration avoiding excessive inflating pressures, but the resultant tidal volumes might be highly variable. Of note, this tidal volume variability may be higher than the accepted standard of care (eg, 6–8 mL/kg) due to the contribution of the patient's spontaneous inspiratory effort.

Inverse Ratio Ventilation

IRV is positive-pressure ventilation with an inspiratory–expiratory (I:E) ratio of greater than 1. The main indication for IRV is the treatment of refractory hypoxemia during severe ARDS. The I:E ratios usually range from 1.2 to 1.5, whereas in IRV, they may be 1:1, 2:1, or higher. The purpose of IRV is to maintain a high mean airway pressure and to hold plateau pressure (Ppl) within a safe range. The prolongation of inspiration allows for recruitment of lung units with a long-time constant which may improve oxygenation.[91] Deep sedation and/or paralysis is commonly required with this mode of ventilation. This application is most commonly used with time-cycled pressure-control ventilation, but it can also be used with volume-cycled ventilation. There is moderate improvement in oxygenation with this mode, and carbon dioxide elimination is preserved or enhanced. The development of auto-PEEP is common in IRV, and it may be responsible for some of the improvements in oxygenation; however, it also increases the risk of barotrauma.

High-Frequency Oscillatory Ventilation

High-frequency oscillatory ventilation (HFOV) is a lung-protective strategy which has been used in both pediatric and adult populations for the treatment of ARDS or as a second-line therapy in the management of ventilated patients with bronchopleural fistulas.[92] Like APRV and IRV, HFOV is usually applied as a rescue measure when conventional mechanical ventilation has failed. HFOV uses low tidal volumes and constant mean airway pressures along with high respiratory rates in order to improve oxygenation and ventilation while eliminating the traumatic "inflate–deflate" cycle that occurs in conventional modes. Commonly, patients receiving HFOV require a greater amount of sedation and neuromuscular blockade, which can subsequently lead to prolonged hospital stays.[93] Complications of HFOV include air trapping and hyperinflation which, if unrecognized, may lead to barotrauma and result in pneumothorax, pneumomediastinum, or pneumopericardium. Importantly, patients on HFOV can have decreased venous return, decreased cardiac output, intraventricular hemorrhage, and increased intrathoracic pressures.

Advanced Modes of Mechanical Ventilation

New modes of mechanical ventilation have been developed to facilitate liberation from ventilators. They emerged from a need for greater control of the ventilator by the patient, better ventilator synchrony, and monitoring of respiratory mechanics during ventilator weaning.[94] The most common modes are volume-assured pressure support ventilation, proportional assist ventilation, neurally adjusted ventilatory assist (NAVA), and adaptive support ventilation (ASV).

Volume-assured pressure support ventilation combines pressure support ventilation with volume-assisted ventilation. By doing so, it decreases the patient's work of breathing, assures a set tidal volume, and optimizes inspiratory flow. Proportional assist ventilation is a form of synchronized ventilator support in which the ventilator generates pressure in proportion to the patient's effort or in proportion to the flow and volume generated by the patient's effort leading to variation in inspiratory pressure.[95] This effect can potentially prevent excessive diaphragm loading and atrophy by disuse. During assisted ventilation, both the patient and ventilator contribute to the pressure required to overcome the elastic and resistive load during breathing. The compliance of the respiratory system and the airway resistance is calculated by ventilator software by means of a brief end-inspiratory occlusion performed randomly every four to ten breaths.[96] Of note, this calculation may be inaccurate in the presence of leaks. When compared with pressure support ventilation, proportional assist ventilation shows benefits regarding ventilator synchrony, weaning success, sleep quality, duration of mechanical ventilation, lung and diaphragm protection, rate of reintubation, but not mortality.[96] NAVA delivers pressure in response to the patient's respiratory drive, measured by the electrical activity of the diaphragm. Patients take full control of the magnitude and timing of the mechanical support provided. NAVA has shown to decrease the risk of lung hyperinflation, respiratory alkalosis, and hemodynamic complications compared with other weaning modes of ventilation.[97] NAVA requires the insertion of a specialized nasogastric catheter that detects the diaphragm activity with electrodes.[98] Compared with other modes of ventilation, NAVA improves ventilator synchrony and duration of mechanical ventilation but not survival.[99] ASV is a closed loop-controlled ventilator mode, which automatically adjusts to optimize the patient's work of breathing. As the patient's respiratory effort starts, ASV delivers pressure supported breaths according to the set minute ventilation; this results in the best combination of tidal volume, respiratory rate, and patient's inspiratory effort. In ASV mode, FiO_2 and PEEP are set manually.[100]

Extracorporeal Membrane Oxygenation

Another modality for advanced management of refractory hypoxemia in severe ARDS is extracorporeal life support (ECLS). In most cases, veno-venous extracorporeal membrane oxygenation is the ECLS modality of choice for patients with isolated respiratory failure. Patients who are experiencing refractory hypoxemia in the setting of concomitant cardiogenic shock may require veno-arterial ECMO support. Similar to prone positioning, this management modality requires specific expertise and is not widely available at all centers. Patients should be considered for ECLS when they have hypoxia in the setting of severe ARDS and traditional supportive measures (low tidal volume ventilation, appropriate PEEP selection, and conservative fluid management) have failed. Additional less invasive therapies should also be attempted if feasible (including NMBAs and prone positioning) before consideration for ECLS.[101] The rationale for ECLS in severe ARDS ($PaO_2/FiO_2 < 80$ mm Hg or pH < 7.25 with a $PaCO_2 \geq 60$ mm Hg) is related to its ability to dramatically improve oxygenation and ventilation while allowing for "lung rest," thus avoiding the more injurious aspects of mechanical ventilation.

Patient selection criteria are not standardized and vary per institution. However, some commonly accepted relative contraindications to ECMO support exist and are usually related to advanced age, limited life-expectancy, irreversible cause of lung injury, prolonged mechanical ventilation, and significant central nervous system

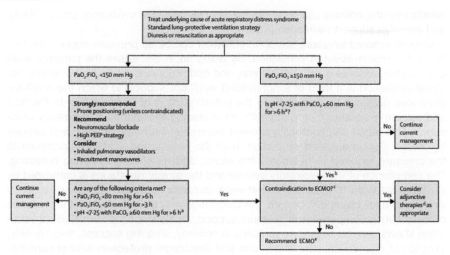

Fig. 2. Algorithm for management of acute respiratory distress syndrome. ECMO, extracorporeal membrane oxygenation; PaCO₂, partial pressure of carbon dioxide in arterial blood; PaO₂:FiO₂, ratio of partial pressure of oxygen in arterial blood to the fractional concentration of oxygen in inspired air; PEEP, positive end-expiratory pressure. [a]With respiratory rate increased to 35 breaths per minute and mechanical ventilation settings adjusted to keep a plateau airway pressure of ≤32 cm of water. [b]Consider neuromuscular blockade. [c]There are no absolute contraindications that are agreed on except end-stage respiratory failure when lung transplantation will not be considered; exclusion criteria used in the EOLIA trial 1 can be taken as a conservative approach to contraindications to ECMO. [d]Eg, neuromuscular blockade, high PEEP strategy, inhaled pulmonary vasodilators, recruitment maneuvers, high-frequency oscillatory, and ventilation. [e]Recommend early ECMO as per EOLIA trial criteria; salvage ECMO, which involves deferral of ECMO initiation until further decompensation (as in the crossovers to ECMO in the EOLIA control group), is not supported by the evidence but might be preferable be preferable to not initiating ECMO at all in such patients. (*From* Abrams D, Ferguson ND, Brochard L et al. ECMO for ARDS: from salvage to standard of care? [published correction appears in Lancet Respir Med. 2019 Feb;7(2):e9]. *Lancet Respir Med* 2019 Feb;7(2):108-110; with permission.)

injury/pathology.[101] The only absolute contraindication for ECLS at this time is a lack of anticipated lung recovery without a plan for or possibility of lung transplantation.[101] Additional relative contraindications and a suggested patient selection algorithm can be found in **Fig. 2**. It is important to identify patients who might benefit from ECLS support early in their ARDS course and rapidly optimize conservative medical therapies in these patients. It is well established that mortality on ECMO increases with prolonged mechanical ventilation before cannulation.[102] To this end, patients under consideration for ECMO support should be transferred to facilities capable of providing this support early in their ARDS course.[101,103]

SUMMARY

PPCs are a common and underrecognized phenomenon that are associated with substantial morbidity, mortality, and increased health care costs. Preoperative recognition of high-risk patients, optimization before surgery, and meticulous intraoperative care are essential to limit PPC occurrence. When PPCs occur, early recognition and evidence-based treatment can limit progression to ARDS and thus avoid the high mortality associated with this condition.

CLINICS CARE POINTS

- Along with lung-protective ventilation, intraoperative infection prevention, judicious volume administration and appropriately chosen/dosed anesthetics can reduce PORF.
- Multifactorial chest physiotherapy programs reduce postoperative pneumonia and are recommended by the CDC.
- Noninvasive ventilation helps with lung re-expansion and weak respiratory effort, thereby reducing risk of tracheal intubation.
- Proning is an important intervention for ARDS that is underutilized - especially in the postoperative population.

REFERENCES

1. Miskovic A, Lumb AB. Postoperative pulmonary complications. Br J Anaesth 2017;118:317–34.
2. Sabate S, Mazo V, Canet J. Predicting postoperative pulmonary complications: implications for outcomes and costs. Curr Opin Anesthesiol 2014;27:201–9.
3. Shander A, Fleisher LA, Barie PS, et al. Clinical and economic burden of postoperative pulmonary complications: patient safety summit on definition, risk-reducing interventions, and preventive strategies. Crit Care Med 2011;39: 2163–72.
4. Thompson DA, Makary MA, Dorman T, et al. Clinical and economic outcomes of hospital acquired pneumonia in intra-abdominal surgery patients. Ann Surg 2006;243(4):547–52.
5. Lawrence VA, Hilsenbeck SG, Noveck H, et al. Medical complications and outcomes after hip fracture repair. Arch Intern Med 2002;162(18):2053–7.
6. Serpa NA, Hemmes SN, Barbas CS, et al. Incidence of mortality and morbidity related to postoperative lung injury in patients who have undergone abdominal or thoracic surgery: a systematic review and meta-analysis. Lancet Respir Med 2014;2(12):1007–15.
7. Canet J, Sabaté S, Mazo V, et al. Development and validation of a score to predict postoperative respiratory failure in a multicentre European cohort. A prospective, observational study. Eur J Anaesthesiol 2015;32:458–70.
8. Attaallah AF, Vallejo MC, Elzamzamy OM, et al. Perioperative risk factors for postoperative respiratory failure. J Perioper Pract 2019;29(3):49–53.
9. Kim M, Brady JE, Li G. Interaction effects of acute kidney injury, acute respiratory failure, and sepsis on 30-day postoperative mortality in patients undergoing high-risk intraabdominal general surgical procedures. Anesth Analg 2015;121: 1536–46.
10. Gupta H, Gupta P, Morrow L, et al. Development and validation of a risk calculator predicting postoperative respiratory failure. Chest 2011;140(5):1207–15.
11. Canet J, Gallart L, Gomar C, et al. Prediction of postoperative pulmonary complications in a population-based surgical cohort. Anesthesiology 2010;113:1338–50.
12. Arozullah AM, Daley J, Henderson WG, et al. Multifactorial risk index for predicting postoperative respiratory failure in men after major noncardiac surgery. The National Veterans Administration Surgical Quality Improvement Program. Ann Surg 2000;232:242–53.
13. Blum JM, Stentz MJ, Dechert R, et al. Preoperative and intraoperative predictors of postoperative acute respiratory distress syndrome in a general surgical population. Anesthesiology 2013;118:19–29.

14. Hua M, Brady JE, Li G. A scoring system to predict unplanned intubation in patients having undergone major surgical procedures. Anesth Analg 2012;115: 88–94.

15. Tusman G, Bohm SH, Warner DO, et al. Atelectasis and perioperative pulmonary complications in high-risk patients. Curr Opin Anaesthesiol 2012;25:1–10.

16. Melo MFV, Eikermann M. Protect the lungs during abdominal surgery it may change the postoperative outcome. Anesthesiology 2013;118:1254–7.

17. Sasaki N, Meyer MJ, Eikermann M. Postoperative respiratory muscle dysfunction: pathophysiology and preventive strategies. Anesthesiology 2013;118: 961–78.

18. Nishino T, Shirahata M, Yonezawa T, et al. Comparison of changes in the hypoglossal and the phrenic nerve activity in response to increasing depth of anesthesia in cats. Anesthesiology 1984;60:19–24.

19. Eikermann M, Vogt FM, Herbstreit F, et al. The predisposition to inspiratory upper airway collapse during partial neuromuscular blockade. Am J Respir Crit Care Med 2007;175:9–15.

20. Ranieri VM, Rubenfeld GD, Thompson BT, et al. Acute respiratory distress syndrome: the Berlin Definition. JAMA 2012;307:2526–33.

21. Litell JM, Gong MN, Talmor D, et al. Acute lung injury: prevention may be the best medicine. Respir Care 2011;56:1546–54.

22. Villar J, Perez-Mendez L, Blanco J, et al. A universal definition of ARDS: the PaO2/FiO2 ratio under a standard ventilatory setting: a prospective, multicenter validation study. Intensive Care Med 2013;39:583–92.

23. Gajic O, Dabbagh O, Park PK, et al. Early identification of patients at risk of acute lung injury: evaluation of lung injury prediction score in a multicenter cohort study. Am J Respir Crit Care Med 2011;183:462–70.

24. Biehl M, Kashiouris MG, Gajic O. Ventilator-induced lung injury: minimizing its impact in patients with or at risk for ARDS. Respir Care 2013;58:927–37.

25. van Kaam AH, Lachmann RA, Herting E, et al. Reducing atelectasis attenuates bacterial growth and translocation in experimental pneumonia. Am J Respir Crit Care Med 2004;169:1046–53.

26. Brueckmann B, Villa-Uribe J, Eikermann M, et al. Development and validation of a score for prediction of postoperative respiratory complications. Anesthesiology 2013;118(6):1276–85.

27. Musallam KM, Rosendaal FR, Zaatari G, et al. Smoking and the risk of mortality and vascular and respiratory events in patients undergoing major surgery. JAMA Surg 2013;148:755–62.

28. Mason DP, Subramanian S, Nowicki ER, et al. Impact of smoking cessation before resection of lung cancer: a Society of Thoracic Surgeons General Thoracic Surgery Database study. Ann Thorac Surg 2009;88:362–70 [Discussion: 70–71].

29. Hemmes SN, Serpa Neto A, Schultz MJ. Intraoperative ventilatory strategies to prevent postoperative pulmonary complications: a meta-analysis. Curr Opin Anaesthesiol 2013;26:126–33.

30. Hedenstierna G. Oxygen and anesthesia: what lung do we deliver to the postoperative ward? Acta Anaesthesiol Scand 2012;56:675–85.

31. Hovaguimian F, Lysakowski C, Elia N, et al. Effect of intraoperative high inspired oxygen fraction on surgical site infection, postoperative nausea and vomiting, and pulmonary function: systematic review and meta-analysis of randomized controlled trials. Anesthesiology 2013;119:303–16.

32. COVIDSurg Collaborative. Mortality and pulmonary complications in patients undergoing surgery with perioperative SARS-CoV-2 infection: an international cohort study. Lancet 2020;396(10243):27–38, published correction appears in Lancet. 2020 Jun 9.

33. Kayani B, Onochie E, Patil V, et al. The effects of COVID-19 on perioperative morbidity and mortality in patients with hip fractures. Bone Joint J 2020; 102-B(9):1136–45.

34. Knisely A, Zhou ZN, Wu J, et al. Perioperative Morbidity and Mortality of Patients With COVID-19 Who Undergo Urgent and Emergent Surgical Procedures. Ann Surg 2021;273(1):34–40.

35. Lei S, Jiang F, Su W, et al. Clinical characteristics and outcomes of patients undergoing surgeries during the incubation period of COVID-19 infection. EClinicalMedicine 2020;21:100331.

36. Haffner MR, Le HV, Saiz AM, et al. Postoperative In-Hospital Morbidity and Mortality of Patients With COVID-19 Infection Compared With Patients Without COVID-19 Infection. JAMA Netw Open 2021;4(4):e215697.

37. ASA and APSF Statement on Perioperative Testing for the COVID-19 Virus. American Society of Anesthesiologists. Available at: https://www.asahq.org/about-asa/newsroom/news-releases/2021/08/asa-and-apsf-statement-on-perioperative-testing-for-the-covid-19-virus. Accessed May 14, 2022.

38. ASA and APSF Joint Statement on Elective Surgery and Anesthesia for Patients after COVID-19 Infection. American Society of Anesthesiologists. Available at: https://www.asahq.org/about-asa/newsroom/news-releases/2022/02/asa-and-apsf-joint-statement-on-elective-surgery-procedures-and-anesthesia-for-patients-after-covid-19-infection. Accessed May 14, 2022.

39. COVIDSurg Collaborative. Delaying surgery for patients with a previous SARS-CoV-2 infection. Br J Surg 2020;107(12):e601–2.

40. Deng JZ, Chan JS, Potter AL, et al. The risk of postoperative complications after major elective surgery in active or resolved COVID-19 in the United States. Ann Surg 2022;275:242–6.

41. El-Boghdadly K, Cook TM, Goodacre T, et al. SARS-CoV-2 infection, COVID-19 and timing of elective surgery: A multidisciplinary consensus statement on behalf of the Association of Anaesthetists, the Centre for Peri-operative Care, the Federation of Surgical Specialty Associations, the Royal College of Anaesthetists and the Royal College of Surgeons of England. Anaesthesia 2021;76: 940–6.

42. COVID-19 Treatment Guidelines Panel. Coronavirus Disease 2019 (COVID-19) Treatment Guidelines. National Institutes of Health. Available at: https://www.covid19treatmentguidelines.nih.gov/. Accessed May 31, 2022.

43. Osadnik CR, Tee VS, Carson-Chahhoud KV, et al. Non-invasive ventilation for the management of acute hypercapnic respiratory failure due to exacerbation of chronic obstructive pulmonary disease. Cochrane Database Syst Rev 2017;7: CD004104.

44. Berbenetz N, Wang Y, Brown J, et al. Non-invasive positive pressure ventilation (CPAP or bilevel NPPV) for cardiogenic pulmonary oedema. Cochrane Database Syst Rev 2019;4(4):CD005351.

45. Chughtai M, Gwam CU, Mohamed N, et al. The Epidemiology and Risk Factors for Postoperative Pneumonia. J Clin Med Res 2017;9(6):466–75.

46. Warner DO. Preventing postoperative pulmonary complications: the role of the anesthesiologist. Anesthesiology 2000;92(5):1467–72.

47. Jaber S, Lescot T, Futier E, et al. Effect of noninvasive ventilation on tracheal re-intubation among patients with hypoxemic respiratory failure following abdominal surgery: a randomized clinical trial. JAMA 2016;315(13):1345–53.

48. Ireland CJ, Chapman TM, Mathew SF, et al. Continuous positive airway pressure (CPAP) during the postoperative period for prevention of postoperative morbidity and mortality following major abdominal surgery. Cochrane Database Syst Rev 2014;2014(8):CD008930.

49. PRISM trial group. Postoperative continuous positive airway pressure to prevent pneumonia, re-intubation, and death after major abdominal surgery (PRISM): a multicentre, open-label, randomised, phase 3 trial. Lancet Respir Med 2021; 9(11):1221–30.

50. Parke RL, Bloch A, McGuinness SP. Effect of Very-High-Flow Nasal Therapy on Airway Pressure and End-Expiratory Lung Impedance in Healthy Volunteers. Respir Care 2015;60(10):1397–403.

51. Hernández G, Vaquero C, Colinas L, et al. Effect of Postextubation High-Flow Nasal Cannula vs Noninvasive Ventilation on Reintubation and Postextubation Respiratory Failure in High-Risk Patients: A Randomized Clinical Trial. JAMA 2016;316(15):1565–74.

52. Ferguson ND, Fan E, Camporota L, et al. The Berlin definition of ARDS: an expanded rationale, justification, and supplementary material. Intensive Care Med 2012;38(10):1573–82 [Epub 2012 Aug 25. Erratum in: Intensive Care Med. 2012 Oct;38(10):1731-1582].

53. Bellani G, Laffey JG, Pham T, et al, ESICM Trials Group. Noninvasive Ventilation of Patients with Acute Respiratory Distress Syndrome. Insights from the LUNG SAFE Study. Am J Respir Crit Care Med 2017;195(1):67–77.

54. Chen L, Zhao H, Alam A, et al. Postoperative remote lung injury and its impact on surgical outcome. BMC Anesthesiol 2019;19:30.

55. National Heart, Lung, and Blood Institute Acute Respiratory Distress Syndrome (ARDS) Clinical Trials Network, Wiedemann HP, Wheeler AP, et al. Comparison of two fluid-management strategies in acute lung injury. N Engl J Med 2006; 354(24):2564–75.

56. Semler MW, Wheeler AP, Thompson BT, et al. Impact of initial central venous pressure on outcomes of conservative versus liberal fluid management in acute respiratory distress syndrome. Crit Care Med 2016;44(4):782–9.

57. Miller Timothy E, Myles Paul S. Perioperative Fluid Therapy for Major Surgery. Anesthesiology 2019;130:825–32.

58. Annane D, Pastores SM, Rochwerg B, et al. Guidelines for the diagnosis and management of critical illness-related corticosteroid insufficiency (CIRCI) in critically ill patients (Part I): Society of Critical Care Medicine (SCCM) and European Society of Intensive Care Medicine (ESICM) 2017. Intensive Care Med 2017;43: 1751–63.

59. Meduri GU, Golden E, Freire AX, et al. Methylprednisolone infusion in early severe ARDS: results of a randomized controlled trial. Chest 2007;131(4):954–63.

60. Villar J, Ferrando C, Martínez D, et al. Dexamethasone treatment for the acute respiratory distress syndrome: a multicentre, randomised controlled trial. Lancet Respir Med 2020;8(3):267–76.

61. Bellani G, Laffey JG, Pham T, et al. Epidemiology, patterns of care, and mortality for patients with acute respiratory distress syndrome in intensive care units in 50 countries. JAMA 2016;315(8):788–800.

62. Buckley MS, Agarwal SK, Garcia-Orr R, et al. Comparison of fixed-dose inhaled epoprostenol and inhaled nitric oxide for acute respiratory distress syndrome in critically ill adults. J Intensive Care Med 2021;36(4):466–76.

63. Gebistorf F, Karam O, Wetterslev J, et al. Inhaled nitric oxide for acute respiratory distress syndrome (ARDS) in children and adults. Cochrane Database Syst Rev 2016;2016(6):CD002787.

64. Torbic H, Szumita PM, Anger KE, et al. Clinical and economic impact of formulary conversion from inhaled Flolan to inhaled Veletri for refractory hypoxemia in critically ill patients. Ann Pharmacother 2016;50(2):106–12.

65. Afshari A, Brok J, Møller AM, et al. Inhaled nitric oxide for acute respiratory distress syndrome and acute lung injury in adults and children: a systematic review with meta-analysis and trial sequential analysis. Anesth Analg 2011;112(6):1411–21.

66. Papazian L, Forel JM, Gacouin A, et al. ACURASYS Study Investigators: Neuromuscular blockers in early acute respiratory distress syndrome. N Engl J Med 2010;363:1107–16.

67. Gainnier M, Roch A, Forel JM, et al. Effect of neuromuscular blocking agents on gas exchange in patients presenting with acute respiratory distress syndrome. Crit Care Med 2004;32:113–9.

68. National Heart, Lung, and Blood Institute PETAL Clinical Trials Network, Moss M, Huang DT, et al. Early Neuromuscular Blockade in the Acute Respiratory Distress Syndrome. N Engl J Med 2019;380(21):1997–2008.

69. Ahmad AM. Essentials of Physiotherapy after Thoracic Surgery: What Physiotherapists Need to Know. A Narrative Review. Korean J Thorac Cardiovasc Surg 2018;51(5):293–307.

70. Svensson-Raskh A, Schandl AR, et al. Mobilization started within 2 hours after abdominal surgery improves peripheral and arterial oxygenation: a single-center randomized controlled trial. Phys Ther 2021;101(5):pzab094.

71. Ambrosino N, Gabbrielli L. Physiotherapy in the perioperative period. Best Pract Res Clin Anaesthesiol 2010;24(2):283–9.

72. Carvalho CR, Paisani DM, Lunardi AC. Incentive spirometry in major surgeries: a systematic review. Rev Bras Fisioter 2011;15(5):343–50.

73. Gosselink R, Schrever K, Cops P, et al. Incentive spirometry does not enhance recovery after thoracic surgery. Crit Care Med 2000;28(3):679–83.

74. Tablan OC, Anderson LJ, Besser R, et al. CDC; Healthcare Infection Control Practices Advisory Committee. Guidelines for preventing health-care-associated pneumonia, 2003: recommendations of CDC and the Healthcare Infection Control Practices Advisory Committee. MMWR Recomm Rep 2004;53(RR-3):1–36.

75. Cassidy MR, Rosenkranz P, McCabe K, et al. Reducing Postoperative Pulmonary Complications With a Multidisciplinary Patient Care Program. JAMA Surg 2013;148(8):740–5.

76. Wren SM, Martin M, Yoon JK, et al. Postoperative pneumonia-prevention program for the inpatient surgical ward. J Am Coll Surg 2010 Apr;210(4):491–5.

77. Lawrence VA, Cornell JE, Smetana GW, et al. Strategies to reduce postoperative pulmonary complications after noncardiothoracic surgery: systematic review for the American College of Physicians. Ann Intern Med 2006;144(8):596–608.

78. Thompson SL, Lisco SJ. Postoperative respiratory failure. Int Anesthesiol Clin 2018;56(1):147–64. Winter.

79. Sud S, Friedrich JO, Taccone P, et al. Prone ventilation reduces mortality in patients with acute respiratory failure and severe hypoxemia: systematic review and meta-analysis. Intensive Care Med 2010;36(4):585–99.
80. Guérin C, Reignier J, Richard JC, et al. Prone positioning in severe acute respiratory distress syndrome. N Engl J Med 2013;368(23):2159–68.
81. Pelosi P, Brazzi L, Gattinoni L. Prone position in acute respiratory distress syndrome. Eur Respir J 2002;20(4):1017–28.
82. Pelosi P, Croci M, Calappi E, et al. Prone positioning improves pulmonary function in obese patients during general anesthesia. Anesth Analg 1996;83(3): 578–83.
83. Nyrén S, Mure M, Jacobsson H, et al. Pulmonary perfusion is more uniform in the prone than in the supine position: scintigraphy in healthy humans. J Appl Physiol (1985) 1999;86(4):1135–41.
84. Albert RK, Hubmayr RD. The prone position eliminates compression of the lungs by the heart. Am J Respir Crit Care Med 2000;161(5):1660–5.
85. Nyrén S, Radell P, Lindahl SG, et al. Lung ventilation and perfusion in prone and supine postures with reference to anesthetized and mechanically ventilated healthy volunteers. Anesthesiology 2010;112(3):682–7.
86. Benoit Z, Wicky S, Fischer JF, et al. The effect of increased FIO(2) before tracheal extubation on postoperative atelectasis. Anesth Analg 2002;95: 1777–81.
87. Dries DJ, Marini JJ. Airway pressure release ventilation. J Burn Care Res 2009; 30(6):929–36.
88. Putensen C, Zech S, Wrigge H, et al. Long term effects of spontaneous breathing during ventilatory support in patients with acute lung injury. Am J Respir Crit Care Med 2001;164(1):43–9.
89. Esan A, Hess DR, Raoof S, et al. Severe hypoxemic respiratory failure: part 1: ventilatory strategies. Chest 2010;137(5):1203–16.
90. Porhomayon J, El-Solh AA, Nader ND. Applications of airway pressure release ventilation. Lung 2010;188(2):87–96.
91. Kotani T, Katayama S, Fukuda S, et al. Pressure-controlled inverse ratio ventilation as a rescue therapy for severe acute respiratory distress syndrome. Springerplus 2016;5(1):716.
92. Vitale D, Patrizio Petrone MD, Marini CP. High-Frequency Oscillatory Ventilation (HFOV) as primary ventilator strategy in the management of severe acute respiratory distress syndrome (ARDS) with Pneumothorax in the Setting of Trauma. Am Surg 2017;83(3):E99.
93. Jarvis S, Burt MK, English W. High frequency oscillatory ventilation. Anaesth Tutorial Week 2012;261:1–11.
94. Amato MB, Barbas CS, Bonassa J, et al. Volume-assured pressure support ventilation (VAPSV). A new approach for reducing muscle workload during acute respiratory failure. Chest 1992;102(4):1225–34.
95. Younes M. Proportional assist ventilation: a new approach to ventilatory support: theory. Am Rev Respir Dis 1992;145:114–20.
96. Vaporidi K. NAVA and PAV+ for lung and diaphragm protection. Curr Opin Crit Care 2020;26(1):41–6.
97. Sinderby C, Navalesi P, Beck J, et al. Neural control of mechanical ventilation in respiratory failure. Nat Med 1999;5:1433–6.
98. Sinderby C, Beck J. Neurally adjusted ventilatory assist (NAVA): an update and summary of experiences. Neth Crit Care 2007;11:243–52.

99. Kacmarek RM, Villar J, Parrilla D, et al. NAVa In Acute respiraTORy failure (NA-VIATOR) Network. Neurally adjusted ventilatory assist in acute respiratory failure: a randomized controlled trial. Intensive Care Med 2020;46(12):2327–37.
100. Taniguchi C, Victor ES, Pieri T, et al. Smart Care™ versus respiratory physiotherapy-driven manual weaning for critically ill adult patients: a randomized controlled trial. Crit Care 2015 Jun 11;19(1):246.
101. Tonna JE, Abrams D, Brodie D, et al. Management of Adult Patients Supported with Venovenous Extracorporeal Membrane Oxygenation (VV ECMO): Guideline from the Extracorporeal Life Support Organization (ELSO). ASAIO J 2021;67(6): 601–10.
102. Brogan T.V., Lequier L., Lorusso R., et al., Extracorporeal life support: the ELSO red book, 5th edition, Extracorporeal Life Support Organization; Ann Arbor, MI, 415–423.
103. Peek GJ, Mugford M, Tiruvoipati R, et al. Efficacy and economic assessment of conventional ventilatory support versus extracorporeal membrane oxygenation for severe adult respiratory failure (CESAR): a multicentre randomised controlled trial. Lancet 2009;374(9698):1351–63 [Epub 2009 Sep 15. Erratum in: Lancet. 2009 Oct 17;374(9698):1330].

Patient Blood Management, Anemia, and Transfusion Optimization Across Surgical Specialties

Michael E. Kiyatkin, MD[a],*, Domagoj Mladinov, MD, PhD[b],
Mary L. Jarzebowski, MD[c], Matthew A. Warner, MD[d]

KEYWORDS

- Perioperative • Anemia • Patient blood management • Transfusion threshold
- Allogenic blood product • Transfusion-associated circulatory overload
- Transfusion-related acute lung injury • Transfusion-related immunomodulation

KEY POINTS

- Preoperative anemia should give pause before elective surgery with at least moderate volume blood loss anticipated.
- Anemia is readily addressable preoperatively, with targeted management improving outcomes and reducing transfusion utilization.
- Management of nonbleeding anemia includes blood conservation, etiology-based treatment, and correction of coagulopathy.
- Except for certain high-risk patients, red blood cell transfusion in patients with nonbleeding anemia should follow a restrictive strategy targeting a hemoglobin concentration of 7 or 8 g/dL.
- Hemoglobin concentrations during acute surgical bleeding do not provide an accurate assessment of red blood cell mass; a more nuanced approach focusing on oxygen delivery and tissue perfusion is warranted.

INTRODUCTION

Anemia and overall blood health are intricately linked with perioperative complications and transfusion utilization. Accordingly, the concept of patient blood management

[a] Department of Anesthesiology, Albert Einstein College of Medicine, Montefiore Medical Center, 111 East 210th Street, Bronx, NY 10467, USA; [b] Department of Anesthesiology, Perioperative and Pain Medicine, Brigham and Women's Hospital, 75 Francis Street, Boston, MA 02115, USA; [c] Department of Anesthesiology, University of Michigan, 1540 East Hospital Drive, Ann Arbor, MI 48109, USA; [d] Department of Anesthesiology and Perioperative Medicine, Mayo Clinic, Rochester, 200 1st Street, Rochester, MN 55905, USA
* Corresponding author.
E-mail address: mkiyatkin@montefiore.org

Anesthesiology Clin 41 (2023) 161–174
https://doi.org/10.1016/j.anclin.2022.10.003

(PBM) has taken center stage as a model of care that should be broadly adopted to improve patient blood health and clinical outcomes. PBM can be defined as "a patient-centered, systematic, evidence-based approach to improve patient outcomes by managing and preserving a patient's own blood, while promoting patient safety and empowerment."[1] This approach emphasizes prevention over treatment and endorses a comprehensive approach to management of anemia and hemostasis derangements, of which blood transfusions are often not the requisite treatment.

In this article, we address key aspects of PBM, focusing on the prevention and treatment of anemia. Although transfusion is often not a first-line therapy for anemia, it remains an essential tool that must be used appropriately to improve patient outcomes while conserving resources and minimizing risk. Hence, a substantial portion is dedicated to discussing how red blood cell (RBC) transfusions may be optimally incorporated into perioperative management strategies. Finally, we outline a vision for the future of PBM, including the research, quality improvement, and administrative steps necessary to achieve and maintain the goals of this care model.

Cause and Treatment of Anemia in Perioperative Medicine

Anemia is typically defined by a hemoglobin concentration less than 13 g/dL in men and less than 12 g/dL in nonpregnant women.[2] Anemia is highly prevalent, reaching up to 50% in surgical populations and elderly hospitalized patients.[3,4] Indeed, approximately one-third of adults present for surgery with untreated anemia, which may be secondary to nutritional deficiencies, inflammatory states (ie, anemia of inflammation or chronic disease), kidney disease, bone marrow failure, hemoglobinopathies, and hemolysis, among other causes. Postoperatively, numerous additional mechanisms contribute to anemia including surgical hemorrhage, blood loss from phlebotomy, and hemodilution. Additionally, inflammation related to surgery and illness creates a state of functional iron deficiency and suppressed erythropoiesis.[5] Importantly, anemia experienced during surgery and critical illness is long-lasting and associated with major adverse outcomes such as readmission, impaired physical function, and mortality.[6–9]

Perioperative anemia management begins with diagnosis of the underlying cause(s) followed by targeted treatment. Iron deficiency is the most common cause. Oral supplementation is inexpensive but often poorly tolerated secondary to gastrointestinal side effects. Although traditionally dosed daily, evidence suggests that alternate day, such as Monday, Wednesday, Friday dosing may result in better absorption and decreased side effects.[10–12] Oral iron should be implemented at least 6 to 8 weeks before elective surgery with expected moderate-to-high blood loss (>500 mL).[13,14] Intravenous (IV) iron is recommended in patients with iron deficiency who are unresponsive or intolerant to oral iron, or when surgery is within 6 weeks.[13] Several formulations allow for a single total dose infusion (eg, 1000 mg iron dextran).[5] For patients with anemia of inflammation, erythropoiesis-stimulating agents (ESAs) may be considered. For example, epoetin may be administered at 600 units/kg weekly with repeat dosing dictated by hemoglobin response.[5] Iron supplementation should be started before ESA therapy to ensure adequate iron stores. The major concern with ESAs is increased risk of thrombotic events, which has been seen with prolonged ESA use targeting high hemoglobin concentrations (>13 g/dL) in patients with chronic kidney disease and malignancy.[15–17] The risks and benefits of perioperative ESAs are best determined by the underlying cause of anemia, individual patient characteristics, procedure type, use of perioperative venous thromboprophylaxis, and severity of anemia. Although recent consensus guidelines suggest that ESAs should not be broadly used in patients with anemia who are undergoing elective surgery,[14] short-term perioperative use improves hemoglobin recovery and decreases transfusion rates in various types of surgery without increasing complication rates.[5,18–21] Folate and vitamin B_{12} deficiencies, although much less common than iron deficiency, may also contribute to perioperative anemia and may generally be treated with oral therapies, with IV or intramuscular therapies reserved for those with severe disease.[22]

Perioperative Blood Conservation and Coagulation Optimization

In addition to preoperative anemia diagnosis and treatment, perioperative PBM efforts must focus on blood conservation strategies. Cell salvage techniques, in which shed blood is filtered and returned to the patient, are broadly applicable for surgeries with moderate-to-high anticipated blood loss and in patients at high risk for perioperative anemia. The availability of leukocyte depletion filters extends cell salvage to high-risk oncologic and obstetric cases. Acute normovolemic hemodilution (ANH) is another transfusion-sparing method most often used in cardiac surgery.[23–25] This consists of autologous blood removal at the beginning of a procedure, volume replacement with crystalloids and/or colloids, and then the return of autologous blood after the completion of the major bleeding insult. Similar to ANH, low central venous pressure techniques entail intraoperative removal of whole blood without crystalloid and/or colloid replacement, thereby reducing blood loss in liver resection surgeries.[26] Finally, low-volume phlebotomy techniques may be used to reduce blood loss during diagnostic sampling by 3-fold to 10-fold.[27]

Additionally, blood loss and exposure to allogeneic blood products can be further reduced through targeted treatment of coagulopathy, optimization of perioperative coagulation status and anticoagulant and antiplatelet medications, and preservation of normal organ function and physiology (eg, body temperature, acid–base status). Antifibrinolytic agents such as tranexamic acid (TXA) have been shown to reduce blood loss during surgery.[28] Although traditionally used only in hemorrhage and high-risk procedures such as cardiac, major orthopedic, and transplantation surgeries, the recently published POISE-III trial randomized more than 9500 adults undergoing a variety of noncardiac surgeries to intraoperative TXA or placebo and revealed a significant reduction in bleeding events (9.1% vs 11.7%) with TXA without an increased risk for adverse cardiovascular events (14.2% vs 13.9%).[29]

A Restrictive Red Blood Cell Transfusion Strategy Is Best

RBC transfusion triggers, or more appropriately "thresholds," have existed since the 1940s, at which time a "10/30 transfusion rule" was recommended specifying hemoglobin and hematocrit thresholds of 10 g/dL and 30%, respectively.[30] The landmark Transfusion Requirements in Critical Care trial challenged this by demonstrating no mortality difference in septic, traumatic, and other critically ill adults transfused with a restrictive hemoglobin threshold of 7 g/dL compared with a liberal threshold of 10 g/dL.[31] Subsequently, numerous trials and meta-analyses in various patient populations similarly noted equivalent or superior outcomes with restrictive transfusion strategies (ie, <7–8 g/dL).[32,33] Accordingly, the Patient Blood Management International Consensus Conference, European Society of Intensive Care Medicine, American Society of Anesthesiologists, Eastern Association for the Surgery of Trauma, and the American Association of Blood Banks all recommend restrictive transfusion for nonbleeding anemia.[14,34–36]

Limitations of Transfusion Thresholds

In nonbleeding anemia, the concept of a transfusion threshold is generally based on the false dichotomy of having to choose between anemia tolerance and transfusion risk. As discussed above, transfusion is not the first-line therapy for nonbleeding anemia. Unfortunately, trials evaluating RBC-based transfusion strategies did not assess the efficacy of hemoglobin threshold-based interventions compared with alternative interventions. Additionally, most existing trials showed limited differences in pre-transfusion hemoglobin concentrations and the total number of transfused units between groups.[37]

Importantly, hemoglobin concentrations during acute surgical bleeding and intravascular volume shifts provide neither an accurate assessment of RBC mass nor an estimate of oxygen carrying capacity. Hence, multiple clinical practice guidelines recommend a more nuanced approach that also considers estimated blood loss, clinical findings suspicious for circulatory shock, and the potential for ongoing hemorrhage.[34–36] Additionally, a distinction should be made between transfusion thresholds and targets. The latter reflect the minimum hemoglobin concentration that should be attained after a transfusion. During acute blood loss, posttransfusion hemoglobin targets may be more appropriate for assessing the adequacy of any transfusion-based resuscitation strategy.[38] In massive hemorrhage, which is classified by numerous definitions (eg, ≥3 units RBCs in ≤1 hour; ≥50% of estimated blood volume in ≤3 hours; ≥1.5 L estimated blood loss; persistent heavy bleeding with evidence of hemorrhagic shock and need for surgery or embolization),[39,40] RBCs are typically administered as part of an empiric ratio-guided strategy (eg, 1:1:1 ratio of plasma, platelets, and RBCs). As summarized in **Fig. 1**, hemoglobin thresholds alone are insufficient to guide transfusion decisions during active bleeding and especially massive hemorrhage, and transfusions should be given to maintain adequate oxygen carrying capacity until hemorrhage is controlled.[39–41] Once it is controlled, however, a judicious hemoglobin threshold approach should be reinstated.

Additional concerns about transfusion thresholds arise from methodologic and patient-specific heterogeneity in clinical trials. Methodologic heterogeneity includes differences in hemoglobin thresholds and compliance with assigned interventions,

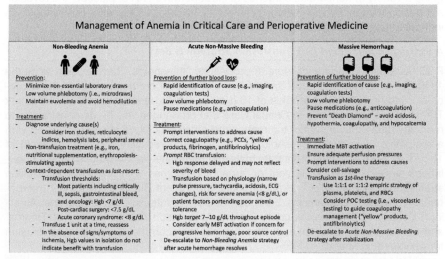

Fig. 1. Recommended management of anemia in perioperative medicine and critical care according to the principles of patient blood management. ECG, electrocardiogram; Hgb, hemoglobin; MBT, massive blood transfusion; PCC, prothrombin complex concentrate; POC, point-of-care; RBC, red blood cell.

which may dilute between-group outcome differences. Regarding patient-specific heterogeneity, it has been broadly postulated that high-risk patients (eg, those with coronary disease, postcardiac surgery) may be less likely to tolerate restrictive transfusion strategies (see **Fig. 1**). Although certain patients are indeed less likely to tolerate anemia, the evidence to support liberal over restrictive transfusion strategies is limited. For example, in those with acute myocardial infarction (MI), the recently completed REALITY trial found that a restrictive strategy ($\leq$8 g/dL) was safe and noninferior compared with a liberal strategy ($\leq$10 g/dL) with respect to major adverse cardiovascular events.[42] Similarly, the recent Transfusion Requirements in Cardiac Surgery III (TRICS III) trial, which included more than 5000 patients undergoing high-risk cardiac surgery, found no significant differences in composite death, MI, stroke, or acute renal failure in patients treated with restrictive (<7.5 g/dL) versus liberal strategies (<9.5 g/dL).[43] Accordingly, the latest systematic reviews recommend a transfusion threshold of 7.5 or less to 8 g/dL for postoperative cardiac surgical patients.[44,45]

Despite evidence broadly supporting restrictive transfusion thresholds, optimal transfusion strategies remain incompletely defined in certain populations. In elderly patients undergoing hip fracture surgery, one meta-analysis suggested increased risk of ischemic organ injury and mortality with restrictive strategies,[45] leading some experts to endorse a higher hemoglobin target of 9 g/dL in this population.[46] Other groups for which optimal transfusion strategies remain undefined include critically ill and surgical oncology patients[47,48] and those with acute neurologic injury,[49,50] with experts generally unable to recommend one transfusion strategy over another. Trials in these and other high-risk patient groups are ongoing. In these high-risk patients, as in all patients, it is critically important to prevent or attenuate anemia development, address underlying causes, and remember that transfusion is not first-line anemia therapy in the absence of active bleeding or evidence of inadequate tissue oxygen delivery.

The key question with regard to hemoglobin concentration is "how low can we go?" before a transfusion is truly indicated. Unfortunately, there are no trials comparing RBC transfusion with no transfusion in patients with acute perioperative anemia. However, from observational studies in Jehovah's Witnesses patients with severe anemia, outcomes are comparable to similarly anemic patients who are able to receive transfusions; increases in perioperative complications are generally not observed until hemoglobin concentration reduces to less than 5 to 6 g/dL.[51–53] In healthy volunteers undergoing acute isovolemic anemia, abrupt decreases in hemoglobin concentrations to 5 g/dL were often well-tolerated with appropriate compensatory increases in cardiac output and oxygen extraction,[54] although approximately 5% of volunteers experienced reversible ECG changes consistent with myocardial ischemia.[55] Considered together, this suggests that many patients are likely to tolerate hemoglobin concentrations less than 7 g/dL with preservation of euvolemia. This supports broadly applying restrictive transfusion strategies in the perioperative setting with the caveat that some patients may tolerate even greater anemia before warranting transfusion, whereas others may display signs of impaired oxygen delivery at higher hemoglobin levels.

Physiologic Transfusion Triggers

Recognizing the limitations of hemoglobin thresholds, there is growing interest in physiology-based triggers for RBC transfusion. Indeed, a recent survey of intensivists revealed that most providers incorporate patient clinical features such as tachycardia alongside hemoglobin concentrations when making transfusion decisions.[56] Two recent trials investigated the utility of incorporating mixed venous oxygen saturation (SvO_2) into transfusion decisions and discovered that an SvO_2-guided strategy resulted in fewer transfusions without increasing ischemic events compared with traditional hemoglobin threshold approaches.[57,58] Another recent observational study examined the arterial-to-venous oxygen saturation (AVO$_2$) difference in transfused patients, finding that transfusion in patients with a larger AVO$_2$ difference was associated with lower mortality, less kidney injury, and faster recovery compared with transfusion in patients with a smaller AVO$_2$ difference.[59] Until more data is available on the safety and efficacy of physiologic transfusion triggers, clinical practice guidelines continue to recommend hemoglobin-based thresholds for nonbleeding anemia.[60]

Complications of Red Blood Cell Transfusion

Allogenic RBC transfusion carries with it the risk of ABO incompatibility, bacterial infection, and autoimmune hemolytic anemia, among others. Additionally, RBC transfusion is associated with multiorgan failure and longer ICU and hospital length of stay as well as increased postoperative venous thromboembolism.[61] It is important to recognize that surgical patients are exposed to a multitude of unique stresses that exacerbate patient-specific risk factors for transfusion-related adverse events (eg, preexisting cardiopulmonary illness, critical illness). Although a comprehensive review of transfusion complications is beyond the scope of this article, we provide a brief overview of 3 key transfusion-related adverse events.

Transfusion-Associated Circulatory Overload

Transfusion-associated circulatory overload (TACO) was the leading cause of transfusion-related deaths in 2014 and 2018, representing 32% of mortalities.[62] Its incidence is likely underreported but is estimated to occur in up to 12% of patients receiving transfusions, including approximately 5% of transfused surgical patients.[63] In an attempt to better define this condition, the Center for Disease Control (CDC) National Healthcare Safety Network recently updated the diagnostic criteria for TACO (**Box 1**), emphasizing the variable temporal association of transfusion with symptom onset (ie, up to 12 hours following transfusion).[64]

The primary hypothesized mechanism behind TACO is circulatory overload due to infusion of pure colloid. It can therefore occur following transfusion of any blood component.[65] There may be a secondary immune-mediated pathogenesis because TACO is accompanied by fever in more than one-third of patients,[66] and its incidence has decreased following implementation of leukoreduction of red cells.[67]

Surgical patients, especially those who are critically ill, are particularly vulnerable to TACO. The following perioperative risk factors have been identified: emergency surgery, preexisting chronic kidney disease, preoperative echocardiographic evidence

---

Box 1
2021 CDC biovigilance network definition of transfusion-associated circulatory overload[64]

New onset or exacerbation of 3 or more of the following within 12 hours of transfusion (#1 and/or #2 are mandatory):
1. Acute respiratory distress (eg, dyspnea, tachypnea, cyanosis, or hypoxemia)
2. Radiographic or clinical evidence of acute or worsening pulmonary edema (eg, crackles on auscultation, orthopnea, cough, S3, or pink frothy sputum)
3. Elevated brain natriuretic peptide (BNP) or NT-pro-BNP relevant biomarker
4. Cardiovascular changes not explained by underlying medical condition (eg, elevated central venous pressure, left heart failure, jugular venous distension, peripheral edema)
5. Evidence of fluid overload

https://www.cdc.gov/nhsn/pdfs/biovigilance/bv-hv-protocol-current.pdf.

of left ventricular dysfunction, and mixed product transfusion.[68] A study of a heterogeneous intensive care population identified these same risk factors plus older age, female sex, and larger transfusion volumes along with an overall positive fluid balance.[69]

PBM strategies should be used perioperatively to minimize risk for TACO, for example, restrictive transfusion strategies and minimization of transfusion volumes. In those with risk factors, slower transfusion rates should be used, and patients should be closely monitored to detect changes in clinical status.[65] If TACO is suspected, transfusion should be stopped if still ongoing. Treatment is largely supportive. Positive pressure ventilation and loop diuretics are commonly used to prevent further pulmonary edema.[70]

Transfusion-Associated Acute Lung Injury

Transfusion-associated acute lung injury (TRALI) presents similarly to TACO but carries higher morbidity and mortality. It represents 26% of transfusion-related deaths.[71] The CDC Biovigilance Network defines TRALI as acute onset posttransfusion respiratory distress and hypoxemia with radiographic evidence of bilateral infiltrates without evidence of circulatory overload (**Box 2**).[72] A 2019 consensus redefinition stratified TRALI into Type I (no patient risk factors for acute respiratory distress syndrome, ARDS) and Type II (underlying risk factors for ARDS or concomitant mild ARDS with acute deterioration following transfusion).[60] Transfusion-associated dyspnea is a related term describing acute respiratory distress within 24 hours of transfusion but not meeting criteria for TACO or TRALI.

Similar to ARDS, TRALI pathogenesis is hypothesized to be "two-hit" mediated, with a primary pulmonary or extrapulmonary insult attracting neutrophils to the pulmonary vasculature followed by a secondary insult driving neutrophil activation.[73,74] Neutrophil-mediated destruction of the alveolar capillary basement membrane allows exudative fluid to flood the alveoli. Neutrophil activation may be immune-mediated or nonimmune mediated. In the immune-mediated subtype, pathogenic antibodies are transfused.[74] This is more common if the donor has been exposed to certain human neutrophil antigens through pregnancy or prior blood transfusion.[75] Alternatively, the nonimmune-mediated subtype may occur from transfusion of other cellular and acellular components (ie, biologic response modifiers), including lipids, platelets, and specific red cell antigens.[74]

Although TRALI has been reported following transfusion of all blood components, it is usually seen following plasma and plasma-containing products, especially from multiparous female donors. For this reason, multiparous donors are preferentially excluded from the plasma donor pool.[76] However, due to transfusion of a larger

---

Box 2
2021 CDC biovigilance network definition of transfusion-associated acute lung injury[64]

All the following criteria should be met:
- No evidence of acute lung injury before transfusion
- Acute lung injury onset during or within 6 hours of cessation of transfusion
- Hypoxemia defined by any of these methods:
  - $Pao_2/Fio_2 < 300$
  - Oxygen saturation less than 90% on room air
  - Other clinical evidence
- Radiographic evidence of bilateral infiltrates
- No evidence of left atrial hypertension (ie, circulatory overload)

https://www.cdc.gov/nhsn/pdfs/biovigilance/bv-hv-protocol-current.pdf.

number of RBC units, most TRALI-related deaths in fact occur following RBC transfusion.[71] Leukoreduction was proposed as a mitigation strategy; however, studies in countries practicing universal leukoreduction have not definitively demonstrated any association with reduced TRALI incidence.[77]

Management of TRALI involves stopping the inciting transfusion, notifying the hospital blood bank, and providing supportive care. A formal transfusion reaction workup should be performed, and the blood supplier must work to identify the donor and initiate appropriate testing for human leukocyte antigen and/or neutrophil antigen antibodies. Although TRALI is a distinct clinical entity from ARDS, ventilatory support is guided by the same lung protective principles.[78] If necessary, the patient may receive additional blood products from other donors.

Transfusion-Related Immunomodulation

Transfusion-related immunomodulation (TRIM) refers to the attenuation of immune function following transfusion of allogenic blood components. This is most likely due to transfusion of leukocytes and leukocyte-derived factors.[79] The mechanism of TRIM is multifaceted including attenuation of monocyte and cytotoxic T-cell activity, activation of suppressor T-cells, inhibition of antitumoral cytokines such as interleukin-2, and release of prostaglandins.[80] Leukoreduction via screen filters effectively reduces the number of leukocytes in a unit of packed RBCs by up to 99.9%, which offers the theoretic benefits of reducing cytokines and other bioactive substances released from leukocytes. However, a Cochrane review of leukoreduced RBC transfusions failed to show any significant improvement in infectious complications.[81]

This immunomodulation is highly relevant for oncologic surgery. Even without transfusion, this surgical setting is characterized by disruption of normal immune homeostasis due to poor preoperative functional and nutritional status, inhaled anesthesia, preoperative anemia, and specific cancer effects. Determining the distinct contribution of transfusion to this complex immune disruption is challenging. A Cochrane review of the association between perioperative RBC transfusion and colorectal cancer recurrence showed a significant association (OR 1.42, 95% CI 1.20–1.67).[82] Other studies similarly noted increased risk of cancer recurrence and reduced disease-free survival in those receiving perioperative RBC transfusions.[82,83]

This complication is also important for surgical site and nosocomial infection. The contribution of TRIM to hospital-acquired infection is unclear, with some studies demonstrating associations between perioperative RBC transfusion and iatrogenic infections such as ventilator-associated pneumonia.[84–86] Although there is definitive evidence, anesthesiologists must continue to weigh the potential benefits of transfusion with the risks of TRIM and subsequent infection in individual patients.

SUMMARY

Recognizing the importance of perioperative blood health optimization and allogeneic transfusion reductions, it is essential to incorporate PBM principles into perioperative care. There are several key steps in this process. First, the presence of preoperative anemia must not go overlooked before elective surgery with at least moderate volume anticipated blood loss (ie, $\geq$500 mL). Anemia is readily addressable before surgery, and targeted management improves hemoglobin concentration and may reduce transfusion utilization during and after surgery.[18,87,88] Second, for patients with acute surgical bleeding, we must promptly identify anatomic sources of bleeding, address underlying abnormalities in hemostasis, and use evidence-based pharmacologic and transfusion therapies. Third, for patients without acute bleeding or critical anemia (ie, anemia accompanied by evidence of oxygen deficiency), we must recognize that a "transfusion-first" paradigm for anemia management is ill-advised and outdated. This is especially true postoperatively, with a multitude of clinical trials showing no benefit of liberal transfusion.

It is imperative that clinicians take action to reduce the risks associated with severe perioperative anemia. Fortunately, preventive, diagnostic, and nontransfusion-based treatment strategies are readily available and accessible for anesthesiologists and perioperative care professionals.[5] Future studies must be designed to evaluate the efficacy of comprehensive PBM strategies in various perioperative settings and diverse patient populations (eg, etiology-directed anemia management before and after surgery, low-volume phlebotomy techniques, staged surgical procedures, blood conservation modalities). Research must be conducted congruently with quality improvement initiatives to identify barriers and facilitators to PBM implementation. Finally, clinicians must promote and support anemia optimization initiatives locally by working with their clinical leaders and administrative professionals to support investment in PBM programs as a common-sense method to improve patient outcomes.

CLINICS CARE POINTS

- Whenever possible, work up causes of anemia and treat accordingly in advance of surgery. This may require days to weeks for full treatment effect.
- For surgeries with expected moderate-to-high blood loss (>500 mL), maximize perioperative blood conservation strategies including cell salvage. One gram of tranexamic acid may be considered for surgical bleeding, however one should consider thrombosis risk given that it is not yet proven to be completely safe.
- For the vast majority of patients with nonbleeding anemia, follow a restrictive transfusion strategy targeting a hemoglobin concentration of 7-8 g/dL.
- During ongoing hemorrhage, hemoglobin concentrations have limited utility and transfusion should be guided by a more nuanced approach that considers estimated blood loss, evidence of shock, and potential for further hemorrhage.
- In massive hemorrhage, a ratio-guided approach should be utilized, most typically 6 units of fresh frozen plasma to 6 units or 1 dose of platelets to 6 units of packed red blood cells.

DISCLOSURE

Dr. Warner is supported by a National Heart, Lung, and Blood Institute of the National Institutes of Health (NIH) grant (K23HL153310). The content of this article is solely the responsibility of the authors and does not represent the official views of the NIH.

REFERENCES

1. Shander A, Hardy JF, Ozawa S, et al. A global definition of patient blood management. Anesth Analg 2022;135(3):476–88.
2. World Health Organization. 2011. Available at: https://apps.who.int/iris/bitstream/handle/10665/85839/WHO_NMH_NHD_MNM_11.1_eng.pdf?sequence=22&isAllowed=y. Accessed June 14, 2022.
3. Migone De Amicis M, Poggiali E, Motta I, et al. Anemia in elderly hospitalized patients: prevalence and clinical impact. Intern Emerg Med 2015;10(5):581–6.

4. Muñoz M, Gómez-Ramírez S, Campos A, et al. Pre-operative anaemia: prevalence, consequences and approaches to management. Blood Transfus 2015; 13(3):370–9.

5. Warner MA, Shore-Lesserson L, Shander A, et al. Perioperative Anemia: Prevention, Diagnosis, and Management Throughout the Spectrum of Perioperative Care. Anesth Analg 2020;130(5):1364–80.

6. van der Laan S, Billah T, Chi C, et al. Anaemia among intensive care unit survivors and association with days alive and at home: an observational study. Anaesthesia 2021;76(10):1352–7.

7. Warner MA, Hanson AC, Frank RD, et al. Prevalence of and Recovery From Anemia Following Hospitalization for Critical Illness Among Adults. JAMA Netw Open 2020;3(9):e2017843.

8. Warner MA, Kor DJ, Frank RD, et al. Anemia in Critically Ill Patients With Acute Respiratory Distress Syndrome and Posthospitalization Physical Outcomes. J Intensive Care Med 2021;36(5):557–65.

9. Warner MA, Hanson AC, Schulte PJ, et al. Early Post-Hospitalization Hemoglobin Recovery and Clinical Outcomes in Survivors of Critical Illness: A Population-Based Cohort Study. J Intensive Care Med 2022;37(8):1067–74.

10. Moretti D, Goede JS, Zeder C, et al. Oral iron supplements increase hepcidin and decrease iron absorption from daily or twice-daily doses in iron-depleted young women. Blood 2015;126(17):1981–9.

11. Stoffel NU, Cercamondi CI, Brittenham G, et al. Iron absorption from oral iron supplements given on consecutive versus alternate days and as single morning doses versus twice-daily split dosing in iron-depleted women: two open-label, randomised controlled trials. Lancet Haematol 2017;4(11):e524–33.

12. Stoffel NU, Zeder C, Brittenham GM, et al. Iron absorption from supplements is greater with alternate day than with consecutive day dosing in iron-deficient anemic women. Haematologica 2020;105(5):1232–9.

13. Muñoz M, Acheson AG, Auerbach M, et al. International consensus statement on the peri-operative management of anaemia and iron deficiency. Anaesthesia 2017;72(2):233–47.

14. Mueller MM, Van Remoortel H, Meybohm P, et al. Patient Blood Management: Recommendations From the 2018 Frankfurt Consensus Conference. JAMA 2019;321(10):983–97.

15. Phrommintikul A, Haas SJ, Elsik M, et al. Mortality and target haemoglobin concentrations in anaemic patients with chronic kidney disease treated with erythropoietin: a meta-analysis. Lancet 2007;369(9559):381–8.

16. Pfeffer MA, Burdmann EA, Chen CY, et al. A trial of darbepoetin alfa in type 2 diabetes and chronic kidney disease. N Engl J Med 2009;361(21):2019–32.

17. Aapro M, Scherhag A, Burger HU. Effect of treatment with epoetin-beta on survival, tumour progression and thromboembolic events in patients with cancer: an updated meta-analysis of 12 randomised controlled studies including 2301 patients. Br J Cancer 2008;99(1):14–22.

18. Spahn DR, Schoenrath F, Spahn GH, et al. Effect of ultra-short-term treatment of patients with iron deficiency or anaemia undergoing cardiac surgery: a prospective randomised trial. Lancet 2019;393(10187):2201–12.

19. Feagan BG, Wong CJ, Kirkley A, et al. Erythropoietin with iron supplementation to prevent allogeneic blood transfusion in total hip joint arthroplasty. A randomized, controlled trial. Ann Intern Med 2000;133(11):845–54.

20. Weltert L, Rondinelli B, Bello R, et al. A single dose of erythropoietin reduces perioperative transfusions in cardiac surgery: results of a prospective single-blind randomized controlled trial. Transfusion 2015;55(7):1644–54.
21. Kosmadakis N, Messaris E, Maris A, et al. Perioperative erythropoietin administration in patients with gastrointestinal tract cancer: prospective randomized double-blind study. Ann Surg 2003;237(3):417–21.
22. Devalia V, Hamilton MS, Molloy AM, et al. Guidelines for the diagnosis and treatment of cobalamin and folate disorders. Br J Haematol 2014;166(4):496–513.
23. Barile L, Fominskiy E, Di Tomasso N, et al. Acute normovolemic hemodilution reduces allogeneic red blood cell transfusion in cardiac surgery: a systematic review and meta-analysis of randomized trials. Anesth Analg 2017;124(3):743–52.
24. Mladinov D, Eudailey KW, Padilla LA, et al. Effects of acute normovolemic hemodilution on post-cardiopulmonary bypass coagulation tests and allogeneic blood transfusion in thoracic aortic repair surgery: An observational cohort study. J Cardiovasc Surg 2021;36(11):4075–82.
25. Mladinov D, Padilla LA, Leahy B, et al. Hemodilution in high-risk cardiac surgery: Laboratory values, physiological parameters, and outcomes. Transfusion 2022; 62(4):826–37.
26. Park L, Gilbert R, Baker L, et al. The safety and efficacy of hypovolemic phlebotomy on blood loss and transfusion in liver surgery: a systematic review and meta-analysis. HPB (Oxford) 2020;22(3):340–50.
27. Shander A, Corwin HL. A narrative review on hospital-acquired anemia: keeping blood where it belongs. Transfus Med Rev 2020;34(3):195–9.
28. Levy JH, Koster A, Quinones QJ, et al. Antifibrinolytic therapy and perioperative considerations. Anesthesiology 2018;128(3):657–70.
29. Devereaux PJ, Marcucci M, Painter TW, et al. Tranexamic acid in patients undergoing noncardiac surgery. N Engl J Med 2022;386(21):1986–97.
30. Adams RC, Lundy JS. Anesthesia in cases of poor surgical risk: some suggestions for decreasing the risk. Anesthesiology 1942;3:603–7.
31. Hebert PC, Wells G, Blajchman MA, et al. A multicenter, randomized, controlled clinical trial of transfusion requirements in critical care. N Engl J Med 1999;340(6): 409–17.
32. Walsh TS, Boyd JA, Watson D, et al. Restrictive versus liberal transfusion strategies for older mechanically ventilated critically ill patients: a randomized pilot trial. Crit Care Med 2013;41(10):2354–63.
33. Holst LB, Haase N, Wetterslev J, et al. Lower versus higher hemoglobin threshold for transfusion in septic shock. N Engl J Med 2014;371(15):1381–91.
34. ASA. Practice guidelines for perioperative blood management: an updated report by the American Society of Anesthesiologists Task Force on Perioperative Blood Management*. Anesthesiology 2015;122(2):241–75.
35. Vlaar AP, Oczkowski S, de Bruin S, et al. Transfusion strategies in non-bleeding critically ill adults: a clinical practice guideline from the European Society of Intensive Care Medicine. Intensive Care Med 2020;46(4):673–96.
36. Napolitano LM, Kurek S, Luchette FA, et al. Clinical practice guideline: red blood cell transfusion in adult trauma and critical care. Crit Care Med 2009;37(12): 3124–57.
37. Trentino KM, Farmer SL, Isbister JP, et al. Restrictive Versus Liberal Transfusion Trials: Are They Asking the Right Question? Anesth Analg 2020;131(6):1950–5.
38. Will ND, Kor DJ, Frank RD, et al. Initial Postoperative Hemoglobin Values and Clinical Outcomes in Transfused Patients Undergoing Noncardiac Surgery. Anesth Analg 2019;129(3):819–29.

39. American College of Surgery. Trauma Quality Improvement Program. Massive Transfusion in Trauma Guidelines. 2014. Available at: https://www.facs.org/media/zcjdtrd1/transfusion_guildelines.pdf. Accessed May 28, 2022.

40. ACOG. Practice Bulletin No. 183: Postpartum Hemorrhage. Obstet Gynecol 2017;130(4):e168–86.

41. Cannon JW, Khan MA, Raja AS, et al. Damage control resuscitation in patients with severe traumatic hemorrhage: A practice management guideline from the Eastern Association for the Surgery of Trauma. J Trauma acute Care Surg 2017;82(3):605–17.

42. Ducrocq G, Gonzalez-Juanatey JR, Puymirat E, et al. Effect of a Restrictive vs Liberal Blood Transfusion Strategy on Major Cardiovascular Events Among Patients With Acute Myocardial Infarction and Anemia: The REALITY Randomized Clinical Trial. JAMA 2021;325(6):552–60.

43. Mazer CD, Whitlock RP, Fergusson DA, et al. Six-Month Outcomes after Restrictive or Liberal Transfusion for Cardiac Surgery. N Engl J Med 2018;379(13): 1224–33.

44. Lasocki S, Pene F, Ait-Oufella H, et al. Management and prevention of anemia (acute bleeding excluded) in adult critical care patients. Ann Intensive Care 2020;10(1):97.

45. Hovaguimian F, Myles PS. Restrictive versus Liberal Transfusion Strategy in the Perioperative and Acute Care Settings: A Context-specific Systematic Review and Meta-analysis of Randomized Controlled Trials. Anesthesiology 2016; 125(1):46–61.

46. Griffiths R, Babu S, Dixon P, et al. Guideline for the management of hip fractures 2020: Guideline by the Association of Anaesthetists. Anaesthesia 2021;76(2): 225–37.

47. Bergamin FS, Almeida JP, Landoni G, et al. Liberal versus restrictive transfusion strategy in critically ill oncologic patients: the transfusion requirements in critically ill oncologic patients randomized controlled trial. Crit Care Med 2017;45(5): 766–73.

48. Tay J, Allan DS, Chatelain E, et al. Liberal Versus Restrictive Red Blood Cell Transfusion Thresholds in Hematopoietic Cell Transplantation: A Randomized, Open Label, Phase III, Noninferiority Trial. J Clin Oncol 2020;38(13):1463–73.

49. Desjardins P, Turgeon AF, Tremblay MH, et al. Hemoglobin levels and transfusions in neurocritically ill patients: a systematic review of comparative studies. Crit Care 2012;16(2):R54.

50. Gobatto ALN, Link MA, Solla DJ, et al. Transfusion requirements after head trauma: a randomized feasibility controlled trial. Crit Care 2019;23(1):89.

51. Carson JL, Noveck H, Berlin JA, et al. Mortality and morbidity in patients with very low postoperative Hb levels who decline blood transfusion. Transfusion 2002; 42(7):812–8.

52. Shander A, Javidroozi M, Naqvi S, et al. An update on mortality and morbidity in patients with very low postoperative hemoglobin levels who decline blood transfusion (CME). Transfusion 2014;54(10 Pt 2):2688–95 ; quiz 2687.

53. Shander A, Javidroozi M, Gianatiempo C, et al. Outcomes of Protocol-Driven Care of Critically Ill Severely Anemic Patients for Whom Blood Transfusion Is Not an Option. Crit Care Med 2016;44(6):1109–15.

54. Weiskopf RB, Viele MK, Feiner J, et al. Human cardiovascular and metabolic response to acute, severe isovolemic anemia. JAMA 1998;279(3):217–21.

55. Leung JM, Weiskopf RB, Feiner J, et al. Electrocardiographic ST-segment changes during acute, severe isovolemic hemodilution in humans. Anesthesiology 2000;93(4):1004–10.
56. de Bruin S, Scheeren TWL, Bakker J, et al. Transfusion practice in the non-bleeding critically ill: an international online survey-the TRACE survey. Crit Care 2019;23(1):309.
57. Zeroual N, Blin C, Saour M, et al. Restrictive Transfusion Strategy after Cardiac Surgery. Anesthesiology 2021;134(3):370–80.
58. Fischer MO, Guinot PG, Debroczi S, et al. Individualised or liberal red blood cell transfusion after cardiac surgery: a randomised controlled trial. Br J Anaesth 2022;128(1):37–44.
59. Fogagnolo A, Taccone FS, Vincent JL, et al. Using arterial-venous oxygen difference to guide red blood cell transfusion strategy. Crit Care 2020;24(1):160.
60. Vlaar APJ, Toy P, Fung M, et al. A consensus redefinition of transfusion-related acute lung injury. Transfusion 2019;59(7):2465–76.
61. Goel R, Patel EU, Cushing MM, et al. Association of Perioperative Red Blood Cell Transfusions With Venous Thromboembolism in a North American Registry. JAMA Surg 2018;153(9):826–33.
62. Fatalities FDA. Reported to FDA Following Blood Collection and Transfusion. 2016. Available at: https://www.fda.gov/files/vaccines%2C%20blood%20%26% 20biologics/published/Fatalities-Reported-to-FDA-Following-Blood-Collection-and-Transfusion–Annual-Summary-for-FY2016.pdf. Accessed May 14, 2022.
63. Bosboom JJ, Klanderman RB, Migdady Y, et al. Transfusion-Associated Circulatory Overload: A Clinical Perspective. Transfus Med Rev 2019;33(2):69–77.
64. National CDC. Healthcare Safety Network Biovigilance Component Hemovigilance Module Surveillance Protocol. In: CDC NHSN biovigilance component. 2021. Available at: https://www.cdc.gov/nhsn/pdfs/biovigilance/bv-hv-protocol-current.pdf. Accessed May 15, 2022.
65. van den Akker TA, Grimes ZM, Friedman MT. Transfusion-associated circulatory overload and transfusion-related acute lung injury. Am J Clin Pathol 2021;156(4): 529–39.
66. Parmar N, Pendergrast J, Lieberman L, et al. The association of fever with transfusion-associated circulatory overload. Vox Sang 2017;112(1):70–8.
67. Blumberg N, Heal JM, Gettings KF, et al. An association between decreased cardiopulmonary complications (transfusion-related acute lung injury and transfusion-associated circulatory overload) and implementation of universal leukoreduction of blood transfusions. Transfusion 2010;50(12):2738–44.
68. Clifford L, Jia Q, Subramanian A, et al. Risk factors and clinical outcomes associated with perioperative transfusion-associated circulatory overload. Anesthesiology 2017;126(3):409–18.
69. Menis M, Anderson SA, Forshee RA, et al. Transfusion-associated circulatory overload (TACO) and potential risk factors among the inpatient US elderly as recorded in Medicare administrative databases during 2011. Vox Sang 2014; 106(2):144–52.
70. Gupta SP, Nand N, Gupta MS, et al. Haemodynamic changes following blood transfusion in cases of chronic severe anemia: increased safety with simultaneous furosemide administration. Angiology 1983;34(11):699–704.
71. US Food and Drug Administration. 2016. Available at: https://www.fda.gov/ media/111226/download. Accessed April 27, 2022.
72. Prevention CfDCa. National Healthcare Safety Network Biovigilance Component, Hemovigilance Module. Surveill Protoc 2021.

73. Peters AL, Van Stein D, Vlaar AP. Antibody-mediated transfusion-related acute lung injury; from discovery to prevention. Br J Haematol 2015;170(5):597–614.

74. McVey MJ, Kapur R, Cserti-Gazdewich C, et al. Transfusion-related Acute Lung Injury in the Perioperative Patient. Anesthesiology 2019;131(3):693–715.

75. Bux J. Transfusion-related acute lung injury (TRALI): a serious adverse event of blood transfusion. Vox Sang 2005;89(1):1–10.

76. Chapman CE, Stainsby D, Jones H, et al. Ten years of hemovigilance reports of transfusion-related acute lung injury in the United Kingdom and the impact of preferential use of male donor plasma. Transfusion 2009;49(3):440–52.

77. Reesink HW, Lee J, Keller A, et al. Measures to prevent transfusion-related acute lung injury (TRALI). Vox Sang 2012;103(3):231–59.

78. Goldberg AD, Kor DJ. State of the art management of transfusion-related acute lung injury (TRALI). Curr Pharm Des 2012;18(22):3273–84.

79. Cata JP, Wang H, Gottumukkala V, et al. Inflammatory response, immunosuppression, and cancer recurrence after perioperative blood transfusions. Br J Anaesth 2013;110(5):690–701.

80. Vamvakas EC. Possible mechanisms of allogeneic blood transfusion-associated postoperative infection. Transfus Med Rev 2002;16(2):144–60.

81. Simancas-Racines D, Osorio D, Martí-Carvajal AJ, et al. Leukoreduction for the prevention of adverse reactions from allogeneic blood transfusion. Cochrane Database Syst Rev 2015;12:CD009745.

82. Amato A, Pescatori M. Perioperative blood transfusions for the recurrence of colorectal cancer. Cochrane Database Syst Rev 2006;1:CD005033.

83. Wu HL, Tai YH, Lin SP, et al. The Impact of Blood Transfusion on Recurrence and Mortality Following Colorectal Cancer Resection: A Propensity Score Analysis of 4,030 Patients. Sci Rep 2018;8(1):13345.

84. Rohde JM, Dimcheff DE, Blumberg N, et al. Health care-associated infection after red blood cell transfusion: a systematic review and meta-analysis. JAMA 2014; 311(13):1317–26.

85. Raghavan M, Marik PE. Anemia, allogenic blood transfusion, and immunomodulation in the critically ill. Chest 2005;127(1):295–307.

86. Weber WP, Zwahlen M, Reck S, et al. The association of preoperative anemia and perioperative allogeneic blood transfusion with the risk of surgical site infection. Transfusion 2009;49(9):1964–70.

87. Guinn NR, Fuller M, Murray S, et al. Treatment through a preoperative anemia clinic is associated with a reduction in perioperative red blood cell transfusion in patients undergoing orthopedic and gynecologic surgery. Transfusion 2022; 62(4):809–16.

88. Richards T, Baikady RR, Clevenger B, et al. Preoperative intravenous iron to treat anaemia before major abdominal surgery (PREVENTT): a randomised, double-blind, controlled trial. Lancet 2020;396(10259):1353–61.

Delirium Prevention and Management in Frail Surgical Patients

Kimberly F. Rengel, MD[a], Lindsay A. Wahl, MD[b],
Archit Sharma, MD, MBA[c], Howard Lee, MD[b],
Christina J. Hayhurst, MD[a],*

KEYWORDS

- Delirium • Frailty • Aging • Cognitive impairment • Preoperative screening

KEY POINTS

- Delirium is a syndrome of acute brain dysfunction that is highly prevalent in surgical populations, particularly older and more frail adults.
- Frailty is a state of increased vulnerability to adverse outcomes after exposure to stress that increases with age and is highly prevalent in surgical populations.
- Patients presenting preoperatively with frailty are at higher risk for cognitive complications including postoperative delirium. Application of validated screening tools for frailty in the preoperative setting may help identify high-risk patients and inform multidisciplinary conversations around surgical care.
- No treatment is available at this time for delirium. The best strategy for avoiding delirium is prevention, and multicomponent bundles have shown the greatest success in reducing incidence and duration of delirium.

INTRODUCTION

Acute brain dysfunction, or delirium, is often thought to be the most common postoperative complication. This syndrome disproportionately affects vulnerable populations such as older adults and is associated with prolonged hospitalization, increased need for readmission, higher mortality up to 5 years after major surgery, and higher cost of care. Because of its widespread impact on patients' hospital course, delirium has

[a] Division of Anesthesiology Critical Care Medicine, Department of Anesthesiology, Vanderbilt University Medical Center, 1211 21st Avenue South, 422 MAB, Nashville, TN 37212, USA;
[b] Department of Anesthesiology, Northwestern University Feinberg School of Medicine, Northwestern Memorial Hospital, 251 East Huron, Suite 5-704, Chicago, IL 60611, USA;
[c] Division of Cardiothoracic Anesthesia, Solid Organ Transplant, and Critical Care, Department of Anesthesia, University of Iowa Carver College of Medicine, 200 Hawkins Drive, 6512 JCP, Iowa City, IA 52242, USA
* Corresponding author.
E-mail address: christina.j.hayhurst@vumc.org

Anesthesiology Clin 41 (2023) 175–189
https://doi.org/10.1016/j.anclin.2022.10.011

drawn the attention of health care providers as a major public health problem.[1–4] Over the past 30 years, attention has been simultaneously drawn to frailty, a syndrome of decreased reserve that predisposes patients to adverse outcomes when exposed to stress. Frailty spans physical, cognitive, and mental health domains and is more prevalent with increasing age but may still be present in younger, high-risk populations. We are increasingly recognizing the large proportion of frail adults who require surgery and their associated increased risk of postoperative complications, prolonged hospital stay, new disability, development of dementia and/or cognitive decline, discharge to a facility other than home, increased health care costs, and mortality.[5–13] Delirium and frailty share many common links and similar outcomes in the perioperative period; however, they remain underrecognized in our surgical population.[14] The purpose of this review is to increase awareness of these conditions and outline tools for screening, risk stratification, prevention, and management of delirium in the perioperative period.

DELIRIUM DEFINITION AND DIAGNOSIS

Delirium is the syndrome that presents in acute brain dysfunction. Hallmark features of delirium outlined in the Diagnostic and Statistical Manual 5th edition (DSM-5) include (1) acute presentation with fluctuation throughout the day, (2) inattention and altered awareness, (3) impaired cognition, (4) evidence that these changes are related to the patient's current medical condition, and (5) absence of a preexisting neurocognitive disorder that better accounts for the symptoms.[15] Delirium can be classified based on the patient's psychomotor symptoms into hyperactive, hypoactive, and mixed subtypes.[16,17] Patients with the hyperactive subtype are agitated, restless, or combative—behaviors commonly associated with delirium. In contrast, patients with hypoactive delirium are lethargic, with slowed speech and mentation. Differentiating hypoactive delirium from sedation, drowsiness, or other organic causes can be challenging without application of an appropriate screening tool; this is particularly true in the postoperative setting where patients may have received several sedating medications. Many patients fluctuate between both hyper- and hypoactive delirium and are classified as having mixed delirium.

The gold standard to diagnose delirium is evaluation by a psychiatric professional using the DSM-5 criteria.[15] Given the lack of feasibility of this resource-intensive evaluation, several validated screening tools have been developed to use at bedside. The Nursing Delirium Symptom Checklist (NuDESC)[18] and Confusion Assessment Method for the Intensive Care Unit (CAM-ICU)[19] have demonstrated greater than 90% specificity to detect delirium in the early postoperative period, although neither tool demonstrates a strong sensitivity for postoperative delirium.[20] A summary of basic principles of these diagnostic tools is outlined in **Box 1**.

DEFINITION AND FRAMEWORKS OF FRAILTY

Increasing age is often associated with changes in health; however, there is a wide variability in risk for adverse events and mortality that is not accounted for by chronological age alone. Frailty emerged over the past 30 years as a construct to identify states of increased vulnerability to adverse events, regardless of age. Frailty is certainly more common with increasing age, but not all older adults become frail. Even though there are two prevailing frameworks for defining frailty that present markedly different theories, there is no consensus as to which framework should be used clinically (**Fig. 1**).[21] The phenotypic or biologic framework defines frailty as "a biologic syndrome of decreased reserve and resistance to stressors, resulting from cumulative

---

Box 1
Delirium Diagnosis

* Diagnostic and Statistical Manual 5th Edition[a]

*Gold Standard
- Disturbance in attention and awareness
- Acute onset with fluctuation in status
- Altered cognition
- Caused by a general medical condition
- Not related to a preexisting neurocognitive disorder

Assessment should be performed by trained neuropsychiatric personnel

Confusion Assessment Method for the ICU[b]
- Feature 1: acute change in mental status from baseline with fluctuation over the past 24 hours
- Feature 2: inattention
- Feature 3: altered consciousness
- Feature 4: disorganized thinking

Assessment may be performed by any trained personnel. Diagnosis requires both features 1 and 2 to be present with either 3 or 4.

Nursing Delirium Screening Checklist[c]
- Disorientation
- Agitation or inappropriate behavior
- Impaired communication
- Altered perception or hallucinations
- Psychomotor slowing

Nursing staff screen patients and score them from 0 to 2 in each of the above categories over the course of a 12-hour shift. Scores ≥ 2 indicate delirium.

[a] Association AP. Diagnostic and statistical manual of mental disorders, fifth edition. Washington, DC.: American Psychiatric Association; 2013. [b] Ely EW, Inouye SK, Bernard GR, et al. Delirium in mechanically ventilated patients: validity and reliability of the confusion assessment method for the intensive care unit (CAM-ICU). JAMA. 2001;286(21):2703-2710. [c] Neufeld KJ, Leoutsakos JS, Sieber FE, et al. Evaluation of two delirium screening tools for detecting post-operative delirium in the elderly. Br J Anaesth. 2013;111(4):7.

---

declines across multiple physiologic systems, causing vulnerability to adverse outcomes."[22] Framework creators hypothesized that dysregulation of energy metabolism and stress response leads to the development of five clinical characteristics: unintentional weight loss of at least 10 pounds in the previous year, self-reported exhaustion, weakness as measured by grip strength, slowed gait speed, and a low level of physical activity. In the initial study of community-dwelling older adults, presence of three or more of these characteristics was predictive of new falls, worsening mobility or new disability in the activities of daily living, hospitalization, and death.[22] The second framework defines frailty as an accumulation of deficits over time. This model measures a "frailty index" by assessing for deficits across more than 30 domains of symptoms, signs, functional impairments, and laboratory abnormalities and dividing the number of deficits present by the total assessed.[23,24] Frail older adults in the community experienced a higher mortality rate during the initial study than those scored as fit using a frailty index.[24] In a comparison of these two frameworks, the phenotypic definition of frailty is easier to implement in a clinical setting and can broadly discriminate between levels of risk, whereas the frailty index is more challenge to translate into the clinical space but provides a more precise identification of risk.[25]

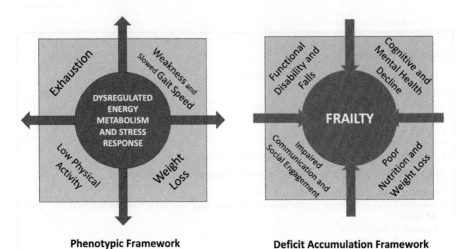

Phenotypic Framework   **Deficit Accumulation Framework**

Fig. 1. Above are depicted the two differing frameworks proposed for frailty. The Phenotypic Framework describes frailty as the physical manifestations resulting from dysregulated energy metabolism and stress response leading to weakness, slowed gait, exhaustion, decrease in physical activity, and weight loss. Conversely, the Defict Accumulation Framework hypothesizes that frailty results from an accumulation of deficits in functional and cognitive ability, the impact of declining health and increasing co-morbidity burden, and environmental factors including nutrition and social engagement.

EPIDEMIOLOGY
Delirium

The occurrence of postoperative delirium varies widely with age, baseline health status, type of procedure, and assessment method.[26] Among older adults requiring major noncardiac surgery, delirium occurs in 13% to 50%[27–29] with the highest rates occurring after orthopedic (12%–51%)[27] and cardiac (11%–52%)[27,30] surgery. Mahanna-Gabriellei and colleagues[12]. found that in patients older than 65 years who underwent major noncardiac surgery, prefrail and frail patients had nearly three times odds of developing delirium than those who were not frail. Similarly, in a smaller pilot trial of older adults requiring cardiac surgery, only 2.6% of nonfrail patients developed postoperative delirium compared with 47.1% of frail patients.[30]

Frailty

Observational studies of prevalence of frailty also range widely. A systematic review of frailty prevalence in community-dwelling older adults ranged from 4.0% to 59.1% with a weighted frailty prevalence of 10.7%.[31] Frailty prevalence is consistently higher, regardless of assessment method, in older surgical patients. Prospective observational studies have reported frailty prevalence of 25.5% in emergency general surgery,[10] 33% in cardiac surgery,[13] and 36.6% (measured by the Modified Frailty Index) to 42.3% (measured by the Clinical Frailty Scale) in elective noncardiac surgery.[11] In a systematic review and meta-analysis of 2281 general surgery patients from 9 observational studies ranging in mean age from 61 to 77 years, 31.3% to 46.8% of patients were prefrail and 10.4% to 37.0% were frail.[32] Although distinct variation exists across surgical specialties and method of measuring frailty, the evidence demonstrates that a significant portion of surgical patients, especially older adults, are frail before surgery and at a higher risk of adverse outcomes. Risk factors commonly associated with frailty include older age, lack of access to private insurance or Medicare, obesity, poor nutrition habits, and depression.[33]

INTERSECTION OF FRAILTY AND DELIRIUM

In a prospective observational study done by Brown and colleagues,[30] the investigators found that in patients older than 55 years requiring cardiac surgery, up to 30.9% were frail. The risk for postoperative delirium was at least 2.1-fold higher in frail patients when compared with nonfrail patients. Similarly, a study performed by Jung and colleagues[34] found that 51.9% to 66.2% of the patients were frail depending on the screening tool, and being frail resulted in 3- to 8-fold increase in the development of postoperative delirium. These results were replicated in a meta-analysis of nine studies of patients aged 65 years or older who required elective, nonemergent inpatient surgery (including both cardiac and noncardiac surgeries); patients with preoperative frailty had an increased odds of developing postoperative delirium (odds ratio [OR] 2.14, confidence interval [CI] 1.43–3.19) compared with nonfrail patients.[29]

SCREENING
Frailty

Screening tools for frailty align with one of the two major frameworks, and details of the individual tools are included in **Table 1**. Tools based on the biologic framework of frailty include the Fried Frailty Phenotype,[22] which was validated in surgical patients and may be referred to as the Hopkins Frailty Score,[6] and the FRAIL scale.[35] The FRAIL scale was developed by the Geriatric Advisory Panel of the International Academy of Nutrition and Aging, and incorporates four components of the frailty phenotype, but replaces activity level with presence of five or more illnesses, accounting for the contribution of both biological changes and deficit accumulation.[35] It is truly intended as a screening tool to identify those at risk for frailty and adverse outcomes who need a more comprehensive assessment. Generalized tools developed based on the deficit accumulation model include the original Frailty Index,[23] and the Clinical Frailty Scale, which simplifies the index into a health care provider's assessment of comorbidities and their effect on the patient's daily life.[36] Deficit accumulation models adapted for and validated in surgical populations include the Risk Analysis Index[37] and the Modified Frailty Index.[38] It is important to note that frailty is a multidimensional syndrome, and screening tools alone cannot identify which areas affect patients the most (i.e. physical frailty, cognitive frailty, poor nutrition); this underlines the need for further workup, where geriatric specialists may be needed to understand the personalized needs of each patient.

Cognitive Screening

Preexisting cognitive impairment is an established risk factor for postoperative delirium,[39,40] and cognitive changes are a major pillar of the frailty syndrome. Joint guidelines issued by the American College of Surgeons and the American Geriatrics Society[41] recommend baseline cognitive screening before surgery; however, subsequent studies have had mixed results. Poor performance on a preoperative Mini-Cog assessment was associated with more postoperative delirium, longer length of stay, and discharge to a location other than home in a cohort of older adults awaiting elective orthopedic surgery.[42] Interestingly, in a large retrospective study of frail elective surgery patients, the Mini-Cog was not sufficiently sensitive to detect significant differences in postoperative adverse outcomes.[43] Similarly, in a prospective cohort of spine surgery patients, the Mini-Cog did not predict postoperative delirium;

Table 1
Frailty assessment tools

Tool	Description
Phenotypic/Biologic Framework	
Fried Frailty Phenotype[a]	Evaluated for presence of 5 criteria:
	• Weight loss ≥10 pounds in 1 year
	• Exhaustion
	• Weakness measured by grip strength
	• Slowed walking speed
	• Low physical activity
	Patients who meet 3 or more criteria are considered frail.
Phenotypic/Biologic Framework AND Deficit Accumulation Framework	
FRAIL Scale[b]	Evaluation in 5 domains:
	• *Fatigue*
	• *Resistance (ability to climb 1 flight of stairs)*
	• *Ambulation (ability to walk 1 block)*
	• *Illnesses (greater than 5 comorbidities)*
	• *Loss of weight (>5% loss of body weight)*
	Scoring: 0 = robust, 1–2 = pre-frail, ≥3 = frail
Deficit Accumulation Framework	
Frailty Index[c]	Original index included 92 items (referred to as deficits) spanning multiple categories including
	• Symptoms (eg, sleep disturbances, memory difficulties, depressed mood)
	• Signs (eg, tremors, weak peripheral pulses)
	• Abnormal laboratory values (eg, calcium, creatinine, urea)
	• Comorbid diseases (eg, diabetes, Parkinson disease)
	• Disabilities (eg, dependence in dressing or bathing)
	Number of deficits is divided by total number of items assessed to give an index from 0 to 1 with values closer to 1 indicating worse frailty.
Clinical Frailty Scale[d]	Physicians evaluate and classify patients as
	1—Very fit
	2—Well
	3—Well, with treated comorbid disease
	4—Apparently vulnerable
	5—Mildly frail
	6—Moderately frail
	7—Severely frail
Risk Analysis Index (RAI)[e]	14 questions assessing 11 variables and 2 statistical interactions including the following:
	Age, Sex, Cancer, Weight Loss, Renal Failure, Congestive Heart Failure, Loss of Appetite, Shortness of Breath, Cognitive Decline, Need for Skilled Nursing, Disability in Activities of Daily Living
	Scored on a scale of 0–81 with a cutoff of ≥ 21 for frailty
Modified Frailty Index (mFI)[f]	A simplification of the frailty index to 11 points relevant to perioperative patients:
	Diabetes mellitus, Not independent functional status, COPD, Congestive heart failure, Myocardial infarction within 6 months, Cardiac problems, Hypertension, Peripheral vascular disease, Clouding or delirium, TIA or CVA, History of CVA with deficit
	Each increasing point is associated with a stepwise increase in morbidity and mortality for perioperative patients.

[a] Fried LP, Tangen CM, Walston J, et al. Frailty in older adults: evidence for a phenotype. J Gerontol A Biol Sci Med Sci. 2001;56(3):M146-156.
[b] Abellan van Kan G, Rolland YM, Morley JE, Vellas B. Frailty: toward a clinical definition. J Am Med Dir Assoc. 2008;9(2):71-72.
[c] Mitnitski AB, Mogilner AJ, Rockwood K. Accumulation of deficits as a proxy measure of aging. ScientificWorldJournal. 2001;1:323-336.
[d] Rockwood K, Song X, MacKnight C, et al. A global clinical measure of fitness and frailty in elderly people. CMAJ. 2005;173(5):489-495.
[e] Hall DE, Arya S, Schmid KK, et al. Development and Initial Validation of the Risk Analysis Index for Measuring Frailty in Surgical Populations. JAMA Surg. 2017;152(2):175-182.
[f] Velanovich V, Antoine H, Swartz A, Peters D, Rubinfeld I. Accumulating deficits model of frailty and postoperative mortality and morbidity: its application to a national database. J Surg Res. 2013;183(1):104-110.

however, poor performance on the Animal Verbal Fluency assessment[44] and frailty based on the FRAIL scale were predictive of postoperative delirium.[45] Even though we lack consensus on the best screening tools, implementing appropriate frailty and cognitive screening in the preoperative period will likely help us to better understand the risk profile of our patients and initiate interdisciplinary discussions on perioperative management, postoperative complications, need for geriatric or palliative care consultation, patient disposition, and therapy needs postoperatively. In addition, there is evidence that screening alone improves postoperative outcomes that may be secondary to the heightened vigilance among the medical team.[46]

DELIRIUM PREVENTION AND MANAGEMENT

It is critically important to note that there is no Food and Drug Administration–approved treatment of delirium. The best strategy is prevention. The management of delirium is highly reliant on symptomatic control with the implementation of multicomponent care bundles, demonstrating the highest success at preventing and minimizing delirium.

Choice of Anesthetic

Current evidence is inconsistent regarding the best anesthetic technique to minimize or prevent postoperative delirium. Many have considered regional or neuraxial anesthesia for older adults over general anesthesia, thinking this may prevent neuronal injury and postoperative delirium. However, a large meta-analysis[47] and a recent large multicenter randomized trial[48] did not find a difference in rates of delirium between regional/neuraxial anesthesia or general anesthesia in older adults requiring surgical repair of hip fracture, a population that generally experiences high rates of both frailty and delirium. The use of total intravenous anesthetic over inhaled anesthetics is another strategy considered by many anesthesiologists in managing patients at high risk of delirium; however, multiple randomized trials have failed to demonstrate a difference in postoperative delirium between these 2 strategies.[49–51] Similarly, trials examining the effect of individual inhaled anesthetic agents have not demonstrated a difference in rates of postoperative delirium between sevoflurane or desflurane.[52,53] Classically, use of medications such as benzodiazepines, gabapentinoids, opiates, and anticholinergics in older patients has been associated with the development of delirium. The impact of preoperative administration of benzodiazepines continues to be debated, with one recent study finding no difference in early postoperative delirium,[54] whereas another study found higher risk in older adults presenting for joint replacement who received both gabapentinoids and preoperative midazolam.[55]

Depth of Anesthesia

Another field of thought postulates that exposure to anesthetic medications contributes to postoperative delirium and unnecessarily high exposure, or anesthetic overdose, will increase the risk. Traditionally, the use of end tidal concentration[56] monitoring of volatile anesthetics fails to provide an accurate assessment of individual patient dose response, and there is not an equivalent monitor in providing intravenous anesthetics in the United States. Processed electroencephalography (EEG) has increasingly been used to monitor brain activity in response to anesthetics to avoid periods of burst suppression indicative of anesthetic overdose and target ideal levels of anesthesia at minimal drug concentrations. Early studies showed promise in reducing postoperative delirium by titrating anesthetic dose using EEG,[57–59] prompting the Fifth International Perioperative Neurotoxicity Working Group to include EEG monitoring in their Best Practices for Postoperative Brain Health in 2018.[60] Subsequently, three large randomized trials that included a variety of noncardiac and cardiac surgeries and both volatile and intravenous anesthetics have not found any difference in the occurrence of postoperative delirium between patients who received EEG-guided anesthesia versus standard of care, despite decreasing anesthetic exposure.[61–63] Despite the lack of evidence that support EEG-titrated anesthetics, this line of work has revealed that certain individuals are more likely to have lower EEG activity and burst suppression at lower levels of anesthesia and are more prone to delirium[59,64,65]; this has led to the "sensitive brain hypothesis" that certain individuals have less cognitive reserve and higher risk of adverse cognitive outcomes—a concept similar to frailty that warrants more examination to determine if there is a correlation between preoperative frailty and the sensitive brain.

Pharmacologic Adjuncts

Investigators have been seeking a pharmacologic adjunct that can easily be added to the current anesthetic regimen in hopes of reducing postoperative delirium. One thought is that impaired cholinergic transmission can lead to the development of delirium. Gamberini and colleagues[66] investigated the administration of cholinesterase inhibitor rivastigmine the day before and 6 days after cardiac surgery, however found no difference in the rates of postoperative delirium between the 2 groups. Dexmedetomidine is a commonly used sedative in critical care medicine that mimics a more natural sleep pattern given its central alpha-2 agonism with additional benefits including analgesic and anti-inflammatory properties. An early study found that adding a dexmedetomidine infusion during general anesthesia for joint replacement surgery reduced postoperative delirium. Subsequently, larger randomized trials across both cardiac and major noncardiac surgery have failed to replicate this finding and demonstrated no difference in postoperative delirium with the addition of dexmedetomidine,[67–69] although in a recent meta-analysis dexmedetomidine did show a tendency to reduce postoperative delirium after cardiac surgery.[70] Ketamine use during the perioperative period has increased with the focus on multimodal, opioid-sparing anesthetics and has raised the interest of delirium researchers for its antiinflammatory properties. In two large, randomized studies, investigators have not been able to demonstrate a reduction in postoperative delirium when comparing low- and high-dose boluses of ketamine at induction with placebo or comparing preoperative ketamine or haloperidol boluses with placebo.[71,72]

Postoperative Adjuncts

There is an important relationship between postoperative delirium and pain, and patients who developed postoperative delirium have also been shown to require higher doses of postoperative opioids.[73] Gabapentin is increasingly used in multimodal pain management pathways to reduce perioperative opioid use. Leung and colleagues[74] randomized 697 patients to a 3-day course of gabapentin versus placebo after major noncardiac surgery and achieved a reduction in opioid consumption in the intervention group but no difference in postoperative delirium between the 2 groups. Acetaminophen also serves as a multimodal pain adjunct and an antiinflammatory agent. In the DEXACET trial, cardiac surgery patients randomized to 48 hours of postoperative intravenous acetaminophen were less likely to develop delirium and had shorter duration of delirium than those in the placebo group.[75] Further studies are needed to examine the efficacy of acetaminophen given orally versus intravenously and in noncardiac surgeries as well. Antipsychotics have often been considered a primary management tool for delirium. The data on use of antipsychotics for prevention of delirium are mixed, but the strongest quality evidence does not support the use of antipsychotics prophylactically to prevent delirium.[76–80] Further, a large trial that randomized ICU patients with delirium to haloperidol, ziprasidone, or placebo found no difference between the three groups in reducing the duration of delirium.[81] Current guidelines from the Society of Critical Care Medicine (SCCM) do still support the use of antipsychotics in hyperactive delirium where patients are at risk of harm to themselves or others, recognizing that this is treating the symptoms and not the delirium itself.[82]

Multicomponent Bundles

Recognizing that delirium and frailty are multifactorial syndromes, bundles addressing multiple risk factors implemented across all care teams are an appealing strategy for mitigating risk of adverse outcomes. The original multicomponent bundle, the Hospital Elder Life Program, was designed to reduce delirium in older adults admitted to the hospital by addressing eight distinct risk factors linked with delirium development including efforts for daily reorientation, cognitive therapy, appropriate sleep hygiene, early mobilization, restoring vision aids, restoring hearing aids and optimizing communication, avoiding dehydration or constipation, and providing feeding assistance.[83] A meta-analysis of 14 implementation studies demonstrated a significant reduction in the incidence of delirium (OR 0.47, 95% CI 0.36–0.59) in addition to a 42% reduction in falls, hospital cost savings, and a reduction in long-term care costs.[84] Applied specifically in the perioperative setting, the bundle reduces delirium and hospital length of stay.[85] The ABCDEF bundle, adapted to address the needs of critically ill patients, includes daily Awakening and Breathing trials, Choice and depth of sedation, Delirium monitoring and management, Early mobility, Family engagement and is associated with less delirium.[86] A large academic medical center created an interdisciplinary protocol for trauma patients identified as frail on admission to the trauma service that incorporated early ambulation, multimodal pain regimens, bowel regimens, nonpharmacologic delirium prevention measures, consults with nutrition and physical therapy, and a geriatric assessment. A before and after implementation trial in 269 patients over 2 years demonstrated a reduction in the odds of developing delirium (OR 0.44, 95% CI 0.22–0.88) and being readmitted within 30 days (OR 0.25, 95% CI 0.07–0.84).[87]

SUMMARY

We are increasingly performing surgical procedures on vulnerable populations with a high prevalence of frailty and risk for postoperative delirium. There is very little evidence that different types of anesthetics make a difference in frail patients developing delirium, and there are no specific medications that have robust evidence for prevention or treatment. Future areas of study could include prehabilitation to reduce cognitive vulnerability. A critical step in preventing delirium and further adverse outcomes is to better understand the baseline characteristics and risk factors for these patients, implement feasible screening strategies for frailty and cognitive dysfunction, and provide prevention measures, particularly for those at highest risk of postoperative delirium.

CLINICS CARE POINTS

- Fraility is a risk factor for post-operative delirium and can be screened for in the pre-operative period.
- There is no evidence to suggest any anesthetic technique is superior to help prevent delirium.
- There are no medications that effectively prevent or treat delirium at this time.
- Perioperative multicomponent bundles can be used to help reduce the incidence of post-operative derlirium.

DISCLOSURE

Dr K.F. Rengel receives support from the Vanderbilt Faculty Research Scholars program.

FUNDING

Dr. Rengel receive funding from the NIH (1R01AG061161-01A1).

REFERENCES

1. Brown CHt, Laflam A, Max L, et al. The impact of delirium after cardiac surgical procedures on postoperative resource use. Ann Thorac Surg 2016;101(5): 1663–9.
2. Brown CHt, LaFlam A, Max L, et al. Delirium after spine surgery in older adults: incidence, risk factors, and outcomes. J Am Geriatr Soc 2016;64(10):2101–8.
3. Moskowitz EE, Overbey DM, Jones TS, et al. Post-operative delirium is associated with increased 5-year mortality. Am J Surg 2017;214(6):1036–8.
4. Witlox J, Eurelings LS, de Jonghe JF, et al. Delirium in elderly patients and the risk of postdischarge mortality, institutionalization, and dementia: a meta-analysis. JAMA 2010;304(4):443–51.
5. Shinall MC Jr, Arya S, Youk A, et al. Association of preoperative patient frailty and operative stress with postoperative mortality. JAMA Surg 2020;155(1): e194620.
6. Makary MA, Segev DL, Pronovost PJ, et al. Frailty as a predictor of surgical outcomes in older patients. J Am Coll Surg 2010;210(6):901–8.
7. Robinson TN, Wallace JI, Wu DS, et al. Accumulated frailty characteristics predict postoperative discharge institutionalization in the geriatric patient. J Am Coll Surg 2011;213(1):37–42 [discussion: 42-34].
8. Robinson TN, Wu DS, Pointer L, et al. Simple frailty score predicts postoperative complications across surgical specialties. Am J Surg 2013;206(4):544–50.
9. Robinson TN, Wu DS, Stiegmann GV, et al. Frailty predicts increased hospital and six-month healthcare cost following colorectal surgery in older adults. Am J Surg 2011;202(5):511–4.

10. McIsaac DI, Moloo H, Bryson GL, et al. The association of frailty with outcomes and resource use after emergency general surgery: a population-based cohort study. Anesth Analg 2017;124(5):1653–61.

11. McIsaac DI, Taljaard M, Bryson GL, et al. Frailty as a predictor of death or new disability after surgery: a prospective cohort study. Ann Surg 2020;271(2):283–9.

12. Mahanna-Gabrielli E, Zhang K, Sieber FE, et al. Frailty is associated with postoperative delirium but not with postoperative cognitive decline in older noncardiac surgery patients. Anesth Analg 2020;130(6):1516–23.

13. Nakano M, Nomura Y, Suffredini G, et al. Functional outcomes of frail patients after cardiac surgery: an observational study. Anesth Analg 2020;130(6):1534–44.

14. Quinlan N, Marcantonio ER, Inouye SK, et al. Vulnerability: the crossroads of frailty and delirium. J Am Geriatr Soc 2011;59(Suppl 2):S262–8.

15. Association AP. Diagnostic and statistical manual of mental disorders. fifth edition. Washington, DC: American Psychiatric Association; 2013.

16. Lipowski ZJ. Transient cognitive disorders (delirium, acute confusional states) in the elderly. Am J Psychiatry 1983;140(11):1426–36.

17. Lipowski ZJ. Delirium in the elderly patient. N Engl J Med 1989;320(9):578–82.

18. Gaudreau JD, Gagnon P, Harel F, et al. Fast, systematic, and continuous delirium assessment in hospitalized patients: the nursing delirium screening scale. J Pain Symptom Manage 2005;29(4):368–75.

19. Ely EW, Inouye SK, Bernard GR, et al. Delirium in mechanically ventilated patients: validity and reliability of the confusion assessment method for the intensive care unit (CAM-ICU). JAMA 2001;286(21):2703–10.

20. Neufeld KJ, Leoutsakos JS, Sieber FE, et al. Evaluation of two delirium screening tools for detecting post-operative delirium in the elderly. Br J Anaesth 2013; 111(4):7.

21. Walston J, Bandeen-Roche K, Buta B, et al. Moving frailty toward clinical practice: NIA intramural frailty science symposium summary. J Am Geriatr Soc 2019;67(8): 1559–64.

22. Fried LP, Tangen CM, Walston J, et al. Frailty in older adults: evidence for a phenotype. J Gerontol A Biol Sci Med Sci 2001;56(3):M146–56.

23. Mitnitski AB, Mogilner AJ, Rockwood K. Accumulation of deficits as a proxy measure of aging. ScientificWorldJournal 2001;1:323–36.

24. Rockwood K, Mitnitski A. Frailty defined by deficit accumulation and geriatric medicine defined by frailty. Clin Geriatr Med 2011;27(1):17–26.

25. Rockwood K, Andrew M, Mitnitski A. A comparison of two approaches to measuring frailty in elderly people. J Gerontol A Biol Sci Med Sci 2007;62(7): 738–43.

26. Brown CHt, Dowdy D. Risk factors for delirium: are systematic reviews enough? Crit Care Med 2015;43(1):232–3.

27. Inouye SK, Westendorp RG, Saczynski JS. Delirium in elderly people. Lancet 2014;383(9920):911–22.

28. Daiello LA, Racine AM, Yun Gou R, et al. Postoperative delirium and postoperative cognitive dysfunction: overlap and divergence. Anesthesiology 2019;131(3): 477–91.

29. Gracie TJ, Caufield-Noll C, Wang NY, et al. The association of preoperative frailty and postoperative delirium: a meta-analysis. Anesth Analg 2021;133(2):314–23.

30. Brown CHt, Max L, LaFlam A, et al. The association between preoperative frailty and postoperative delirium after cardiac surgery. Anesth Analg 2016;123(2): 430–5.

31. Collard RM, Boter H, Schoevers RA, et al. Prevalence of frailty in community-dwelling older persons: a systematic review. J Am Geriatr Soc 2012;60(8): 1487–92.

32. Hewitt J, Long S, Carter B, et al. The prevalence of frailty and its association with clinical outcomes in general surgery: a systematic review and meta-analysis. Age Ageing 2018;47(6):793–800.

33. Feng Z, Lugtenberg M, Franse C, et al. Risk factors and protective factors associated with incident or increase of frailty among community-dwelling older adults: A systematic review of longitudinal studies. PLoS One 2017;12(6):e0178383.

34. Jung P, Pereira MA, Hiebert B, et al. The impact of frailty on postoperative delirium in cardiac surgery patients. J Thorac Cardiovasc Surg 2015;149(3): 869–75, e861-862.

35. Abellan van Kan G, Rolland YM, Morley JE, et al. Frailty: toward a clinical definition. J Am Med Dir Assoc 2008;9(2):71–2.

36. Rockwood K, Song X, MacKnight C, et al. A global clinical measure of fitness and frailty in elderly people. CMAJ 2005;173(5):489–95.

37. Hall DE, Arya S, Schmid KK, et al. Development and Initial Validation of the Risk Analysis Index for Measuring Frailty in Surgical Populations. JAMA Surg 2017; 152(2):175–82.

38. Velanovich V, Antoine H, Swartz A, et al. Accumulating deficits model of frailty and postoperative mortality and morbidity: its application to a national database. J Surg Res 2013;183(1):104–10.

39. Vasilevskis EE, Han JH, Hughes CG, et al. Epidemiology and risk factors for delirium across hospital settings. Best Pract Res Clin Anaesthesiol 2012;26(3): 277–87.

40. Ansaloni L, Catena F, Chattat R, et al. Risk factors and incidence of postoperative delirium in elderly patients after elective and emergency surgery. Br J Surg 2010; 97(2):273–80.

41. Chow WB, Rosenthal RA, Merkow RP, et al. Optimal preoperative assessment of the geriatric surgical patient: a best practices guideline from the American College of Surgeons National Surgical Quality Improvement Program and the American Geriatrics Society. J Am Coll Surg 2012;215(4):453–66.

42. Culley DJ, Flaherty D, Fahey MC, et al. Poor performance on a preoperative cognitive screening test predicts postoperative complications in older orthopedic surgical patients. Anesthesiology 2017;127(5):765–74.

43. O'Reilly-Shah VN, Hemani S, Davari P, et al. A preoperative cognitive screening test predicts increased length of stay in a frail population: a retrospective case-control study. Anesth Analg 2019;129(5):1283–90.

44. Long LS, Wolpaw JT, Leung JM. Sensitivity and specificity of the animal fluency test for predicting postoperative delirium. Can J Anaesth 2015;62(6):603–8.

45. Susano MJ, Grasfield RH, Friese M, et al. Brief preoperative screening for frailty and cognitive impairment predicts delirium after spine surgery. Anesthesiology 2020;133(6):1184–91.

46. Hall DE, Arya S, Schmid KK, et al. Association of a frailty screening initiative with postoperative survival at 30, 180, and 365 days. JAMA Surg 2017;152(3):233–40.

47. Guay J, Parker MJ, Gajendragadkar PR, et al. Anaesthesia for hip fracture surgery in adults. Cochrane Database Syst Rev 2016;2:CD000521.

48. Neuman MD, Feng R, Carson JL, et al. Spinal anesthesia or general anesthesia for hip surgery in older adults. N Engl J Med 2021;385(22):2025–35.

49. Miller D, Lewis SR, Pritchard MW, et al. Intravenous versus inhalational maintenance of anaesthesia for postoperative cognitive outcomes in elderly people undergoing non-cardiac surgery. Cochrane Database Syst Rev 2018;8:CD012317.

50. Royse CF, Andrews DT, Newman SN, et al. The influence of propofol or desflurane on postoperative cognitive dysfunction in patients undergoing coronary artery bypass surgery. Anaesthesia 2011;66(6):455–64.

51. Tanaka P, Goodman S, Sommer BR, et al. The effect of desflurane versus propofol anesthesia on postoperative delirium in elderly obese patients undergoing total knee replacement: a randomized, controlled, double-blinded clinical trial. J Clin Anesth 2017;39:17–22.

52. Magni G, Rosa IL, Melillo G, et al. A comparison between sevoflurane and desflurane anesthesia in patients undergoing craniotomy for supratentorial intracranial surgery. Anesth Analg 2009;109(2):567–71.

53. Meineke M, Applegate RL 2nd, Rasmussen T, et al. Cognitive dysfunction following desflurane versus sevoflurane general anesthesia in elderly patients: a randomized controlled trial. Med Gas Res 2014;4(1):6.

54. Wang ML, Min J, Sands LP, et al. Midazolam premedication immediately before surgery is not associated with early postoperative delirium. Anesth Analg 2021; 133(3):765–71.

55. Athanassoglou V, Cozowicz C, Zhong H, et al. Association of perioperative midazolam use and complications: a population-based analysis. Reg Anesth Pain Med 2022;47(4):228–33.

56. Hendrickx JFA, De Wolf AM. End-tidal anesthetic concentration: monitoring, interpretation, and clinical application. Anesthesiology 2022;136(6):985–96.

57. Radtke FM, Franck M, Lendner J, et al. Monitoring depth of anaesthesia in a randomized trial decreases the rate of postoperative delirium but not postoperative cognitive dysfunction. Br J Anaesth 2013;110(Suppl 1):i98–105.

58. Chan MT, Cheng BC, Lee TM, et al. BIS-guided anesthesia decreases postoperative delirium and cognitive decline. J Neurosurg Anesthesiol 2013;25(1):33–42.

59. Whitlock EL, Torres BA, Lin N, et al. Postoperative delirium in a substudy of cardiothoracic surgical patients in the BAG-RECALL clinical trial. Anesth Analg 2014;118(4):809–17.

60. Berger M, Schenning KJ, Brown CHt, et al. Best practices for postoperative brain health: recommendations from the fifth international perioperative neurotoxicity working group. Anesth Analg 2018;127(6):1406–13.

61. Wildes TS, Mickle AM, Ben Abdallah A, et al. Effect of electroencephalography-guided anesthetic administration on postoperative delirium among older adults undergoing major surgery: the ENGAGES randomized clinical trial. JAMA 2019;321(5):473–83.

62. Tang CJ, Jin Z, Sands LP, et al. ADAPT-2: a randomized clinical trial to reduce intraoperative eeg suppression in older surgical patients undergoing major noncardiac surgery. Anesth Analg 2020;131(4):1228–36.

63. Besch G, Vettoretti L, Claveau M, et al. Early post-operative cognitive dysfunction after closed-loop versus manual target controlled-infusion of propofol and remifentanil in patients undergoing elective major non-cardiac surgery: protocol of the randomized controlled single-blind POCD-ELA trial. Medicine (Baltimore) 2018;97(40):e12558.

64. Fritz BA, Kalarickal PL, Maybrier HR, et al. Intraoperative electroencephalogram suppression predicts postoperative delirium. Anesth Analg 2016;122(1):234–42.

65. Fritz BA, Maybrier HR, Avidan MS. Intraoperative electroencephalogram suppression at lower volatile anaesthetic concentrations predicts postoperative delirium occurring in the intensive care unit. Br J Anaesth 2018;121(1):241–8.

66. Gamberini M, Bolliger D, Lurati Buse GA, et al. Rivastigmine for the prevention of postoperative delirium in elderly patients undergoing elective cardiac surgery–a randomized controlled trial. Crit Care Med 2009;37(5):1762–8.

67. Deiner S, Luo X, Lin HM, et al. Intraoperative infusion of dexmedetomidine for prevention of postoperative delirium and cognitive dysfunction in elderly patients undergoing major elective noncardiac surgery: a randomized clinical trial. JAMA Surg 2017;152(8):e171505.

68. Li X, Yang J, Nie XL, et al. Impact of dexmedetomidine on the incidence of delirium in elderly patients after cardiac surgery: A randomized controlled trial. PLoS One 2017;12(2):e0170757.

69. Turan A, Duncan A, Leung S, et al. Dexmedetomidine for reduction of atrial fibrillation and delirium after cardiac surgery (DECADE): a randomised placebo-controlled trial. Lancet 2020;396(10245):177–85.

70. Li P, Li LX, Zhao ZZ, et al. Dexmedetomidine reduces the incidence of postoperative delirium after cardiac surgery: a meta-analysis of randomized controlled trials. BMC Anesthesiol 2021;21(1):153.

71. Avidan MS, Maybrier HR, Abdallah AB, et al. Intraoperative ketamine for prevention of postoperative delirium or pain after major surgery in older adults: an international, multicentre, double-blind, randomised clinical trial. Lancet 2017; 390(10091):267–75.

72. Hollinger A, Rust CA, Riegger H, et al. Ketamine vs. haloperidol for prevention of cognitive dysfunction and postoperative delirium: A phase IV multicentre randomised placebo-controlled double-blind clinical trial. J Clin Anesth 2021;68: 110099.

73. Vaurio LE, Sands LP, Wang Y, et al. Postoperative delirium: the importance of pain and pain management. Anesth Analg 2006;102(4):1267–73.

74. Leung JM, Sands LP, Chen N, et al. Perioperative gabapentin does not reduce postoperative delirium in older surgical patients: a randomized clinical trial. Anesthesiology 2017;127(4):633–44.

75. Subramaniam B, Shankar P, Shaefi S, et al. Effect of intravenous acetaminophen vs placebo combined with propofol or dexmedetomidine on postoperative delirium among older patients following cardiac surgery: the DEXACET randomized clinical trial. JAMA 2019;321(7):686–96.

76. Fukata S, Kawabata Y, Fujisiro K, et al. Haloperidol prophylaxis does not prevent postoperative delirium in elderly patients: a randomized, open-label prospective trial. Surg Today 2014;44(12):2305–13.

77. Wang W, Li HL, Wang DX, et al. Haloperidol prophylaxis decreases delirium incidence in elderly patients after noncardiac surgery: a randomized controlled trial. Crit Care Med 2012;40(3):731–9.

78. Prakanrattana U, Prapaitrakool S. Efficacy of risperidone for prevention of postoperative delirium in cardiac surgery. Anaesth Intensive Care 2007;35(5):714–9.

79. Kalisvaart KJ, de Jonghe JF, Bogaards MJ, et al. Haloperidol prophylaxis for elderly hip-surgery patients at risk for delirium: a randomized placebo-controlled study. J Am Geriatr Soc 2005;53(10):1658–66.

80. Page VJ, Ely EW, Gates S, et al. Effect of intravenous haloperidol on the duration of delirium and coma in critically ill patients (Hope-ICU): a randomised, double-blind, placebo-controlled trial. Lancet Respir Med 2013;1(7):515–23.

81. Girard TD, Exline MC, Carson SS, et al. Haloperidol and ziprasidone for treatment of delirium in critical illness. N Engl J Med 2018;379:2506–16.
82. Devlin JW, Skrobik Y, Gelinas C, et al. Clinical practice guidelines for the prevention and management of pain, agitation/sedation, delirium, immobility, and sleep disruption in adult patients in the ICU. Crit Care Med 2018;46(9):e825–73.
83. Inouye SK, Bogardus ST Jr, Charpentier PA, et al. A multicomponent intervention to prevent delirium in hospitalized older patients. N Engl J Med 1999;340(9): 669–76.
84. Hshieh TT, Yang T, Gartaganis SL, et al. Hospital elder life program: systematic review and meta-analysis of effectiveness. Am J Geriatr Psychiatry 2018; 26(10):1015–33.
85. Chen CC, Li HC, Liang JT, et al. Effect of a modified hospital elder life program on delirium and length of hospital stay in patients undergoing abdominal surgery: a cluster randomized clinical trial. JAMA Surg 2017;152(9):827–34.
86. Barnes-Daly MA, Phillips G, Ely EW. Improving hospital survival and reducing brain dysfunction at seven california community hospitals: implementing PAD guidelines Via the ABCDEF bundle in 6,064 patients. Crit Care Med 2017; 45(2):171–8.
87. Bryant EA, Tulebaev S, Castillo-Angeles M, et al. Frailty identification and care pathway: an interdisciplinary approach to care for older trauma patients. J Am Coll Surg 2019;228(6):852–859 e851.

Perioperative Fluid Management and Volume Assessment

Jennifer Elia, MD[a],*, Murtaza Diwan, MD[b],
Ranjit Deshpande, MD, FCCM, MBBS[c], Jason C. Brainard, MD, FCCM[d],
Kunal Karamchandani, MD, FCCP, FCCM[e]

KEYWORDS

- Fluid management • Fluid responsiveness • Frank-Starling curve
- Goal-directed therapy • Dynamic parameters

KEY POINTS

- Specific hemodynamic goals during the perioperative period include maintaining adequate blood volume and perfusion pressure to ensure optimal tissue blood flow and oxygen delivery.
- Identifying patients likely to benefit from fluid administration during the perioperative period is important to avoid the deleterious effects associated with either hypovolemia or excess fluid administration.
- Using the differences in stroke volume that occur during the respiratory cycle, dynamic parameters can assess the likelihood that a patient will be fluid responsive.
- There is much literature comparing balanced crystalloids to normal saline, but ongoing controversy exists regarding which fluids to use for intraoperative fluid administration.
- At present, most evidence points to a reduction in perioperative morbidity with the use of goal-directed fluid therapy.

INTRODUCTION

Despite significant advances in medical care, postoperative morbidity and mortality remain high, especially after urgent and emergent procedures. Fluid therapy is an integral component of perioperative care and helps maintain or restore effective

[a] Department of Anesthesiology, University of California, Irvine School of Medicine, 101 The City Drive South, Building 53-225, Orange, CA 92868, USA; [b] Department of Anesthesiology, University of Michigan, 1500 East Medical Center Drive, Ann Arbor, MI 48109, USA; [c] Department of Anesthesiology, Yale School of Medicine, 333Cedars Street, TMP 3, New Haven, CT 06510, USA; [d] Department of Anesthesiology, University of Colorado, University of Colorado Hospital, 12401 East 17th Avenue, Mail Stop B113, Aurora, CO 80045, USA; [e] Department of Anesthesiology and Pain Management, University of Texas, Southwestern Medical Center, 5323 Harry Hines Boulevard, Dallas, TX 75390, USA
* Corresponding author.
E-mail address: jelia@hs.uci.edu

Anesthesiology Clin 41 (2023) 191–209
https://doi.org/10.1016/j.anclin.2022.10.010   anesthesiology.theclinics.com
1932-2275/23/© 2022 Elsevier Inc. All rights reserved.

circulating blood volume. The principal goal of fluid management is to optimize cardiac preload, thus maximizing stroke volume (SV) to maintain adequate organ perfusion. Although the importance of fluid therapy during the perioperative period has been established, controversy exists on what kind of fluid therapy is ideal. Also, there is wide variability in practice both at the individual and institutional levels. Perioperative morbidity is linked to the amount of intravenous fluid administered; insufficient or excess fluid therapy can lead to postoperative complications.[1–3] One of the biggest challenges with fluid management during the perioperative period is estimation of a patient's volume status and volume responsiveness. Accurate assessment of volume status is necessary for appropriate and judicious utilization of fluid therapy. Similarly, it is important to assess a patient's volume responsiveness, because only patients who are volume responsive will have an increase in their SV with fluid administration. Both static and dynamic indicators of fluid responsiveness have been widely studied. Although dynamic indicators are more accurate, static parameters are easier to measure. Intraoperative fluid therapy should then be tailored to patient- and situation-specific scenarios. This review (1) discusses the overarching goals of perioperative fluid management, (2) reviews the physiology of fluid responsiveness as well as the parameters that can be used to assess fluid responsiveness, and (3) provides evidence-based recommendations on intraoperative fluid management.

Goals of Perioperative Fluid Management

Specific hemodynamic goals during the perioperative period include maintaining adequate blood volume and perfusion pressure to ensure optimal tissue blood flow and oxygen delivery. Fluid infusions directly increase intravascular volume, and subsequently improve global and regional perfusion as well as blood pressure if the heart is preload responsive; this often improves oxygen delivery and tissue oxygenation. Intravenous infusion of fluid directly expands plasma volume with transient or sustained effect that varies based on the osmotic properties of the fluid, blood flow distribution, type and level of anesthesia, vascular endothelial integrity, and the physiologic state. However, these changes are influenced by the individual patient's cardiac and peripheral vascular status. Hypovolemia is common during the perioperative period, especially if mechanical bowel preparation has been instituted.[4] Although the benefits of bowel preparation are unclear, it has been shown to cause preoperative dehydration, by inducing functional hypovolemia.[5,6] Also, insensible losses related to induction of anesthesia and surgical exposure, as well as blood and other bodily fluid losses lead to a decrease in effective circulatory blood volume.[7,8] Fluid therapy is often used to replenish this decreased effective circulating blood volume.

Preoperative Fasting

Dehydration before elective surgery is common and is compounded by increased fasting times.[9] Historically, the increased risk of aspiration, as described by Mendelson[10] led to "nil by mouth after midnight" becoming the standard recommendation for fasting before surgery requiring general anesthesia. It was assumed that fasting resulted in low gastric residual volume, and the lack of stimulus for gastric acid production would cause the pH of the stomach fluid to be higher and therefore less damaging to the lungs in the event of aspiration. However, there is credible evidence that shorter preoperative fasting times are not associated with an increased risk of aspiration or with larger volumes of gastric content.[11] In addition, prolonged fasting does not reliably result in an empty stomach or fluid with a higher pH because no significant difference in gastric fluid volume or pH is observed in patients given oral fluids around 2 hours before an operation.[12–14] Hence, both European and American guidelines promote the intake of clear fluids up to 2 hours before elective surgery.[15,16] The recent change in fasting guidelines for children—allowing children to drink clear fluids up until 1 hour before induction of anesthesia—has led to a renewed interest toward adopting a 1-hour clear fluid fasting guideline for all age groups.[17,18]

Fluid Responsiveness

Identifying patients likely to benefit from fluid administration during the perioperative period is important to avoid the deleterious effects associated with excess fluid administration. In this regard, the concept of "fluid responsiveness" is vital to understand. The Frank-Starling curve relates left ventricular (LV) performance (measured as ventricular SV or cardiac output [CO]) with preload (measured as LV end-diastolic volume or pressure). Based on the Frank-Starling relationship, the ventricular output increases as preload (end-diastolic pressure) increases.[19] On the curve of a normally functioning heart, cardiac performance increases continuously as preload increases, followed by an apparent plateau, wherein the transition occurs from a fluid-responsive to fluid-nonresponsive state. At this point, fluid administration serves no useful purpose and is likely to be harmful.[20] It has been demonstrated that only about 50% of hemodynamically unstable patients are fluid responsive.[21] Thus, only patients who are fluid responsive should be resuscitated with fluid boluses.

ASSESSMENT OF FLUID RESPONSIVENESS WITH STATIC PARAMETERS

Traditional static predictors for fluid responsiveness include vital signs, such as heart rate and blood pressure, urine output, and cardiovascular filling pressures, which include central venous pressure (CVP) and pulmonary artery occlusion pressure (PAOP). Clinical signs, including tachycardia and urine output, are neither sensitive nor specific indices for predicting fluid responsiveness and have thus been removed from almost all clinical recommendations and goal-directed therapy algorithms,[22,23] including the updated 2016 and 2021 recommendations from the European Society of Intensive Care Medicine and Society of Critical Care Medicine.[24] Cardiovascular filling pressures, including CVP and PAOP, have likewise been shown to be inaccurate predictors of preload and fluid responsiveness[21,25]; this is true both for static pressure measurements and for dynamic changes in CVP and PAOP. Many factors, including vascular resistance, intrathoracic pressure, and ventricular compliance, all prevent direct correlation of these filling pressures to volume responsiveness.[23,26,27] The failure of static or dynamic CVP and PAOP measurements to predict positive hemodynamic response (increased SV) to a fluid challenge has been demonstrated.[26] Thus, static parameters, including clinical signs and cardiovascular filling pressures should not be used to predict volume responsiveness.

ASSESSMENT OF FLUID RESPONSIVENESS WITH DYNAMIC PARAMETERS

Some dynamic parameters, such as systolic pressure variation (SPV), pulse pressure variation (PPV), stroke volume variation (SVV), and pulse oximetry (plethysmography) variation are, in fact, useful measurements in predicting the response to fluid administration and have been shown to be superior to static measurements. It is important to understand the Frank-Starling law to better understand and illustrate these concepts.

The Frank-Starling Curve and Mechanical Ventilation

A patient who is fluid responsive should experience an increase in SV and subsequent improvement in end-organ perfusion when fluid is administered. If fluid administration does not improve SV, benefit is unlikely, and harm is probable. This fact is construed from the Frank-Starling principle, which describes the relationship between increase in preload and associated increase in LV SV, until there is a point at which the preload is most optimal (**Fig. 1**). Once this optimal point is reached on the curve, an increase in fluid administration has little effect on the SV. The patient's cardiac physiology now relates to the "flat" portion of the Frank-Starling curve indicating there will be no response to further fluid administration.

There are cyclic changes in the loading parameters of the left and right sides of the heart that are caused by positive pressure ventilation (**Fig. 2**). During inspiration, the right ventricular (RV) SV decreases and LV SV increases. During expiration, the opposite is observed where RV SV increases and LV SV decreases. Although these cyclic changes are observed with mechanical ventilation in all patients, they may be accentuated in patients who are hypovolemic. Thus, the degree of respiratory changes in SV may be an accurate indicator of fluid responsiveness.[28]

The pulmonary artery catheter (PAC) has long been the gold standard for the assessment of fluid status and responsiveness. Filling pressures including CVP, pulmonary artery pressure, pulmonary capillary wedge pressure, and the CO derived by the PAC have been traditionally used to guide fluid management. As an invasive procedure, complications include infection, pneumothorax, hemothorax, air embolism, bleeding, arrhythmias, malposition, and vessel injury. Unfortunately, the PAC is often misused, or its data inaccurately interpreted, and multiple studies have demonstrated that the values derived from a PAC do not accurately predict fluid responsiveness.[29]

In hemodynamically unstable patients, however, dynamic parameters can be used to assess volume responsiveness by evaluating the differences in SV that occur during the respiratory cycle. SPV, PPV, SVV, and pulse oximetry variation have all been shown to be highly predictive of fluid responsiveness.[30]

Systolic Pressure Variation

The SPV is the difference between the maximal and minimal systolic blood pressure (SBP) following a positive pressure breath. SVP consists of the sum of an early

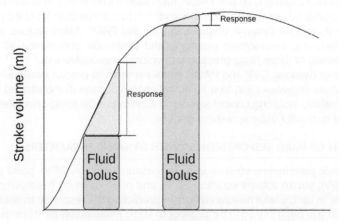

Left ventricular end-diastolic pressure (preload)

Fig. 1. The Frank-Starling curve. The Frank-Starling Curve illustrates the relationship between left ventricular end-diastolic volume (or preload) and left ventricular stroke volume. On the steeper part of the curve, fluid administration will result in an associated increase in stroke volume. On the flatter part of the curve, fluid administration has little effect on stroke volume.

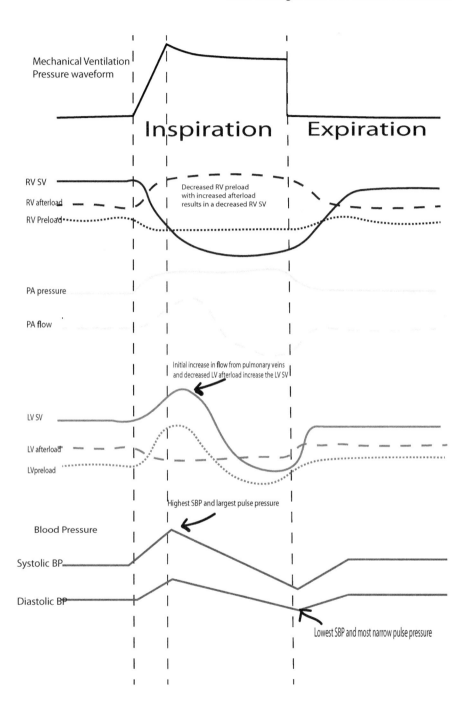

Mechanical Ventilation
Pressure waveform

Inspiration | Expiration

RV SV

RV afterload

RV Preload

Decreased RV preload
with increased afterload
results in a decreased RV SV

PA pressure

PA flow

Initial increase in flow from pulmonary veins
and decreased LV afterload increase the LV SV

LV SV

LV afterload

LVpreload

Highest SBP and largest pulse pressure

Blood Pressure

Systolic BP

Diastolic BP

Lowest SBP and most narrow pulse pressure

inspiratory augmentation of the SBP and the later decrease in SBP. The SPV can be calculated with an arterial line and is calculated by the following equation:

$$SPV = \frac{SBP_{max} - SBP_{min}}{(SBP_{max} + SBP_{min})/2}$$

An increase in SPV happens during hypovolemia, and the extent to which the SBP changes with the variation in pleural pressure can be used to assess LV preload and predict fluid responsiveness. If LV preload is insufficient and there is a large ventilation-mediated change in the SBP, the patient is likely on the ascending portion of the Frank-Starling curve, indicating that administration of volume and increase in preload will increase SV and blood pressure. An SPV of greater than 10 mm Hg suggests that the patient may be fluid responsive.[31,32] SPV has shown to be an accurate predictor of fluid responsiveness in patients with hypotension, and compared with static preload indicators such as CVP, it may be a superior marker of fluid responsiveness.[33] Tavernier and colleagues,[34] for example, showed that SPV is a sensitive indicator of fluid responsiveness in patients with sepsis-induced hypotension.

Pulse Pressure Variation

PPV is an alternative parameter derived from the arterial waveform. Pulse pressure (PP) is defined as the difference between the systolic and diastolic arterial blood pressure. The maximal pulse pressure (PP_{max}) and minimal pulse pressure (PP_{min}) are determined over the same respiratory cycle. PPV greater than approximately 13% correlates with an increased likelihood of fluid responsiveness.[30] PPV is calculated by the following equation:

$$PPV\ (\%) = \frac{PP_{max} - PP_{min}}{(PP_{max} + PP_{min})/2} \times 100$$

In Marik and colleagues'[30] meta-analysis of 22 studies, PPV was shown to be highly predictive and accurate in determining fluid responsiveness in critically ill patients. Importantly, PPV was more accurate than traditional static indices that have historically been used. Lopes and colleagues[35] showed that minimizing PPV by fluid resuscitation intraoperatively improved postoperative outcomes, whereas Michard and colleagues[36] showed that PPV was superior to SPV in the assessment of fluid responsiveness in mechanically ventilated patients with septic shock. This observation could be because SPV not only may accurately reflect the LV SV variations but also may be influenced by the direct transmission of pleural pressure to the thoracic aorta.[37]

It is often difficult to assess whether a spontaneously breathing patient would benefit from fluid administration. In contrast to mechanical ventilation, spontaneous breathing generates negative intrathoracic pressure during inspiration resulting in

Fig. 2. Effects of mechanical ventilation on filling pressures and blood pressure. This figure depicts the physiologic changes occurring during the phases of mechanical ventilation (*top portion*). Right ventricular (RV) stroke volume (SV) and preload (*blue*) decrease during inspiration, whereas afterload is increased. Similarly, the pulmonary artery (PA) pressure (*yellow*) increases during the inspiratory phase. PA flow initially increases but decreases before the expiratory phase begins. Left ventricular (LV) SV and preload (*orange*) also initially increase during inspiration due to increased flow from the pulmonary veins and decreased LV afterload. As a result, systolic and diastolic blood pressure (*red*) increase during the initial part of inspiration and reach the lowest point shortly after the expiratory phase begins.

reduced left heart filling and SV. Alterations in preload secondary to respiration are thus too small to be able to detect any variation in blood pressure or SV, making SPV and PPV less useful in these patients.[38]

Plethysmographic Variability Index

Invasive blood pressure monitoring is necessary to calculate both SPV and PPV. The noninvasive measurement of respiratory variations in the plethysmographic (pulse oximetry) waveform can also indicate a patient's fluid status.[39] The plethysmographic variability index (PVi) provides a continuous measurement of the variability of the plethysmograph during the respiratory cycle, measuring changes in the arterial and venous vessels. In systole, there is an increase in the amount of hemoglobin present in the fingertip and this leads to a decrease in light absorption. The opposite is noted during diastole, thus allowing pulse oximetry to serve as a noninvasive method to evaluate the arterial pulse. The PVi is a dynamic index between 0 and 100 with higher values indicating increased variability, signaling a higher likelihood that a patient may be fluid responsive.[40,41] There is a strong correlation between respiratory variations in pulse oximetry and respiratory variations in arterial PP (SPV and PPV),[42] suggesting that PVi can be used as a surrogate to determine fluid responsiveness. The calculation of the variation, however, usually requires offline recording and analysis, which makes it difficult for real-time utilization.

Stroke Volume Variation

SVV is the difference between the maximal and minimal SV during the respiratory cycle divided by the mean SV. SV can be measured using echocardiography. Reliability of SV measurements by echocardiography is limited by operator variability. Zhang and colleagues[43] published a meta-analysis in 2011 that found that SVV was a good predictor of fluid responsiveness with a sensitivity of 81% and specificity of 80%.

$$SVV(\%) = \frac{SV_{max} - SV_{min}}{SV_{mean}} \times 100$$

SVV can also be obtained with newer modalities that measure SV and CO, such as beat-to-beat pulse contour analysis calibrated by thermodilution. These devices use arterial lines with a thermistor. Different devices use slightly different algorithms in their calculations to determine CO (common devices include the FloTrac/Vigileo [Edwards Lifesciences, Irvine, CA, USA], PiCCO [Pulse Index Contour Cardiac Output, Getinge, Wayne, NJ, USA], and LiDCO [Lithium Dilution Cardiac Output, Masimo, Irvine, CA, USA]). These devices provide a less invasive method compared with PAC-derived measurements of CO and have been shown to measure similar mean CO values, although the dynamic trends among the devices are inconsistent.[44]

The PiCCO system was the first arterial pulse contour device that was used to measure CO in clinical practice. This device has a proprietary algorithm that assumes that the area under the systolic part of the aortic pressure waveform corresponds to SV; this is correlated to the patient's SV with calibration by transpulmonary thermodilution, and thus there is a thermistor-tipped catheter in the artery along with a central venous catheter that is used to inject cold water boluses. The PiCCO Plus system allows for the additional measurement of PPV as well. The LiDCO Plus is an alternative pulse contour method that works on the principle of power conservation in a system and uses a lithium dilution method. This method shows a linear correlation between the new power and vascular flow, and it has been shown to be a reliable assessment of CO in the absence of major hemodynamic changes. The LiDCO rapid device is another alternative that does not require frequent calibration and is similar to the Flo-Trac/Vigileo device. Both devices provide continuous SVV and PPV measurements. The FloTrac device requires a special transducer that can be attached to any standard arterial line and displays the data derived from a proprietary algorithm on a dedicated monitor. The monitor displays continuous CO measurements without the need for any further calibration.

A major drawback of using SVV to assess fluid responsiveness is the need for specific devices and components to gather and interpret the data. In this regard, PPV may be advantageous because it requires only an arterial line for measurements. SVV requires complex computation and additional devices that increase the likelihood of error.[36] At present, there is insufficient evidence to support the routine use of any one of these devices[45] and further studies are needed to determine their cost-effectiveness as well as accuracy in varied clinical scenarios.

Limitations

Dynamic parameters of fluid responsiveness have several limitations that may limit their usage across all clinical settings. First, these measures need to be used in mechanically ventilated patients who are not spontaneously breathing. The tidal volume must be at least 8 mL/kg with a positive end expiratory pressure less than 5 mm Hg. The patient must be in normal sinus rhythm, with an enclosed chest cavity, and normal intra-abdominal pressure. Low arterial compliance and RV or LV failure also make the parameters less reliable. Despite these limitations, the clinical utility of these dynamic parameters is quite high, and in the correct clinical setting, they provide valuable information in the assessment and treatment of hemodynamically unstable patients.

Echocardiography

Both transesophageal and transthoracic echocardiography (TTE) can be used to assess dynamic changes in the RV and LV that indicate hypovolemia. The subaortic velocity-time integral can measure SV and thus be used to assess volume responsiveness. In addition, the measurement of end-diastolic volume can be used as a surrogate for preload.

Ultrasonographic assessment of the inferior vena cava (IVC) is another modality commonly used to evaluate fluid status and gauge fluid responsiveness. IVC diameter and collapsibility (variations associated with respiration) have been shown to accurately estimate CVP and right atrial pressure, particularly in spontaneously breathing patients.[46] Diagnostic accuracy is less consistent in patients who are mechanically ventilated, making this assessment less useful for patients under general anesthesia. A recent meta-analysis, however, revealed that IVC assessment did not seem to reliably correlate with fluid responsiveness.[47] This finding was true for both spontaneously breathing and mechanically ventilated patients, although the investigators note a great deal of heterogeneity in the included studies. In contrast, earlier meta-analyses found respiratory variation of IVC diameter a good predictor of fluid responsiveness, even in mechanically ventilated patients.[48–50]

Although TTE is portable and noninvasive, limitations include accessibility, operator proficiency, and the need for repeated studies to assess dynamic changes associated with volume administration. Access to the patient's chest may be limited, and TTE may not be possible in many circumstances. The risks and costs associated with transesophageal echocardiography preclude its routine use for assessment of fluid responsiveness. In summary, current evidence supporting echocardiographic assessment of IVC variation is unclear, prompting clinicians to use this modality in conjunction with other clinical markers and to understand the limitations.[51]

INTRAOPERATIVE FLUID MANAGEMENT

As our understanding of perioperative fluid therapy evolves, intraoperative fluid therapy goals likewise change with available evidence. As stated earlier, the goal of fluid therapy is to optimize end-organ perfusion because both fluid overload and hypovolemia can lead to significant morbidity and mortality. Intraoperative fluids can broadly be divided into crystalloids and colloids. Blood product administration, also considered colloids, is discussed in another article in this issue. The composition of commonly available fluids is shown in **Table 1**.

Crystalloids: Balanced Solutions Versus Normal Saline

Crystalloid solutions are composed of water and electrolytes. These solutions can be further classified on the tonicity or on the strong ion difference (SID), defined as the

Table 1
Composition of commonly used fluids

Fluid	mOsm/L	pH	Na	Cl	K	Mg	Ca	Dextrose	Organic Anion	SID
Hypertonic										
3% Saline	1026	5.0	513	513	0	0	0	0	-	0
Isotonic										
0.9% Saline	308	5	154	154	0	0	0	0	-	0
Lactated Ringers	273	6.5	130	109	4	0	3	0	Lactate	27
Plasma-Lyte A	294	7.4	140	98	5	3	0	0	Acetate (27) Gluconate (23)	27–50
Plasma-Lyte 148 (Normosol-R)	294	5.5	145	98	5	3	0	0	Acetate (27) Gluconate (23)	27–50
Hypotonic										
Plasmalyte-56 in 5% dextrose	363	3.5–6	40	40	13	3	0	5	Acetate	
0.45% Sodium Chloride + 2.5% dextrose	280	4.5	77	77	0	0	0	25	-	
5% Dextrose in water	252	4	0	0	0	0	0	50	-	
0.45% Sodium chloride	154	5.6	77	77	0	0	0	0	-	

Colloid	mOsm/L	pH	Na	Cl	K	Mg	Ca	Dextrose	COP	SID
25% Albumin (human)			130–160						200–275	
5% Albumin (human)	255	6.7–7.3	130–160	100–130					23	

Abbreviations: Ca, calcium (mmol/L); Cl, chloride (mmol/L); COP, colloid osmotic pressure (mm Hg); K, potassium (mmol/L); Mg, magnesium (mmol/L); mOsm/L, osmolarity; Na, sodium (mmol/L); SID, strong ion difference.

difference between positively and negatively charged strong ions in plasma. Balanced crystalloids are solutions that maintain or normalize acid-base balance through their SID and are hence iso-osmotic and isotonic to plasma. Fluids having a normal or sub-normal chloride content may also be classified as balanced solutions. Commonly used 0.9% normal saline (NS) is an unbalanced isotonic crystalloid because its SID is 0 and has a nonphysiologic chloride concentration.

There is much literature comparing balanced crystalloids to NS. Yet, controversy exists regarding the ideal fluid for intraoperative adminstration.[52,53] Although balanced crystalloids have been associated with decreased risk of major adverse kidney events,[54] the recent PLUS (Plasma-Lyte 148 versus Saline, n = 5037) trial showed no overall mortality difference when using either balanced fluids or NS.[55] Similarly, the SPLIT (Saline vs Plasma-Lyte 148 for ICU fluid Therapy, n = 2278) trial found no difference in incidence of acute kidney injury in patients receiving either buffered solutions or NS in the intensive care unit (ICU), although this study may have been underpowered.[56] The recently published BaSICS (Balanced Solutions in Intensive Care Study, n = 10,520) trial also corroborates these findings, showing no difference in 90-day mortality with the use of either fluid in critically ill patients.[57] In contrast, the SMART (Isotonic Solutions and Major Adverse Renal Events, n = 15,802) trial found the use of balanced crystalloids in critically ill patients to result in lower rate of death, renal replacement therapy, or renal dysfunction when compared with saline.[58] Data are still lacking when it comes to choosing the particular organic anion to buffer the crystalloid (lactate vs acetate).[59] Concep-tually, the use of balanced solutions in patients who need a significant amount of intravenous fluids seems like an appropriate choice. Serum chloride is one of the parameters that could help guide the choice between NS and a balanced crystalloid.[60]

Crystalloids Versus Colloids

Albumin is the most widely used and most studied colloid in the current setting. The SAFE (Saline vs Albumin Fluid Evaluation) trial published in 2004 randomly assigned 6997 patients in the ICU to receive either 4% albumin or NS for fluid resuscitation.[61] Overall, no differences were observed between groups with regard to mortality or other secondary outcomes. Subgroup analysis, however, revealed a significant differ-ence in mortality among trauma patients who suffered a traumatic brain injury (TBI). Investigators later published the SAFE-TBI study, a posthoc analysis further evalu-ating the outcomes of the included patients with TBI.[62] The investigators again demonstrated a higher mortality rate, both at 28 days and 24 months, as well as fewer favorable neurologic outcomes for patients who received albumin.

Additional subgroup analysis of the SAFE trial revealed a higher relative risk of death in patients with severe sepsis who received saline for resuscitation. The ALBIOS (AL-Bumin Italian Outcome Sepsis) trial further evaluated patients with severe sepsis, randomly assigning 1818 patients to receive 20% albumin with crystalloids or crystal-loids alone.[63] The investigators found no difference in mortality or any of their second-ary outcomes. A posthoc analysis based on patient severity with septic shock receiving albumin to correct hypoalbuminemia, however, did show a decreased risk of mortality.[63]

In the cardiac surgery population, there are some data to suggest that albumin administration might increase the incidence of acute kidney injury.[64] A larger retro-spective study did not corroborate these findings and in fact showed an association between albumin administration and improved in-hospital mortality.[65] Randomized tri-als are needed to appropriately address the implications of albumin use in this population. Given the lack of proven benefit and higher cost, crystalloids are still considered first line for resuscitation. However, there is a recommendation to consider albumin in patients who have received large-volume crystalloid resuscitation, as described in the newest Surviving Sepsis Guidelines.[24]

LIBERAL VERSUS RESTRICTIVE FLUID MANAGEMENT

There has been much variability in the practice of intraoperative fluid administration over the past 2 decades.[66] Historically, replacement of both preoperative fasting deficits and intraoperative volume losses accounted for high intraoperative fluid administration. Outcomes related to intraoperative fluid management began surfacing more than 20 years ago, prompting changes in practice and further research into the topic.[67–70] Liberal fluid techniques were associated with increased perioperative morbidity, hospital costs, and length of stay (LOS).[71] Since then, many trials were conducted to compare liberal versus restrictive fluid strategies. Owing to the variability in study designs, however, it is difficult to precisely define what constitutes each fluid strategy. The most widely understood definition of restrictive and liberal fluid management comes from Brandstrup and colleagues[68] in which the liberal fluid administration group gained 4 kg by the first postoperative day compared with 1 kg weight gain in the restrictive group. In addition, the types of fluids administered differ among studies with some strategies using colloid solutions preferentially over crystalloids, and vice versa.

Evidence for Liberal Versus Restrictive Fluid Strategies

The recently conducted RELIEF (Restrictive vs Liberal Fluid Therapy in Major Abdominal Surgery) trial was the largest randomized controlled trial (RCT) evaluating fluid strategies in high-risk patients undergoing major abdominal surgery. The results showed a restrictive fluid strategy was noninferior to liberal fluid administration in terms of overall 1-year survival, but patients in the restrictive group had a higher incidence of acute kidney injury.[72] Median amount of intraoperative crystalloid administration was 1677 mL in the restrictive group versus 3000 mL in the liberal group (median cumulative fluids at 24 hours postsurgery was 3671 mL vs 6146 mL). In a subsequent meta-analysis including 18 RCTs, Messina and colleagues[73] found no difference in early or late postoperative mortality between liberal and restrictive fluid strategies in patients undergoing elective abdominal surgery. The median intraoperative fluid administered was 1925 mL in the restrictive group and 3878 mL in the liberal group. Pooled results from 8 studies, however, showed an association of major renal events with a restrictive fluid approach.

These studies show the evidence to be rather inconclusive when comparing the 2 fluid replacement strategies. Despite this, many national societies have advocated for a more restrictive fluid strategy. In addition, Enhanced Recovery After Surgery (ERAS) programs have included restrictive fluid strategies in their pathways, advocating for a "zero-balance" fluid goal.[74,75] Furthermore, for high-risk surgical patients, ERAS guidelines support the use of goal-directed fluid therapy techniques, a concept that is discussed in more detail in later sections.[76,77] A uniformly restrictive approach to intraoperative fluid management fails to consider baseline comorbidities and ongoing fluid losses, both of which are actively managed in the operating room.

GOAL-DIRECTED FLUID THERAPY

The concept of perioperative goal-directed therapy (GDT) has been proposed to provide objective goals for fluid administration during the perioperative period. By using assessments of dynamic parameters based on the patient's hemodynamics and CO, fluid therapy can be augmented in real time. This strategy is thus tailored individually to address each patient's clinical need and help optimize oxygen delivery and tissue perfusion. A predefined algorithm is generally used to determine when a fluid bolus may be necessary (**Fig. 3**). If SVV, for example, remains greater than 13% for 5 to 10 minutes, this may be an indication that the patient may benefit from additional fluid administration. A small bolus of either crystalloid or colloid can then be given to assess the response on SVV and improvement in hemodynamics. If blood pressure remains low with no change in SVV, the patient is likely not fluid responsive (or on the "flat" portion of the Frank-Starling curve) and may instead benefit from vasopressors or inotropes to augment the hemodynamics.

Evidence for Goal-Directed Fluid Therapy

As with the differing fluid strategies described earlier, the evidence for GDT is somewhat ambiguous. In a 2012 meta-analysis of 34 RCTs, Corcoran and colleagues[78] found that GDT was associated with a reduction in perioperative complications. The trials reviewed included 23 studies that compared GDT with normal care and 11 studies that compared liberal with restrictive fluid administration. When comparing these 2 cohorts, they found similar amounts of fluid administered in the GDT and liberal fluid groups, but that liberal use of fluids without the aid of dynamic parameters was associated with increased LOS, time to return of bowel function, and risk of pneumonia. Similarly, Benes and colleagues[79] found decreased postoperative morbidity (reductions in cardiovascular, abdominal, and infectious complications) and ICU LOS with GDT.

Results of the OPTIMISE (Optimization of Cardiovascular Management to Improve Surgical Outcomes) trial, however, did not corroborate these findings. The study was a large RCT comparing GDT with normal care in patients undergoing major gastrointestinal surgery.[80] The investigators found no significant differences in 30-day

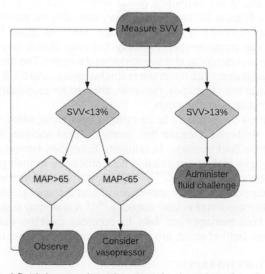

Fig. 3. Goal-directed fluid therapy algorithm. Sample algorithm of goal-directed fluid therapy based on stroke volume variation (SVV). If SVV maintains greater than 13% for more than 5 to 10 minutes, a fluid bolus can be administered. Fluid challenge may consist of 250 mL bolus of crystalloid or colloid. MAP, mean arterial pressure.

complications or mortality between groups, thus questioning the utility of GDT. When the investigators analyzed this trial in the context of 37 other trials, they found GDT to be associated with reduced incidence of postoperative infection and decrease in hospital LOS.

A recent meta-analysis concluded that GDT reduced overall postoperative complications but had no effect on perioperative mortality.[81] There was little difference between the amount of fluids actually administered intraoperatively between the GDT and control subgroups (GDT subgroup received a mean of 1632 mL crystalloids and 1053 mL colloids, whereas the control group received a mean of 1977 mL crystalloids and 758 mL colloids).[81] This observation reiterates the findings of Corcoran and colleagues,[78] emphasizing that hemodynamic-driven fluid therapy through GDT leads to improved outcomes over a strategy without the use of these guiding parameters. Notably, there is great heterogeneity in many of these studies making it difficult to truly compare interventions and outcomes. The devices, algorithms, hemodynamic targets, and fluid type all differ greatly, making overall generalizability low.[82,83] At present, most evidence points to a reduction in perioperative morbidity with the use of GDT. Cost-benefit analyses have also shown GDT to be a cost-effective modality, further advocating for this intervention in a high-risk surgical population.[84] Large randomized trials are needed to further solidify the evidence and show definitive benefits of GDT.

PERIOPERATIVE DERESUSCITATION

A discussion around fluid administration during the perioperative period would be incomplete without a brief overview of "deresuscitation." First coined in 2014, deresuscitation involves the active and aggressive fluid removal in the postoperative period with diuretics or renal replacement therapy[85]; this follows the initial phases of fluid therapy as described by the ROSE concept (**Fig. 4**): Resuscitation, Optimization, Stabilization, and Evacuation (deresuscitation). This model described by Malbrain and colleagues[86] was created to illustrate the dynamic phases of fluid therapy. Fluid overload can lead to increased morbidity and should thus be addressed in the postoperative period when deemed appropriate. There is also some evidence that diuresis favors recruitment of the microcirculation.[87] Multiple approaches have been

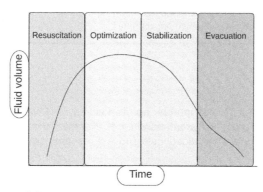

Fig. 4. The 4 phases of fluid therapy as described by the ROSE concept. Resuscitation is marked by fluid administration to achieve hemodynamic goals followed by optimization phase, aiming for a neutral fluid balance. The stabilization phase is marked by organ-specific support, beginning to achieve a negative fluid balance, which is further continued in the evacuation phase. The time frame of this cycle can range from days to weeks.

described for deresuscitation such as albumin-aided diuresis, but more evidence is needed to determine the timing and goals of deresuscitation. Furthermore, it is essential to define clinical end points, goals for vasopressor use, assessment of renal function, and daily reevaluation and adjustment based on patient response.[85]

SUMMARY

Optimizing perioperative fluid therapy is important to improve surgical morbidity and mortality. Even though extensive research has been done on this topic, controversy still exists on the ideal methods to assess which patients would benefit from fluid administration and how much fluid is needed to avoid postoperative complications while at the same time improving tissue oxygenation. The debate between liberal versus conservative fluid administration strategies continues, and well-conducted large-scale trials with clearly-defined fluid administration plans and outcomes are eagerly awaited. Similarly, the choice of fluid during the perioperative period remains a topic of discussion. Crystalloids are preferred as the initial choice, and colloids such as albumin are reserved for procedures with significant blood loss to avoid excessive administration of crystalloids. Recent evidence from the critical care setting strongly points toward a benefit for choosing balanced fluids over NS. GDT-based algorithmic approaches toward fluid administration have shown improvements in outcomes in recent trials and need further exploration. Furthermore, the concept of perioperative "fluid deresuscitation" also needs to be evaluated before recommending routine use in the perioperative setting.

CLINICS CARE POINTS

- Dynamic parameters of volume assessment, such as SVV or PPV, can help guide fluid management during the perioperative period.

- In patients who require significant amounts of intravenous fluids, balanced crystalloid solutions may be more appropriate than NS.

- Neither a restrictive nor a liberal fluid strategy has been shown to improve outcomes, but hemodynamic-driven GDT with the use of dynamic indices may lead to improvement in perioperative outcomes.

- Fluid overload can lead to increased morbidity and should thus be addressed in the postoperative period when deemed appropriate.

DISCLOSURE

J. Elia: no disclosures; R. Deshpande: no disclosures; M. Diwan: no disclosures; J. Brainard: no disclosures; K. Karamchandani: K. Karamchandani is on the scientific advisory board of Eagle pharmaceuticals and is a research advisor for Philips.

REFERENCES

1. Bellamy MC. Wet, dry or something else? Br J Anaesth 2006;97:755–7.
2. Doherty M, Buggy DJ. Intraoperative fluids: how much is too much? Br J Anaesth 2012;109:69–79.
3. Holte K, Sharrock NE, Kehlet H. Pathophysiology and clinical implications of perioperative fluid excess. Br J Anaesth 2002;89:622–32.

4. Junghans T, Neuss H, Strohauer M, et al. Hypovolemia after traditional preoperative care in patients undergoing colonic surgery is underrepresented in conventional hemodynamic monitoring. Int J Colorectal Dis 2006;21:693–7.
5. Güenaga KF, Matos D, Wille-Jørgensen P. Mechanical bowel preparation for elective colorectal surgery. Cochrane Database Syst Rev 2011;9:CD001544.
6. Holte K. Pathophysiology and clinical implications of peroperative fluid management in elective surgery. Dan Med Bull 2010;57:B4156.
7. Reithner L, Johansson H, Strouth L. Insensible perspiration during anaesthesia and surgery. Acta Anaesthesiol Scand 1980;24:362–6.
8. Lamke LO, Nilsson GE, Reithner HL. Water loss by evaporation from the abdominal cavity during surgery. Acta Chir Scand 1977;143:279–84.
9. Danielsson EJD, Lejbman I, Åkeson J. Fluid deficits during prolonged overnight fasting in young healthy adults. Acta Anaesthesiol Scand 2019;63:195–9.
10. Mendelson CL. The aspiration of stomach contents into the lungs during obstetric anesthesia. Am J Obstet Gynecol 1946;52:191–205.
11. Brady M, Kinn S, Stuart P. Preoperative fasting for adults to prevent perioperative complications. Cochrane Database Syst Rev 2003;4:CD004423.
12. Maltby JR, Sutherland AD, Sale JP, et al. Preoperative oral fluids: is a five-hour fast justified prior to elective surgery? Anesth Analg 1986;65:1112–6.
13. Okabe T, Terashima H, Sakamoto A. A comparison of gastric emptying of soluble solid meals and clear fluids matched for volume and energy content: a pilot crossover study. Anaesthesia 2017;72:1344–50.
14. Van de Putte P, Vernieuwe L, Jerjir A, et al. When fasted is not empty: a retrospective cohort study of gastric content in fasted surgical patientsdagger. Br J Anaesth 2017;118:363–71.
15. Practice guidelines for preoperative fasting and the use of pharmacologic agents to reduce the risk of pulmonary aspiration: application to healthy patients undergoing elective procedures: an updated report by the american society of anesthesiologists task force on preoperative fasting and the use of pharmacologic agents to reduce the risk of pulmonary aspiration. Anesthesiology 2017;126:376–93.
16. Smith I, Kranke P, Murat I, et al, European Society of A. Perioperative fasting in adults and children: guidelines from the European Society of Anaesthesiology. Eur J Anaesthesiol 2011;28:556–69.
17. Thomas M, Morrison C, Newton R, et al. Consensus statement on clear fluids fasting for elective pediatric general anesthesia. Paediatr Anaesth 2018;28:411–4.
18. Morrison CE, Ritchie-McLean S, Jha A, et al. Two hours too long: time to review fasting guidelines for clear fluids. Br J Anaesth 2020;S0007-0912(19):31004–9.
19. Han JC, Pham T, Taberner AJ, et al. Solving a century-old conundrum underlying cardiac force-length relations. Am J Physiol Heart Circ Physiol 2019;316:H781–93.
20. Marik PE, Monnet X, Teboul JL. Hemodynamic parameters to guide fluid therapy. Ann Intensive Care 2011;1:1.
21. Marik PE, Cavallazzi R. Does the central venous pressure predict fluid responsiveness? An updated meta-analysis and a plea for some common sense. Crit Care Med 2013;41:1774–81.
22. Vincent JL, Weil MH. Fluid challenge revisited. Crit Care Med 2006;34:1333–7.
23. Michard F, Teboul JL. Predicting fluid responsiveness in ICU patients: a critical analysis of the evidence. Chest 2002;121:2000–8.

24. Evans L, Rhodes A, Alhazzani W, et al. Surviving Sepsis Campaign: International Guidelines for management of sepsis and septic shock 2021. Crit Care Med 2021;49:e1063–143.
25. Bentzer P, Griesdale DE, Boyd J, et al. Will This Hemodynamically Unstable Patient Respond to a Bolus of Intravenous Fluids? JAMA 2016;316:1298–309.
26. Kumar A, Anel R, Bunnell E, et al. Pulmonary artery occlusion pressure and central venous pressure fail to predict ventricular filling volume, cardiac performance, or the response to volume infusion in normal subjects. Crit Care Med 2004;32:691–9.
27. Osman D, Ridel C, Ray P, et al. Cardiac filling pressures are not appropriate to predict hemodynamic response to volume challenge. Crit Care Med 2007; 35:64–8.
28. Michard F, Teboul JL. Using heart-lung interactions to assess fluid responsiveness during mechanical ventilation. Crit Care 2000;4:282–9.
29. Sibbald WJ, Keenan SP. Show me the evidence: a critical appraisal of the Pulmonary Artery Catheter Consensus Conference and other musings on how critical care practitioners need to improve the way we conduct business. Crit Care Med 1997;25:2060–3.
30. Marik PE, Cavallazzi R, Vasu T, et al. Dynamic changes in arterial waveform derived variables and fluid responsiveness in mechanically ventilated patients: a systematic review of the literature. Crit Care Med 2009;37:2642–7.
31. Mathis MR, Schechtman SA, Engoren MC, et al. Arterial Pressure Variation in Elective Noncardiac Surgery: Identifying Reference Distributions and Modifying Factors. Anesthesiology 2017;126:249–59.
32. Dorje P, Tremper KK. Systolic pressure variation: a dynamic measure of the adequacy of intravascular volume, Issue 3 edition. Seminars in Anesthesia. Perioper Med Pain 2005;24(3):147–53.
33. Perel A, Pizov R, Cotev S. Systolic blood pressure variation is a sensitive indicator of hypovolemia in ventilated dogs subjected to graded hemorrhage. Anesthesiology 1987;67:498–502.
34. Tavernier B, Makhotine O, Lebuffe G, et al. Systolic pressure variation as a guide to fluid therapy in patients with sepsis-induced hypotension. Anesthesiology 1998;89:1313–21.
35. Lopes MR, Oliveira MA, Pereira VO, et al. Goal-directed fluid management based on pulse pressure variation monitoring during high-risk surgery: a pilot randomized controlled trial. Crit Care 2007;11:R100.
36. Michard F, Boussat S, Chemla D, et al. Relation between respiratory changes in arterial pulse pressure and fluid responsiveness in septic patients with acute circulatory failure. Am J Respir Crit Care Med 2000;162:134–8.
37. Denault AY, Gasior TA, Gorcsan J, et al. Determinants of aortic pressure variation during positive-pressure ventilation in man. Chest 1999;116:176–86.
38. Soubrier S, Saulnier F, Hubert H, et al. Can dynamic indicators help the prediction of fluid responsiveness in spontaneously breathing critically ill patients? Intensive Care Med 2007;33:1117–24.
39. Partridge BL. Use of pulse oximetry as a noninvasive indicator of intravascular volume status. J Clin Monit 1987;3:263–8.
40. Chu H, Wang Y, Sun Y, et al. Accuracy of pleth variability index to predict fluid responsiveness in mechanically ventilated patients: a systematic review and meta-analysis. J Clin Monit Comput 2016;30:265–74.
41. Cannesson M, Desebbe O, Rosamel P, et al. Pleth variability index to monitor the respiratory variations in the pulse oximeter plethysmographic waveform

amplitude and predict fluid responsiveness in the operating theatre. Br J Anaesth 2008;101:200–6.

42. Cannesson M, Besnard C, Durand PG, et al. Relation between respiratory variations in pulse oximetry plethysmographic waveform amplitude and arterial pulse pressure in ventilated patients. Crit Care 2005;9:R562–8.

43. Zhang Z, Lu B, Sheng X, et al. Accuracy of stroke volume variation in predicting fluid responsiveness: a systematic review and meta-analysis. J Anesth 2011;25:904–16.

44. Hadian M, Kim HK, Severyn DA, et al. Cross-comparison of cardiac output trending accuracy of LiDCO, PiCCO, FloTrac and pulmonary artery catheters. Crit Care 2010;14:R212.

45. Uchino S, Bellomo R, Morimatsu H, et al. Pulmonary artery catheter versus pulse contour analysis: a prospective epidemiological study. Crit Care 2006;10:R174.

46. Ciozda W, Kedan I, Kehl DW, et al. The efficacy of sonographic measurement of inferior vena cava diameter as an estimate of central venous pressure. Cardiovasc Ultrasound 2016;14:33.

47. Orso D, Paoli I, Piani T, et al. Accuracy of ultrasonographic measurements of inferior vena cava to determine fluid responsiveness: a systematic review and meta-analysis. J Intensive Care Med 2020;35:354–63.

48. Long E, Oakley E, Duke T, et al. PRiEDIC: Does respiratory variation in inferior vena cava diameter predict fluid responsiveness: a systematic review and meta-analysis. Shock 2017;47:550–9.

49. Si X. Meta-analysis of ventilated versus spontaneously breathing patients in predicting fluid responsiveness by inferior vena cava variation. In: Cao D, Xu H, Guan X, editors. International journal of clinical medicine. 2018.

50. Zhang Z, Xu X, Ye S, et al. Ultrasonographic measurement of the respiratory variation in the inferior vena cava diameter is predictive of fluid responsiveness in critically ill patients: systematic review and meta-analysis. Ultrasound Med Biol 2014;40:845–53.

51. Via G, Tavazzi G, Price S. Ten situations where inferior vena cava ultrasound may fail to accurately predict fluid responsiveness: a physiologically based point of view. Intensive Care Med 2016;42:1164–7.

52. Antequera Martin AM, Barea Mendoza JA, Muriel A, et al. Buffered solutions versus 0.9% saline for resuscitation in critically ill adults and children. Cochrane Database Syst Rev 2019;7:CD012247.

53. Gottlieb M, Petrak V, Binkley C. Are balanced crystalloid solutions better than normal saline solution for the resuscitation of children and adult patients? Ann Emerg Med 2020;75:532–4.

54. Self WH, Semler MW, Wanderer JP, et al. Investigators S-E: balanced crystalloids versus saline in noncritically ill adults. N Engl J Med 2018;378:819–28.

55. Finfer S, Micallef S, Hammond N, et al. Australian New zealand intensive care society clinical trials g: balanced multielectrolyte solution versus saline in critically ill adults. N Engl J Med 2022;386:815–26.

56. Young P, Bailey M, Beasley R, et al. Effect of a buffered crystalloid solution vs saline on acute kidney injury among patients in the intensive care unit: the split randomized clinical trial. JAMA 2015;314:1701–10.

57. Zampieri FG, Machado FR, Biondi RS, et al. Effect of intravenous fluid treatment with a balanced solution vs 0.9% saline solution on mortality in critically ill patients: the basics randomized clinical trial. JAMA 2021;326(9):1–12.

58. Semler MW, Self WH, Wanderer JP, et al. balanced crystalloids versus saline in critically ill adults. N Engl J Med 2018;378:829–39.

59. Pfortmueller CA, Faeh L, Muller M, et al. Fluid management in patients undergoing cardiac surgery: effects of an acetate- versus lactate-buffered balanced infusion solution on hemodynamic stability (HEMACETAT). Crit Care 2019;23:159.
60. Malbrain M, Langer T, Annane D, et al. Intravenous fluid therapy in the perioperative and critical care setting: executive summary of the international fluid academy (IFA). Ann Intensive Care 2020;10:64.
61. Finfer S, Bellomo R, Boyce N, et al. A comparison of albumin and saline for fluid resuscitation in the intensive care unit. N Engl J Med 2004;350:2247–56.
62. Myburgh J, Cooper DJ, Finfer S, et al. Saline or albumin for fluid resuscitation in patients with traumatic brain injury. N Engl J Med 2007;357:874–84.
63. Caironi P, Tognoni G, Masson S, et al. Albumin replacement in patients with severe sepsis or septic shock. N Engl J Med 2014;370:1412–21.
64. Frenette AJ, Bouchard J, Bernier P, et al. Albumin administration is associated with acute kidney injury in cardiac surgery: a propensity score analysis. Crit Care 2014;18:602.
65. Kingeter AJ, Raghunathan K, Munson SH, et al. Association between albumin administration and survival in cardiac surgery: a retrospective cohort study. Can J Anaesth 2018;65:1218–27.
66. Thacker JK, Mountford WK, Ernst FR, et al. perioperative fluid utilization variability and association with outcomes: considerations for enhanced recovery efforts in sample us surgical populations. Ann Surg 2016;263:502–10.
67. Tambyraja AL, Sengupta F, MacGregor AB, et al. Patterns and clinical outcomes associated with routine intravenous sodium and fluid administration after colorectal resection. World J Surg 2004;28:1046–51 ; discussion 1051-2.
68. Brandstrup B, Tønnesen H, Beier-Holgersen R, et al. Therapy DSGoPF: effects of intravenous fluid restriction on postoperative complications: comparison of two perioperative fluid regimens: a randomized assessor-blinded multicenter trial. Ann Surg 2003;238:641–8.
69. Lobo DN, Bostock KA, Neal KR, et al. Effect of salt and water balance on recovery of gastrointestinal function after elective colonic resection: a randomised controlled trial. Lancet 2002;359:1812–8.
70. Nisanevich V, Felsenstein I, Almogy G, et al. Effect of intraoperative fluid management on outcome after intraabdominal surgery. Anesthesiology 2005;103:25–32.
71. Shin CH, Long DR, McLean D, et al. Effects of intraoperative fluid management on postoperative outcomes: a hospital registry study. Ann Surg 2018;267:1084–92.
72. Myles PS, Bellomo R, Corcoran T, et al. Restrictive versus Liberal Fluid Therapy for Major Abdominal Surgery. N Engl J Med 2018;378:2263–74.
73. Messina A, Robba C, Calabro L, et al. Perioperative liberal versus restrictive fluid strategies and postoperative outcomes: a systematic review and metanalysis on randomised-controlled trials in major abdominal elective surgery. Crit Care 2021;25:205.
74. Gustafsson UO, Scott MJ, Hubner M, et al. Guidelines for perioperative care in elective colorectal surgery: enhanced recovery after surgery (ERAS. World J Surg 2019;43:659–95.
75. Melloul E, Lassen K, Roulin D, et al. Guidelines for perioperative care for pancreatoduodenectomy: enhanced recovery after surgery (ERAS) recommendations 2019. World J Surg 2020;44:2056–84.
76. Nelson G, Bakkum-Gamez J, Kalogera E, et al. Guidelines for perioperative care in gynecologic/oncology: enhanced recovery after surgery (ERAS) society recommendations-2019 update. Int J Gynecol Cancer 2019;29:651–68.

77. Engelman DT, Ben Ali W, Williams JB, et al. Guidelines for perioperative care in cardiac surgery: enhanced recovery after surgery society recommendations. JAMA Surg 2019;154:755–66.
78. Corcoran T, Rhodes JE, Clarke S, et al. Perioperative fluid management strategies in major surgery: a stratified meta-analysis. Anesth Analg 2012;114:640–51.
79. Benes J, Giglio M, Brienza N, et al. The effects of goal-directed fluid therapy based on dynamic parameters on post-surgical outcome: a meta-analysis of randomized controlled trials. Crit Care 2014;18:584.
80. Pearse RM, Harrison DA, MacDonald N, et al. Effect of a perioperative, cardiac output-guided hemodynamic therapy algorithm on outcomes following major gastrointestinal surgery: a randomized clinical trial and systematic review. JAMA 2014;311:2181–90.
81. Messina A, Robba C, Calabro L, et al. Association between perioperative fluid administration and postoperative outcomes: a 20-year systematic review and a meta-analysis of randomized goal-directed trials in major visceral/noncardiac surgery. Crit Care 2021;25:43.
82. Chong MA, Wang Y, Berbenetz NM, et al. Does goal-directed haemodynamic and fluid therapy improve peri-operative outcomes?: A systematic review and meta-analysis. Eur J Anaesthesiol 2018;35:469–83.
83. Wrzosek A, Jakowicka-Wordliczek J, Zajaczkowska R, et al. Perioperative restrictive versus goal-directed fluid therapy for adults undergoing major non-cardiac surgery. Cochrane Database Syst Rev 2019;12:CD012767.
84. Ebm CC, Sutton L, Rhodes A, et al. Cost-effectiveness in goal-directed therapy: are the dollars spent worth the value? J Cardiothorac Vasc Anesth 2014;28:1660–6.
85. Malbrain MLNG, Langer T, Annane D, et al. Intravenous fluid therapy in the perioperative and critical care setting: executive summary of the International Fluid Academy (IFA). Ann Intensive Care 2020;10:64.
86. Malbrain MLNG, Van Regenmortel N, Saugel B, et al. Principles of fluid management and stewardship in septic shock: it is time to consider the four D's and the four phases of fluid therapy. Ann Intensive Care 2018;8:66.
87. Uz Z, Ince C, Guerci P, et al. Recruitment of sublingual microcirculation using handheld incident dark field imaging as a routine measurement tool during the postoperative de-escalation phase-a pilot study in post ICU cardiac surgery patients. Perioper Med (Lond) 2018;7:18.

Acute Kidney Injury and Renal Replacement Therapy

A Review and Update for the Perioperative Physician

Christopher W. Tam, MD[a],*, Shreyajit R. Kumar, MD[b],
Jarva Chow, MD, MS MPH[c]

KEYWORDS

- Acute kidney injury • Intensive care unit • Length of stay
- Acute dialysis quality initiative • RIFLE • Hyperthermic intraperitoneal chemotherapy
- Acute renal failure

KEY POINTS

- Acute kidney injury is a common postoperative complication with significant associated morbidity and mortality.
- Standardized definitions and diagnosis criteria (e.g. RIFLE Criteria, AKIN, KDIGO) are flawed.
- Biomarkers may be able to detect and allow the early diagnosis of AKI, however, further research is needed.
- Understanding indications of intraoperative renal replacement therapy is necessary to manage patients with severe electrolyte abnormalities, massive fluid overload or uremia.

INTRODUCTION

Perioperative acute kidney injury (AKI) is an underrecognized complication affecting patients undergoing cardiac and noncardiac surgery. Postoperative AKI is estimated to occur in 18% to 47% of patients.[1] Intensive care unit (ICU) patients admitted after elective surgery incur a 52% incidence of AKI in the first week of admission, with an even higher incidence in patients admitted after emergency surgery.[1,2] Mortality increases with worsening RIFLE classification, an acronym denoting a multilevel classification system inclusive of the complete spectrum of acute renal dysfunction: *Risk* of

[a] Department of Anesthesiology, Montefiore Medical Center, 111 East 210th Street, Bronx, NY 10467, USA; [b] Department of Anesthesiology, Weill Cornell Medical Center, New York Presbyterian-Hospital, 525 East 68th Street, New York, NY 10065, USA; [c] Department of Anesthesia and Critical Care, University of Chicago, 5841 South Maryland Avenue, Chicago, IL 60637, USA
* Corresponding author.
E-mail address: CTam@montefiore.org

Anesthesiology Clin 41 (2023) 211–230
https://doi.org/10.1016/j.anclin.2022.10.004
1932-2275/23/© 2022 Elsevier Inc. All rights reserved.
anesthesiology.theclinics.com

renal dysfunction, *Injury* to the kidney, *Failure* or *Loss* of kidney function, and *End-stage* kidney disease.[3] Mortality rates in one systematic review were 18.9% in patients qualifying for risk, 36.1% in Injury and 46% in failure.[3] AKI results in increased hospital length of stay (LOS) and increased health-care expenditure.[4–6] Identifying patients at higher risk for postoperative AKI and using a multidisciplinary approach to management and treatment may lead to reduction in both LOS and health-care costs. Biomarkers may facilitate earlier detection and allow proactive nephroprotection.

DIAGNOSIS

AKI is characterized by a rapid decline in kidney function, alongside a buildup of nitrogenous waste products. This definition, however, is fraught by a lack of consensus in the literature. This has resulted in a wide spectrum of reported incidence of AKI and has presented an obstacle for comparative research.[7] The Acute Dialysis Quality Initiative (ADQI) standardized the definition of acute renal failure (ARF) by developing the risk, injury, failure, loss, and end-stage renal disease (RIFLE) criteria in 2004.[8] This is a multilevel schematic, classifying the severity of a patient's renal failure based on changes in discrete variables (serum creatinine, urine output) during a 1-week period (**Fig. 1**).[9] As a patient's classification worsens, the in-hospital mortality increases.[10] The RIFLE criteria was the initial step in creating a concise definition for ARF. It is, however, an imperfect system that may miss early stages of renal failure and may not report an accurate incidence of ARF.[7,10] In 2007, the Acute Kidney Injury Network (AKIN) updated the definition of ARF based on new evidence that minute changes in creatinine had a profound association with mortality[10,11] (see **Fig. 1**). This AKIN criteria enhanced sensitivity by lowering the change in serum creatinine to 0.3 mg/dL within 48 hours as a marker for the presence of AKI.[9] The AKIN group also proposed the use of the term *injury* rather than *failure* to encompass overall disease progression.[9] The 3 stages of AKIN correlate with RIFLE classification. Stage 1 is analogous to *Risk*, whereas stage 2 is similar to *Injury* and stage 3 parallels *Failure*. Furthermore, the AKIN criteria omitted the *Loss* and *End-stage* category of the RIFLE criteria, as these reflect AKI outcomes rather than AKI diagnosis.[9] The RIFLE and AKIN criteria have been validated in multiple studies but neither has proven

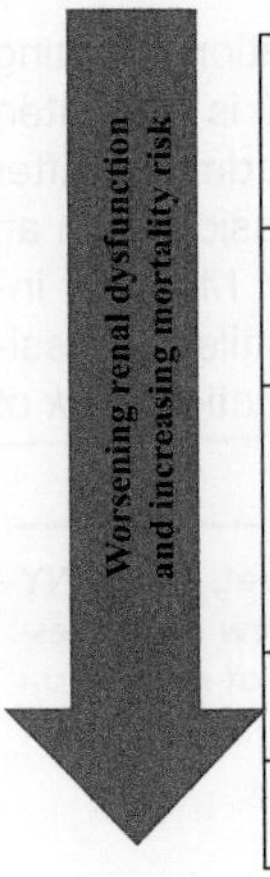

	RIFLE- 2004	AKIN- 2007	KDIGO-2012
'**R**'isk/Stage 1	Serum Creatinine 1.5x baseline within 7 d or > 25% decrease GFR +/- UOP<0.5 ml/kg/hr x 6 h	Serum Creatinine 1.5–2x baseline within 7 d or ≥0.3 mg/dL increase within 48 hours +/- UOP<0.5 ml/kg/hr x 6 hours	Serum Creatinine 1.5–1.9x baseline within 7 d or ≥0.3 mg/dL increase within 48 h +/ - UOP<0.5 ml/kg/hr x 6 h
'**I**'njury/Stage 2	Serum Creatinine 2x baseline or >50% decrease GFR +/- UOP<0.5 ml/kg/hr x 12 h	Serum Creatinine 2-3x baseline +/- UOP<0.5 ml/kg/hr x 12 h	Serum Creatinine 2–2.9x baseline +/- UOP<0.5 ml/kg/hr x 12 h
'**F**'ailure/Stage 3	Serum Creatinine 3x baseline or >75% decrease GFR or Creatinine ≥4 +/- UOP<0.3 ml/kg/hr x 24 hours or anuria x 12 h	Serum Creatinine >3x baseline or Serum Creatinine ≥4 or start of RRT +/- UOP<0.3 ml/kg/hr x 24 h or anuria x 12 h	Serum Creatinine 3x baseline or increase serum creatinine ≥4 (≥0.3 mg/dL increase in 48 h or 1.5x above baseline) or start of RRT +/- UOP<0.3 ml/kg/hr x 24 h or anuria x 12 h
'**L**'oss	>4 wk loss of renal function		
'**E**'nd-stage Renal Disease (ESRD)	>3 mo loss of renal function		

Fig. 1. RIFLE versus AKIN versus KDIGO classification.[8,10,12]

superior in risk stratification or mortality reduction.[8] In 2012, the Kidney Disease: Improving Global Outcomes group (KDIGO) published a third classification criterion: a summation RIFLE and AKIN[12] (see **Fig. 1**). This diagnosed AKI by an increase in serum creatinine of 0.3 mg/dL or greater within 48 hours (AKIN) and a 50% or greater increase in baseline serum creatinine within 7 days (RIFLE).[13] The broader definition aimed to improve sensitivity and facilitate early AKI diagnosis. A large retrospective study evaluated the prognostic accuracy of all 3 classification systems and found that RIFLE and KDIGO were superior to AKIN in AKI detection and in-hospital mortality prediction.[14]

These standardized AKI definitions are flawed and may not reflect real-time renal function. Hourly urine output may fluctuate due to nonrenal causes such as cardiogenic shock and nonoliguric ATN (urine output may be normal despite significant renal injury).[8] Serum creatinine, a surrogate for glomerular filtration rate (GFR), is a similarly flawed marker of real-time renal function[8] and is a delayed marker of real-time GFR. Significant renal injury can incur before a creatinine increase and can be further influenced by volume status.[15] Urine output and serum creatinine remain easily accessible until further refinements in biomarker research are discovered.

PATHOPHYSIOLOGY

Causes of AKI have historically been subdivided into prerenal, intrarenal, or postrenal causes. However, AKI is often a continuum as prerenal injury progresses to intrinsic AKI.[16] Overall, AKI is a complex process mediated by hypoperfusion, inflammation, and neuroendocrine activation. Systemic inflammation results from an interplay of renal microcirculatory dysfunction, renin-angiotensin-aldosterone system, oxidative stress, and cytokine-induced endothelial and tubular injury. Additionally, endogenous vasoconstrictors decrease afferent arteriole renal flow, resulting in renal tubular ischemia and diminished oxygen.[17–21]

Drugs also damage various portions of the nephron, with the tubules experiencing the greatest exposure. Injury patterns are varied and include intratubular crystal deposition, immune dysregulation, acute glomerular injury, vasoconstrictive vascular damage, thrombotic microangiopathy, mitochondrial injury, and oxidative stress.[17,22] Nonsteroidal anti-inflammatory drugs (NSAIDs) and proton pump inhibitors are implicated in drug-induced acute tubulointerstitial nephritis.[17] Crystal precipitation is seen from ciprofloxacin, vancomycin, and several antivirals. Myoglobin and hemoglobin can also act as endotoxins.[17,22]

Table 1 Risk factors[19–22,24–26]	
Age	Major Surgery
Gender	Surgical duration
Preoperative renal function	Emergency surgery
Diabetes	Respiratory insufficiency
Obesity	Peripheral vascular disease
Hypertension	Congestive heart failure
Anemia	Sepsis
Transfusions	Medication use (ie, renin angiotensin aldosterone blockade, diuretics, ACEI, antimicrobials)
Chronic liver disease and ascites	Intraoperative hypotension
Hypoalbuminemia	
Hyponatremia	

Vancomycin, frequently used for surgical prophylaxis, is a well-known nephrotoxin. AKI generally occurs 4 to 8 days after therapy causing proximal tubular injury, acute tubular necrosis (ATN), and drug-induced acute tubulointerstitial nephritis.[17,22,23] Osmotic activity from polysaccharides, starch infusions, and mannitol may result in epithelial cell swelling, tubular lumen occlusion, and AKI from osmotic nephropathy.[17,24]

RISK FACTORS
Patient-Specific Risks

Risk factors for perioperative AKI include age, gender, preoperative renal function, surgical factors, obesity, and hypertension (**Table 1**).[19–22,24–28] Risk factors for persistent advanced chronic kidney disease (CKD) overlaps significantly with general AKI: preoperative renal function, diabetes mellitus, and hypertension. Slower recovery from AKI is also associated with worse outcomes.[25,26]

Modifiable risk factors such as preoperative medication use, weight, and intraoperative hemodynamics, and medication exposure may mitigate postoperative AKI.[19] Obesity, for example, is commensurate with oxidative stress, proinflammatory cytokines, and endothelial dysfunction.[19]

Medication Factors

Aminoglycosides result in a dose-dependent reduction in kidney function in 10% to 25% of patients.[17,22,29] Fluoroquinolones, beta lactams, and vancomycin cause acute glomerulonephritis, acute interstitial nephritis, and ATN.[17,22,29] Piperacillin-tazobactam combination therapy significantly increases the incidence of AKI: 2 to 3 times higher than with vancomycin alone.[22,30] Intensive hydration may mitigate nephrotoxicity by decreasing the drug concentration in proximal tubules and peritubular circulation.[22]

Intraoperative Management

Avoiding intraoperative hypotension is vital to preventing postoperative AKI.[18,26,31] In patients at risk for developing AKI, mild intraoperative hypotension with mean arterial pressure (MAP) less than 55 mm Hg for 10 minutes or MAP less than 60 mm Hg for 20 minutes or greater is a significant risk factor for the development of AKI.[32–34] Ahuja, and colleagues demonstrated that systolic blood pressures less than 90 mm Hg were also associated with postoperative AKI.[35]

Surgery-Specific Factors

Major surgery (cardiac, vascular, lung and liver transplant, and major abdominal procedures) carries an increased risk for postoperative AKI.[18,20,36–43] Patients with higher American Society of Anesthesiologists' Physical Status Classification and emergency surgery further increase this risk.[10,11]

There are many well-documented reasons for postcardiac surgery AKI, including hypoperfusion, nonpulsatile perfusion, hemodilution, hypothermia, and inflammation. Risk of perioperative AKI varies between 1% and 3% in patients undergoing coronary artery bypass grafting and 27% to 29% in patients undergoing aortic valve replacement.[44–46] Cardiopulmonary bypass (CPB) causes inflammation and mechanical injury to circulating erythrocytes, intraoperative hemolysis, release of free hemoglobin, and direct injury to the renal epithelium.[19–21] Hemodilution contributes to decreased oxygen carrying capacity and renal ischemia. Prolonged duration of CPB or aortic cross-clamping and cardiac ischemia-reperfusion all cause renal ischemia.[21,44]

The risk of AKI is significantly greater in surgeries involving the aorta.[21,47,48] Cross-clamping the aorta is required in suprarenal and infrarenal abdominal aortic aneurysm (AAA) repairs, both of which decrease renal blood flow (RBF), increase renovascular resistance and are associated with AKI. Aortic cross-clamping releases nephrotoxic proinflammatory mediators and cytokines. Finally, endovascular techniques are associated with less AKI than open AAA repair but there is contrast dye exposure and a higher risk of embolic complications.[47,48]

Risk factors for abdominal surgery include intraoperative blood transfusions, emergency surgery, intraoperative hemodynamic instability, use of vasopressors and diuretics, and increase in intra-abdominal pressure.[19,20,49] Incidence of postoperative AKI following cytoreductive surgery and hyperthermic intraperitoneal chemotherapy (HIPEC) varies and is cited to be up to 48%.[50] The strongest correlation is between cisplatin-containing HIPEC and AKI. Prerenal state secondary to hyperthermia-induced splanchnic vasodilation may also contribute.[50] Finally, patients receiving angiotensin receptor blockers were at increased risk of developing HIPEC-induced AKI.[50,51]

RISK STRATIFICATION AND BIOMARKERS

Current AKI diagnostic methods are incomplete. Intraoperative and postoperative urine outputs do not correlate well with AKI, and changes in serum creatinine levels lag in AKI until days after insult. Most AKI reflects tubular epithelium injury, and creatinine measures GFR—a poor indicator of tubular function. Volume status, nutrition, steroids, and muscle trauma can all alter creatinine levels. Biomarkers may be able to detect AKI earlier and more accurately; however, their use is not yet widespread[19,20] (**Box 1**).

Urinary neutrophil gelatinase-associated lipocalin (NGAL) is excreted into the plasma and urine within 3 hours of injury, peaks at 6 hours, and remains in circulation for 5 days. However, as a proinflammatory biomarker, its use is limited in patients with a proinflammatory state (ie, sepsis). Cystatin C is a protease inhibitor that detects AKI earlier than creatinine and has demonstrated good predictability for mortality in cardiac surgery patients.[18,44] Urinary KIM-1 is released from tubules during ischemia-reperfusion and predicts dialysis requirement, mortality, and may distinguish ischemic AKI from prerenal azotemia and CKD.[44] TIMP-2 and IGFBP7 are released from the renal tubules during cell cycle arrest and are promising diagnostic biomarkers.[18,19,21]

The furosemide stress test (FST) uses a single weight-based dose of furosemide and measures subsequent urine output during 2 hours to predict the progression to severe AKI.[52,53] Urine output less than 200 mL in the first 2 hours after furosemide administration strongly correlates with disease progression. Studies looking at FST have demonstrated equal or better efficacy predicting AKI and need for renal replacement therapy (RRT) as compared with other biomarkers.[19,52–55]

Box 1
Biomarkers for acute kidney injury[18–20,44,139]

NGAL

KIM-1

Cystatin C

TIMP-2

IGFBP-7

L-FABP

ACUTE KIDNEY INJURY AND PERIOPERATIVE CONSIDERATIONS

The mechanism of perioperative AKI is multifactorial. It encompasses patient comorbidities, surgical factors, intraoperative anesthetic management and pharmacologic therapies. The perioperative physician must balance these considerations to maintain homeostasis, and mitigate the risk of postoperative AKI.

Perioperative Hemodynamic Management

Intraoperative considerations that may cause perioperative AKI include hemodynamic perturbations, anemia, and fluid management. Maintaining end-organ perfusion is the primary hemodynamic goal in preventing AKI. Surgery and anesthesia both contribute to hypotension and hypovolemia.[56] Although literature regarding blood pressure targets for optimal renal perfusion are scant, a MAP of 65 to 70 mm Hg (in patients without comorbid hypertension) and 80 to 85 mm Hg (in patients with hypertension) have been the benchmark for preventing AKI.[57] Recent literature has proposed that perfusion pressure may be a more accurate marker in preventing AKI.[58] Diastolic perfusion pressure (DPP) (DPP = diastolic arterial pressure [DAP] – central venous pressure [CVP]) and mean perfusion pressure (MPP) (MPP = MAP-CVP) have both been evaluated and better correlate with postoperative AKI than MAP alone.[58,59] Saito and colleagues demonstrated that reductions in DAP, MPP, and DPP were more closely associated with AKI than MAP in postoperative cardiac surgical patients.[58,59] Additional studies have demonstrated similar outcomes where perfusion pressure or diastolic arterial pressure is more suggestive of developing AKI than MAP.[58,60,61] Further research is necessary to confirm which perfusion pressure is optimal in perioperative AKI evaluation.

Fluid Therapy

Maintaining intravascular volume and adequate end-organ perfusion is challenging during the intraoperative period. Surgical blood loss, insensible losses, third-spacing of intravascular fluid secondary to inflammation, and preload reduction from positive pressure ventilation all contribute to intraoperative fluid loss.[56] There are many options for fluid resuscitation, including crystalloids, such as normal saline or balanced solutions, as well as colloids, such as starches, albumin, dextrans, and gelatins.[57] Balanced solutions (eg, lactated ringers, Plasmalyte) are correlated with less postoperative AKI.[57] Hyperchloremia from normal saline may reduce RBF due to vasoconstriction and has consistently demonstrated increased correlation with postoperative AKI.[62,63] When normal saline is used, monitoring serum chloride levels may help mitigate the risk of hyperchloremia-induced AKI.[20,57] Several large randomized controlled trials in critically ill patients have not demonstrated a difference in mortality between the colloid versus the crystalloid groups.[64,65] Synthetic colloids have potential adverse effects, including not only increased AKI but also coagulopathy and allergic reactions, and have largely been phased out of clinical use.[57,66–73] Albumin, a colloid extracted from humans, has been effective for volume expansion without adverse effects aside from specific populations (ie, traumatic brain injury patients) and cost.

Anemia

Perioperative anemia reduces oxygen carrying capacity, which can lead to renal medullary hypoxia, ultimately causing AKI. Preoperative anemia with hemoglobin less than 8 mg/dL and a postoperative decrement of more than 4 mg/dL are associated with an increased risk of postoperative AKI in noncardiac surgical patients.[20,74] Yet, blood transfusions are also associated with AKI. It remains uncertain if the increased risk is related to surgical complexity, other confounders, or the transfused blood.[20,74] Further research is required to determine best practices to optimize preoperative hemoglobin in elective surgical cases to reduce the risk of postoperative AKI.

Contrast-Induced Acute Kidney Injury

Contrast-induced AKI (CI-AKI) is a major cause of hospital-acquired AKI with significant short-term and long-term sequelae. According to a meta-analysis of 29 studies, contrast-induced AKI has an incidence ranging from 4.4% to 22.1%.[75,76] The exact incidence is unclear and preventative therapy with isotonic intravenous fluids may significantly reduce the incidence.[76,77] The mechanism of CI-AKI is multifactorial; iodinated contrast causes renal vasoconstriction, increases the viscosity of blood flow through the kidney medulla, and is also cytotoxic to renal tubular cells.[78,79] In addition, risk factors including diabetes mellitus, CKD, and NSAIDs can all further increase incidence of AKI.[79] There is no particular treatment of CI-AKI. However, the risk can be reduced by using iso-osmolar contrast agents and hydrating with isotonic fluids.[80] The use of other preventative therapies such as N-acetylcysteine and sodium bicarbonate infusions has not shown to be beneficial.[81,82]

PREVENTION

Although AKI is associated with significant short-term and long-term morbidity and mortality, preventative strategies are limited and require additional research. Interventions evaluated in the prevention of perioperative AKI include pharmacologic interventions, hemodynamic control, glycemic control, remote ischemic preconditioning (RIPC), and KDIGO bundling.[57]

Pharmacologic Interventions

Renal vasodilator therapy has not been particularly effective for the prevention or treatment of AKI. Low dose, or renal-dose, dopamine has been studied extensively.[57] It was thought that dopamine would improve RBF by selective renal arterial vasodilation in clinical scenarios where renal vasoconstriction would occur.[57] However, meta-analyses have not supported this notion. Dopamine has not shown to prevent or treat AKI, and in one study, dopamine may have worsened renal perfusion and outcome.[83–85]

Fenoldopam is a dopamine A_1 specific receptor agonist that causes systemic and renal vascular dilation that increases RBF to the cortex and medullary regions. This drug was studied in both the critical care and cardiac surgical population to prevent the risk of postoperative AKI.[57] The evidence for the routine use of fenoldopam for AKI prevention is not supported, with studies demonstrating both benefit and no difference in incidence of AKI, need for RRT, and mortality.[86–88] The largest randomized controlled trial (RCT) conducted to evaluate risk reduction of RRT in postoperative cardiac surgical patients was terminated early due to futility; the authors found that fenoldopam did neither reduce the need for RRT nor reduce the risk of 30-day mortality.[89] Furthermore, it is conceivable that the systemic hypotension associated with fenoldopam may worsen renal perfusion.

Levosimendan is an inodilator that increases troponin-c sensitivity to calcium and is used to augment cardiac contractility in patients with heart failure. Levosimendan also causes systemic vasodilation and increases RBF and GFR by dilating the afferent arterioles.[90,91] In addition, it also has anti-inflammatory, antiapoptotic, and antioxidative properties that may further reduce AKI risk.[92–94] In several large trials involving post-cardiac surgery patients, levosimendan did not reduce the incidence of AKI compared with placebo.[95–97] Similarly, levosimendan use in critically ill patients with sepsis did not result in less severe end-organ dysfunction or lower mortality compared with placebo.[98] Based on current evidence, the routine use of levosimendan for preventative or therapeutic intervention is not recommended.

Interestingly, dexmedetomidine, an α_2-selective agonist, has demonstrated renoprotective properties.[1] Based on animal studies, dexmedetomidine has cytoprotective properties, inhibiting apoptosis of proximal tubular cells during hypoperfusion.[99] This preventative effect was further seen in several trials involving cardiac surgical patients, where the incidence of AKI was significantly reduced when dexmedetomidine was used postoperatively or following the induction of anesthesia.[100,101] Two recent meta-analyses also found that dexmedetomidine, when used before CPB, seemed to be most effective in preventing postoperative AKI among patients undergoing cardiac surgery.[102,103] However, a recent RCT evaluating the effects of dexmedetomidine on postoperative atrial fibrillation and delirium did not demonstrate decreased postoperative AKI.[104] Postoperative AKI was a secondary outcome measure in the study, so it is possible that the study was not adequately powered to evaluate for postoperative AKI.[104] Further data is necessary before recommending dexmedetomidine for routine preventative use.

Remote Ischemic Preconditioning

RIPC has been extensively evaluated for the prevention of postoperative AKI in the cardiac surgical population. Although the mechanism by which ischemic preconditioning prevents AKI is not entirely understood, it likely involves neuronal and humoral signaling pathways in preventing cell death.[1,105] The evidence for the routine use of RIPC in the prevention of postoperative AKI is lacking. A recent Cochrane Review found minimal to no benefit with RIPC, no reduction in postoperative AKI, need for dialysis, serum creatinine, length of hospital stay, or mortality.[105] Overall, RIPC is not recommended for preventative use among patients undergoing cardiac or vascular surgery, where renal ischemic reperfusion injury can occur.[105]

Kidney Disease: Improving Global Outcomes Bundle

The KDIGO foundation created a treatment bundle to ensure optimal renal protection by incorporating evidence-based strategies such as maintaining volume status and perfusion pressure, maintaining euglycemia, discontinuing and avoiding nephrotoxic agents, and close monitoring of serum creatinine and urine output.[1]

Optimizing volume status entails the use of intravenous fluid resuscitation and, as mentioned earlier, isotonic crystalloid is the fluid of choice.[20] Determining a patient's volume may be a challenging task. Despite this, it is recommended that the patient's urine output be maintained at least 0.5 mL/kg/h as a marker of renal perfusion and function.[20] In clinical scenarios where oliguria may ensue, management strategies such as a fluid challenge, straight leg raise, noninvasive cardiac output monitors, or using point-of-care ultrasound may help determine cardiac function, cardiac output, stroke volume, and volume status.[106]

With the current available evidence, maintaining a MAP of 65 to 70 mm Hg in normotensive patients and 80 to 85 mm Hg in hypertensive patients is necessary for optimal renal perfusion pressure.[107] The ideal vasopressor of choice for renal perfusion preservation is unknown. All of the available vasopressors (including dopamine at higher doses), norepinephrine, vasopressin, and phenylephrine, are associated with renal afferent arteriole vasoconstriction, leading to renal hypoperfusion.[107] AT II is a hormone that has vasoconstrictive properties, where in recent years has become available as a synthetic agent. According to the ATHOS-3 trial, the use of AT II as an adjunct vasopressor to catecholamine refractory hypotension resulted in a 45% absolute increase in MAP (MAP increase $\geq$10 mm Hg or MAP >75 mm Hg) compared with placebo.[108] In addition, a post hoc analysis of the ATHOS-3 trial demonstrated that the AT II group had faster renal recovery, where patients on RRT were liberated sooner than the placebo group.[109] Nevertheless, AT II remains an adjunct vasopressor until more evidence is acquired to determine the mortality benefit.

Glycemic control has been evaluated extensively in both the medical and surgical patient population. It has shown to improve patient outcomes with a reduction in morbidity and mortality. A randomized trial that took place in the Belgian city of Leuven and nicknamed the Leuven Surgical Trial studied the effects of tight glycemic control in critically ill surgical patients.[110] The authors found that tight glycemic control (80–110 mg/dL) improved survival from the ICU and incidence of AKI by approximately 50% compared with conventional therapy.[110] The NICE-SUGAR trial compared tight glycemic control (80–110 mg/dL) versus more liberal management (<180 mg/dL) in an RCT that included medical and surgical ICU patients.[111] The study results showed tight glycemic control had a higher 90-day mortality compared with the more liberal arm due to high incidence of hypoglycemia.[111] Incidence of AKI, however, was not different between the 2 groups.[111] Based on the results of these 2 trials, it is recommended to target a blood glucose of less than 180 mg/dL to decrease the risk of AKI in critically ill patients.

MANAGEMENT

Identifying patients at risk for AKI while optimizing preventative measures is the mainstay initial therapy for AKI. As mentioned earlier, avoiding nephrotoxic agents, optimizing perfusion pressure and volume status, avoiding hyperglycemia, limiting exposure to and using iso-osmolar contrast agents are preventative and therapeutic measures for AKI. In patients who are at risk for renal injury, serial monitoring of serum creatinine and urine output should be used for the detection of AKI. In clinical scenarios with advanced AKI, the underlying cause of AKI should be identified and treated accordingly. If possible, medications should be renally dosed and close observations of laboratory values (eg, electrolytes, blood urea nitrogen, creatinine, and metabolic acidosis) and the patient's clinical status is warranted to determine if RRT should be initiated.[80]

Indications for Renal Replacement Therapy

The optimal timing for the initiation of RRT is a frequently debated clinical conundrum with inconclusive and insufficient evidence in the literature to provide a consensus.[112] The ongoing controversy regarding early versus late initiation of RRT is beyond the scope of this review article. However, according to the ADQI and KDIGO guidelines, the timing of RRT initiation lacks standardization and remains a subjective and objective decision made based on the clinical presentation of the patient in a case-by-case manner along with the expert discretion of the physician.[113,114] Historically, RRT timing coincides with severe renal dysfunction (ie, stage 3 AKI according to the KDIGO classification), with the onset of clinical symptoms and signs of renal failure (eg, uremic encephalopathy, pericarditis, fatigue, anorexia), symptomatic metabolic acidosis, azotemia, volume overload, and electrolyte abnormalities[114,115] (**Box 2**). In addition, RRT can be initiated in nonrenal-related clinical scenarios and without the presence of severe renal dysfunction such as with toxin poisoning and fluid overload[116] (see **Box 2**).

Box 2
Renal and nonrenal indications for RRT

Renal Indications
1. Electrolyte abnormalities (eg, hyperkalemia, K > 6 mmol/L) refractory to medication therapy
2. Uremic metabolic acidosis
3. Uremia with associate clinical symptoms (eg, pericarditis, encephalopathy, bleeding)
4. Fluid overload refractory to diuretic therapy

Nonrenal Indications
1. Controlling body-temperature
2. Removing inflammatory cytokines (eg, sepsis)
3. Removing radiocontrast
4. Massive fluid overload
5. Drug and toxin removal
   a. Metformin
   b. Lithium
   c. Antiepileptics (eg, phenytoin, carbamazepine, valproic acid, barbiturates)
   d. Antibiotics (eg, cefepime, vancomycin)
   e. Dabigatran
   f. β-blockers (eg, atenolol, metoprolol)
   g. Alcohols (eg, methanol, ethylene glycol)
   h. Salicylates
   i. Acetaminophen

In general, small, nonprotein bound, hydrophilic and low volume of distribution medications or toxins are easier to be cleared by RRT. RRT does not remove common medications of poisoning including benzodiazepines, tricyclic antidepressants, and other recreational drugs. Acetaminophen is dialyzable; however, N-acetylcysteine therapy (NAC) is quite effective and often RRT is not necessary. The efficacy and benefits of cytokine removal by RRT is debatable and currently not in widespread practice for clinical scenarios such as sepsis due to lack of mortality benefit.[116,120,124,134–138,140]

Types of Renal Replacement Therapy

There are 3 main modalities of RRT, including peritoneal dialysis (PD), intermittent hemodialysis (IHD), and continuous renal replacement therapy (CRRT).[117] Prolonged intermittent renal replacement therapy such as sustained low-efficiency dialysis (SLED) is a hybrid form of IHD.[118,119] The choice of RRT modality depends on hospital resource availability as well as patient hemodynamic stability. In the clinical situation of AKI in the ICU setting, CRRT is often the most effective and hemodynamically stable approach.[120]

PD has been used for the treatment of AKI since 1946 and was an effective and hemodynamically stable form of dialysis in the ICU that was tolerated well by the critically ill patient population.[121] PD functions by infusing a high-gradient solvent into the peritoneal cavity and the peritoneum is the natural semipermeable membrane that filters uremic solutes and toxins and fluid removal.[122] The dialysate, which is composed of varying concentrations of dextrose can be tailored based on the clinical scenario of the patient to achieve homeostasis.[122] Nevertheless, it is less used than CRRT and IHD despite the lack of evidence of survival superiority.[123] PD is not commonly used in the acute setting in modern medicine due to impracticalities, where a surgical procedure is necessary for catheter insertion and the effective functionality of PD also depends on the patient having regular bowel motility.[124] In addition, volume removal and solute clearance is unpredictable.[125] Furthermore, the use of PD is associated with complications including hyperglycemia, peritonitis, protein loss, and mechanical complications of the catheter (eg, catheter migration, mechanical kinking, flow dysfunction).[123] Although PD requires less staffing, costs significantly less than extracorporeal RRT, and may reduce RRT time while having similar mortality rates when compared with extracorporeal RRT, further research will be needed to elucidate outcomes and the role of PD in AKI.[123,125]

IHD is used in patients with CKD and in hemodynamically stable patients with severe AKI. IHD lasts for 3 to 4 hours, and due to high blood and dialysate flow rates, it can rapidly correct metabolic and electrolyte abnormalities such as uremic metabolic acidosis, hyperkalemia, and water-soluble poisonings.[115,120] In addition, IHD is widely available, less expensive than CRRT and an effective hemodialysis modality.[115,126] SLED is a hybrid therapy that is a prolonged form of IHD lasting 8 to 12 hours.[115] SLED is effective in fluid and solute removal and is generally well tolerated with critically ill patients given it is more hemodynamically stable than IHD.[115] A recent systematic review and meta-analysis of RRT therapies for AKI among ICU patients did not demonstrate superiority with in-hospital mortality or dialysis dependence between IHD, CRRT, and SLED.[127] However, IHD is associated with an increased risk of hypotension due to rapid fluid removal and large fluid shifts and is often not the RRT modality of choice for critically ill patients. Nevertheless, higher powered RCTs are necessary to better define the utility of various RRT modalities.

CRRT is the most widely used modality of RRT for critically ill patients in the ICU. It is a hemodynamically stable process that uses lower blood and dialysate flow rates for more gradual correction of metabolic and electrolyte abnormalities as well as fluid removal, typically during a 24-hour continuous period via a temporary dialysis catheter[117] (**Box 3**). CRRT includes the processes of convection, diffusion, or a combination of both for solute clearance.[120] CRRT is categorized by the process of solute clearance. Continuous hemodialysis and continuous venovenous hemodialysis use the process of diffusion. Continuous hemofiltration and continuous venovenous hemofiltration use the mechanism of convection. Continuous hemodiafiltration and continuous venovenous hemodiafiltration incorporate a combination of both mechanisms.[120] Similar to IHD, medication dosing adjustments are necessary in patients undergoing CRRT. Continuous arteriovenous RRT has been used in the past; however,

---

Box 3
Recommended sites for temporary dialysis catheter placement in order of preference from the KDIGO 2012 clinical practice guideline[12]

Recommended Sites for Temporary Dialysis Catheter Placement
1. Right internal jugular vein
2. Right or left femoral vein
3. Left internal jugular vein
4. Subclavian vein

The right internal jugular vein (RIJV) is preferred based on anatomic location where it is a direct path to the caval atrial junction, has less risks for placement complications, infections, and thrombosis. If the RIJV is not an option, then one of the femoral veins is used but close observation is needed due to increased risk for catheter-associated infection. The left internal jugular vein (LIJV) is the third option and may be a difficult placement due to tortuosity of the catheter path into the caval atrial junction. The subclavian vein on the patient's dominant side is the last option due to risk of central stenosis and the nondominant side is typically used for arteriovenous fistula creation.[12]*Abbreviations:* ACEI, angtiotensin-converting enzyme inhibitor; AKI, acute kidney injury; ARB, angiotensin receptor blocker; CKD, chronic kidney disease; CPB, cardiopulmonary bypass; IGFBP7, insulin-like growth factor binding factor 7; KIM-1, kidney injury molecule 1; L-FABP, Liver-type fatty acid binding protein; MAP, mean arterial pressure; TIMP-2, tissue inhibitor of metalloproteinase-2.

this has largely been replaced by continuous venovenous RRT due to a lower risk of vascular injury.[128] Slow continuous ultrafiltration (SCUF) is a type of CRRT therapy that uses hemofiltration mainly for fluid removal.[118] SCUF is not a modality of choice for patients with uremia because it has minimal solute clearance. Medications do not need to be adjusted if this mechanism is used.[120] Clinically, SCUF is a useful option in hypervolemic patients with cardiogenic shock and cardiorenal syndrome who are not responsive to diuretic therapy.[118]

Intraoperative RRT has been used predominantly in the liver transplant patient population and has become an integral part of intraoperative management for a successful surgery and survival of the patient.[117,129] Intraoperative RRT has also been reportedly used in cases involving emergency intracranial surgery and emergent surgeries with severe electrolyte abnormalities.[117,130,131] Preoperative AKI is associated with an increased risk of perioperatively mortality among patients undergoing liver transplantation.[129] There are no guidelines for indications of intraoperative RRT and the decision is made in conjunction with the transplant surgeon, anesthesiologist, and nephrologist. In general, indications for intraoperative RRT reported in the literature include hyperkalemia (>5 mmol/L), metabolic acidosis, volume overload, high-risk surgical candidates with AKI and high risk of perioperative complications (ie, high model for end-stage liver disease [MELD] scores), and preoperative RRT via the modalities of CRRT or SLED.[129] The utilization of intraoperative RRT also varies on the expertise, resources, and feasibility (eg, operating room capabilities, nursing personnel) of the hospital center.[117] Nevertheless, evidence for the aforementioned theoretic benefit of intraoperative RRT to support use in the operating room is variable in the literature. A recent meta-analysis found that patients who were at higher perioperative risk with higher MELD scores and required intraoperative RRT did not have a significant difference in short-term mortality when compared with patients with lower MELD and did not need RRT.[132] However, a retrospective study evaluated outcomes among liver transplant patients and found that those who required preoperative RRT had the same incidence of metabolic acidosis and hyperkalemia than those who did not require preoperative RRT but had a higher 30-day mortality and were more likely to receive blood products.[133] Further trials are needed to determine the risks, benefits, and feasibility of intraoperative RRT.

SUMMARY

AKI is a common perioperative complication that has significant implications on postsurgical outcomes. The understanding of AKI diagnosis and management continue to evolve alongside novel discoveries. It is important to be up-to-date on the effects of surgery on kidney function and to tailor management in an individualized and vigilant manner.

CLINICS CARE POINTS

- Postoperative kidney injury is clinically significant and understanding the pathophysiology related to it by the perioperative physician may prevent this postoperative morbidity.

- Preventing acute kidney injury is the mainstay treatment, however, additional work will need to be done to determine early stage diagnosis of this morbidity.

- Intraoperative renal replacement therapy has had increased prevalence in recent years and thorough understanding of the indications, function and intraoperative implications is important for the anesthesiologist in order to effectively manage the patient.

FUNDING STATEMENT

Support was provided solely from Institutional and Departmental Sources.

ACKNOWLEDGMENTS

The authors would like to thank the Department of Anesthesiology faculty for their assistance with article revisions.

DECLARATIONS OF INTEREST

None.

REFERENCES

1. Meersch M, Schmidt C, Zarbock A. Perioperative acute kidney injury: an under-recognized problem. Anesth Analg 2017;125:1223–32.
2. Uchino S, Kellum JA, Bellomo R, et al. Acute renal failure in critically ill patients: a multinational, multicenter study. JAMA 2005;294(7):813–8.
3. Ricci Z, Cruz D, Ronco C. The rifle criteria and mortality in acute kidney injury: a systematic review. Kidney Int 2008;73(5):538–46.
4. Zarbock A, Koyner JL, Hoste EAJ, et al. Update on perioperative acute kidney injury. Anesth Analg 2018;127:1236–45.
5. Wallace MA. Anatomy and physiology of the kidney. AORN J 1998;68(5):799–820.
6. Dalal R, Bruss ZS, Sehdev JS. Physiology, renal blood flow and filtration. [Updated 2021 Jul 26]. In: StatPearls [Internet]. Treasure Island (FL): StatPearls Publishing; 2022. Available from: https://www.ncbi.nlm.nih.gov/books/NBK482248/.
7. Pakula AM, Skinner RA. Acute kidney injury in the critically ill patient: a current review of literature. J Intensive Care Med 2016;31(5):319–24.
8. Bellomo R, Ronco C, Kellum JA, et al. Acute renal failure- definition, outcome measures, animal models, fluid therapy and information technology needs: the second international consensus conference of the acute dialysis quality initiative (ADQI) group. Crit Care 2004;8:R204–12.
9. Mehta RL, Kellum JA, Shah SV, et al. Acute kidney injury network: report of an initiative to improve outcomes in acute kidney injury. Crit Care 2007;11(2):R31.
10. Bagshaw SM, George C, Dinu I, et al. A multi-centre evaluation of the rifle criteria for early acute kidney injury in critically ill patients. Nephrol Dial Transpl 2008;23:1203–10.
11. Lassnigg A, Schmidlin D, Mouhieddine M, et al. Minimal changes of serum creatinine predict prognosis in patients after cardiothoracic surgery: a prospective cohort study. J Am Soc Nephrol 2004;15:1597–605.
12. Kidney disease: improving global outcomes (KDIGO) acute kidney injury work group: KDIGO clinical practice guideline for acute kidney injury. Kidney Int 2012;21:138.
13. Kellum JA, Lameire N, for the KDIGO AKI Guideline Work Group. Diagnosis, evaluation, and management of acute kidney injury: a KDIGO summary (Part 1). Crit Care 2013;17:204.
14. Fuji T, Uchino S, Takinami M, et al. Validation of the kidney disease improving global outcomes criteria for AKI and comparison of three criteria in hospitalized patients. Clin J Am Soc Nephrol 2014;9:848–54.

15. Schetz M, Schortgen F. Ten shortcomings of the current definition of AKI. Intensive Care Med 2017;43(6):911–3.
16. Moore PK, Hsu RK, Liu KD. Management of acute kidney injury: core curriculum 2018. Am J Kidney Dis 2018;72(1):136–48.
17. Kwiatkowska E, Domański L, Dziedziejko V, et al. The Mechanism of Drug Nephrotoxicity and the Methods for Preventing Kidney Damage. Int J Mol Sci 2021; 22(11):6109.
18. Ojo B, Campbell CH. Perioperative Acute Kidney Injury: Impact and Recent Update. Curr Opin Anaesthesiol 2022;35(2):215–23.
19. Gumbert SD, Kork F, Jackson ML, et al. Perioperative Acute Kidney Injury. Anesthesiology 2020;132(1):180–204.
20. Goren O, Matot I. Perioperative acute kidney injury. Br J Anaesth 2015; 115(Suppl 2):ii3–14.
21. Cole SP. Stratification and Risk Reduction of Perioperative Acute Kidney Injury: An Update. Anesthesiol Clin 2018;36(4):539–51.
22. Morales-Alvarez MC. Nephrotoxicity of Antimicrobials and Antibiotics. Adv Chronic Kidney Dis 2020;27(1):31–7.
23. Lodise TP, Patel N, Lomaestro BM, et al. Relationship between Initial Vancomycin Concentration Time Profile and Nephrotoxicity among Hospitalized Patients. Clin Infect Dis 2009;49:507–14.
24. Lin SY, Tang SC, Tsai LK, et al. Incidence and Risk Factors for Acute Kidney Injury Following Mannitol Infusion in Patients With Acute Stroke: A Retrospective Cohort Study. Medicine (Baltimore) 2015;94(47):e2032.
25. Chen JJ, Kuo G, Hung CC, et al. Risk factors and Prognosis Assessment for Acute Kidney Injury: The 2020 Consensus of the Taiwan AKI Task Force. J Formos Med Assoc 2021;120(7):1424–33.
26. Kobayashi Y, Yamaoka K. Analysis of Intraoperative Modifiable Factors to Prevent Acute Kidney Injury After Elective Noncardiac Surgery: Intraoperative Hypotension and Crystalloid Administration Related to Acute Kidney Injury. JA Clin Rep 2021;7(1):27.
27. Matot I, Dery E, Bulgov Y, et al. Fluid Management During Video-assisted Thoracoscopic Surgery for Lung Resection: A Randomized, Controlled Trial of Effects on Urinary Output and Postoperative Renal Function. J Thorac Cardiovasc Surg 2013;146:461–6.
28. Matot I, Paskaleva R, Eid L, et al. Effect of the Volume of Fluids Administered on Intraoperative Oliguria in Laparoscopic Bariatric Surgery: A Randomized Controlled Trial. Arch Surg 2012;147:228–34.
29. McWilliam SJ, Antoine DJ, Smyth RL, et al. Aminoglycoside-induced Nephrotoxicity in Children. Pediatr Nephrol 2017;32:2015–25.
30. Burgess LD, Drew RH. Comparison of the Incidence of Vancomycin-induced Nephrotoxicity in Hospitalized Patients with and without Concomitant Piperacillin-Tazobactam. Pharmacotherapy 2014;34(7):670–6.
31. Brienza N, Giglio MT, Marucci M, et al. Does Perioperative Hemodynamic Optimization Protect Renal Function in Surgical Patients? A Meta-analytic Study. Crit Care Med 2009;37(6):2079–90.
32. Sun LY, Wijeysundera DN, Tait GA, et al. Association of Intraoperative Hypotension with Acute Kidney Injury after Elective Noncardiac Surgery. Anesthesiology 2015;123(3):515–23.
33. Mathis MR, Naik BI, Freundlich RE, et al. Preoperative Risk and the Association Between Hypotension and Postoperative Acute Kidney Injury. Anesthesiology 2020;132:461–75.

34. Walsh M, Devereaux PJ, Garg AX, et al. Relationship Between Intraoperative Mean Arterial Pressure and Clinical Outcomes after Noncardiac Surgery: Toward an Empirical Definition of Hypotension. Anesthesiology 2013;119:507–15.
35. Ahuja S, Mascha EJ, Yang D, et al. Associations of Intraoperative Radial Arterial Systolic, Diastolic, Mean, and Pulse Pressures with Myocardial and Acute Kidney Injury after Noncardiac Surgery: A Retrospective Cohort Analysis. Anesthesiology 2020;132(2):291–306.
36. Nie S, Tang L, Zhang W, et al. Are There Modifiable Risk Factors to Improve AKI? Biomed Res Int 2017;2017:5605634.
37. Ishani A, Xue JL, Himmelfarb J, et al. Acute Kidney Injury Increases Risk of ESRD Among Elderly. J Am Soc Nephrol 2009;20:223e8.
38. Coca SG, Singanamala S, Parikh CR. Chronic Kidney Disease after Acute Kidney Injury: a Systematic Review and Meta-analysis. Kidney Int 2012;81(5):442e8.
39. Sawhney S, Mitchell M, Marks A, et al. Long-term Prognosis after Acute Kidney Injury (AKI): What is the Role of Baseline Kidney Function and Recovery? A Systematic Review. BMJ Open 2015;5:e006497.
40. Bucaloiu ID, Kirchner HL, Norfolk ER, et al. Increased Risk of Death and de novo Chronic Kidney Disease Following Reversible Acute Kidney Injury. Kidney Int 2012;81:477e85.
41. Gautam SC, Brooks CH, Balogun RA, et al. Predictors and Outcomes of Post-Hospitalization Dialysis Dependent Acute Kidney Injury. Nephron 2015;131:185e90.
42. Berkowitz RJ, Engoren MC, Mentz G, et al. Intraoperative Risk Factors of Acute Kidney Injury after Liver Transplantation. Liver Transpl 2022;28(7):1207–23.
43. Wajda-Pokrontka M, Nadziakiewicz P, Krauchuk A, et al. Incidence and Perioperative Risk Factors of Acute Kidney Injury Among Lung Transplant Recipients. Transpl Proc 2022;54(4):1120–3 [published online ahead of print, 2022 Apr 11].
44. Ortega-Loubon C, Fernández-Molina M, Carrascal-Hinojal Y, et al. Cardiac surgery-associated acute kidney injury. Ann Card Anaesth 2016;19(4):687–98.
45. Chawla LS, Zhao Y, Lough FC, et al. Off-pump versus On-pump Coronary Artery Bypass Grafting Outcomes Stratified by Preoperative Renal Function. J Am Soc Nephrol 2012;23(8):1389–97.
46. Shroyer AL, Grover FL, Hattler B, et al. On-pump versus Off-pump Coronary-Artery Bypass Surgery. N Engl J Med 2009;361(19):1827–37.
47. Yang B, Fung A, Pac-Soo C, et al. Vascular Surgery-related Organ Injury and Protective Strategies: Update and Future Prospects. Br J Anaesth 2016;117(Suppl 2):ii32–43.
48. Gamulin Z, Forster A, Morel D, et al. Effects of Infrarenal Aortic Cross-clamping on Renal Hemodynamics in Humans. Anesthesiology 1984;61(4):394–9.
49. Hu L, Gao L, Zhang D, et al. The incidence, risk factors and outcomes of acute kidney injury in critically ill patients undergoing emergency surgery: a prospective observational study. BMC Nephrol 2022;23(1):42.
50. Liesenfeld LF, Wagner B, Hillebrecht HC, et al. HIPEC-Induced Acute Kidney Injury: A Retrospective Clinical Study and Preclinical Model. Ann Surg Oncol 2022;29(1):139–51.
51. Hakeam HA, Breakiet M, ett al Azzam A. The Incidence of Cisplatin Nephrotoxicity Post-Hyperthermic Intraperitoneal Chemotherapy (HIPEC) and Cytoreductive Surgery. Ren Fail 2014;36(10):1486–91.

52. Koyner JL, Davison DL, Brasha-Mitchell E, et al. Furosemide Stress Test and Biomarkers for the Prediction of AKI Severity. J Am Soc Nephrol 2015;26: 2023–31.

53. Chawla LS, Davison DL, Brasha-Mitchell E, et al. Development and Standardization of a Furosemide Stress Test to Predict the Severity of Acute Kidney Injury. Crit Care 2013;17(5):R207.

54. Chen JJ, Chang CH, Huang YT, et al. Furosemide Stress Test as a Predictive Marker of Acute Kidney Injury Progression or Renal Replacement Therapy: A Systemic Review and Meta-analysis. Crit Care 2020;24(1):202.

55. Wei C, Zhang L, Feng Y, et al. Machine Learning Model for Predicting Acute Kidney injury Progression in Critically Ill Patients. BMC Med Inform Decis Mak 2022; 22(1):17.

56. Grocott MPW, Mythen MG, Gan TJ. Perioperative Fluid Management and Clinical Outcomes in Adults. Anesth Analg 2005;100:1093–106.

57. Joannidis M, Druml W, Forni LG, et al. Prevention of Acute Kidney Injury and Protection of Renal Function in the Intensive Care Unit: Update 2017: Expert Opinion of the Working Group on Prevention, AKI section, European Society of Intensive Care Medicine. Intensive Care Med 2017;43(6):730–49.

58. Sato R, Luthe SK, Nasu M. Blood Pressure and Acute Kidney Injury. Crit Care 2017;21:28.

59. Saito S, Uchino S, Takinami M, et al. Postoperative Blood Pressure Deficit and Acute Kidney Injury Progression in Vasopressor-dependent Cardiovascular Surgery Patients. Crit Care 2016;20:74.

60. Legrand M, Dupuis C, Simon C, et al. Association Between Systemic Hemodynamics and Septic Acute Kidney Injury in Critically Ill Patients: A Retrospective Observational Study. Crit Care 2013;17:R278.

61. Wong BT, Chan MJ, Glassford NJ, et al. Mean Arterial Pressure and Mean Perfusion Pressure Deficit in Septic Acute Kidney Injury. J Crit Care 2015;30:975–81.

62. Chowdhury AH, Cox EF, Francis ST, et al. A Randomized, Controlled, Double-blind Crossover Study on the Effects of 2-L Infusions of 0.9% Saline and Plasma-lyte 148 on Renal Blood Flow Velocity and Renal Cortical Tissue Perfusion in Healthy Volunteers. Ann Surg 2012;256:18–24.

63. Nadeem Λ, Salahuddin N, El Hazmi A, et al. Chloride-liberal Fluids are Associated with Acute Kidney Injury after Liver Transplantation. Crit Care 2014;18:625.

64. Annane D, Siami S, Jaber S, et al. Effects of Fluid Resuscitation with Colloids vs. Crystalloids on Mortality in Critically Ill Patients Presenting with Hypovolemic Shock. JAMA 2013;310(7):1809–17.

65. Finfer S, Bellomo R, Boyce N, et al. A Comparison of Albumin and Saline for Fluid Resuscitation in the Intensive Care Unit. N Engl J Med 2004;350(22): 2247–56.

66. Myburgh JA, Finfer S, Bellomo R, et al. Hydroxyethyl Starch or Saline for Fluid Resuscitation in Intensive Care. N Engl J Med 2012;367:1901–11.

67. Perner A, Haase N, Guttormsen AB, et al. Hydroxyethyl Starch 130/0.42 versus Ringer's acetate in Severe Sepsis. N Engl J Med 2012;367:124–34.

68. Gattas DJ, Dan A, Myburgh J, et al. Fluid Resuscitation with 6% Hydroxyethyl Starch (130/0.4 and 130/0.42) in acutely ill patients: systematic review of effects on mortality and treatment with renal replacement therapy. Intensive Care Med 2013;39:558–68.

69. Beyer R, Harmening U, Rittmeyer O, et al. Use of modified fluid gelatin and hydroxyethyl starch for colloidal volume replacement in major orthopaedic surgery. Br J Anaesth 1997;78:44–50.

70. Schortgen F, Lacherade JC, Bruneel F, et al. Effects of Hydroxyethylstarch and gelatin on Renal Function in Severe Sepsis: A Multicentre Randomised Study. Lancet 2001;357:911–6.

71. Mardel SN, Saunders FM, Allen H, et al. Reduced Quality of Clot Formation with Gelatin-based Plasma Substitutes. Br J Anaesth 1998;80:204–7.

72. Kurnik BR, Singer F, Groh WC. Case report: dextran-induced acute anuric renal failure. Am J Med Sci 1991;302:28–30.

73. Laxenaire MC, Charpentier C, Feldman L. Anaphylactoid Reactions to Colloid Plasma Substitutes: Incidence, Risk Factors, Mechanisms. A French Multicenter Prospective Study. Ann Fr Anesth Reanim 1994;13:301–10.

74. Walsh M, Garg AX, Devereaux PJ, et al. The Association Between Perioperative Hemoglobin and Acute Kidney Injury in Patients Having Noncardiac Surgery. Anesth Analg 2013;117:924–31.

75. Eng J, Wilson RF, Subramaniam RM, et al. Comparative Effect of contrast media type on the incidence of contrast-induced nephropathy: a systematic review and meta-analysis. Ann Intern Med 2016;164:417–24.

76. Fähling M, Seelinger E, Patzak A, et al. Understanding and Preventing Contrast-induced Acute Kidney Injury. Nat Rev Nephrol 2017;13(3):169–80.

77. Liss P, Persson PB, Hansell P, et al. Renal Failure in 57,925 Patients Undergoing Coronary Procedures Using Iso-osmolar or low-osmolar Contrast Media. Kidney Int 2006;70:1811–7.

78. Persson PB, Hansell P, Liss P. Pathophysiology of Contrast Medium-induced Nephropathy. Kidney Int 2005;68:14–22.

79. Waheed S, Choi MJ. Trials and Tribulations of Diagnosing and Preventing Contrast-induced Acute Kidney Injury. J Thorac Cardiovasc Surg 2021;162(5):1581–6.

80. Bellomo R, Kellum JA, Ronco C. Acute Kidney Injury. Lancet 2012;380:756–66.

81. Bagshaw SM, McAlister FA, Manns BJ, et al. Acetylcysteine in the Prevention of Contrast-Induced Nephropathy: A case study of the pitfalls in the evolution of evidence. Arch Intern Med 2006;166:161–6.

82. Brar SS, Shen AY, Jorgensen MB, et al. Sodium Bicarbonate vs Sodium Chloride for the Prevention of Contrast Medium-Induced Nephropathy in Patients Undergoing Coronary Angiography: A Randomized Trial. JAMA 2008;300:1038–46.

83. Lauschke A, Teichgraber UKM, Frei U, et al. 'Low dose' Dopamine Worsens Renal Perfusion in Patients with Acute Renal Failure. Kidney Int 2006;69:1669–74.

84. Friedrich JO, Adhikari N, Herridge MS, et al. Meta-analysis: Low-dose Dopamine Increases Urine Output but Does Not Prevent Renal Dysfunction or Death. Ann Intern Med 2005;142:510–24.

85. Holmes CL, Walley KR. Bad Medicine: Low-Dose Dopamine in the ICU. Chest 2003;123:1266–75.

86. Landoni G, Biondi-Zoccai GG, Frati E, et al. Beneficial Impact of Fenoldopam in Critically Ill Patients with or at Risk for Acute Renal Failure: A Meta-analysis of Randomized Clinical Trials. Am J Kidney Dis 2007;49:56–68.

87. Ranucci M, De Benedetti D, Bianchini C, et al. Effects of Fenoldopam Infusion in Complex Cardiac Surgical Operations: A Prospective, Randomized, Double-blind placebo-Controlled Study. Minerva Anestesiol 2010;76(4):249–59.

88. Zangrillo A, Biondi-Zoccai GG, Frati E, et al. Fenoldopam and Acute Renal Failure in Cardiac Surgery: A Meta-analysis of Randomized Placebo-controlled Trials. J Cardiothorac Vasc Anesth 2012;26:407–13.

89. Bove T, Zangrillo A, Guarracino F, et al. Effect of Fenoldopam on Use of Renal Replacement Therapy Among Patients With Acute Kidney Injury After Cardiac Surgery: A Randomized Trial. JAMA 2014;312(21):2244–54.

90. Bragadottir G, Redfors B, Ricksten SE. Effects of Levosimendan on Glomerular Filtration Rate, Renal Blood Flow and Renal Oxygenation after Cardiac Surgery with Cardiopulmonary Bypass: A Randomized Placebo-controlled Study. Crit Care Med 2013;41(10):2328–35.

91. Lannemyr L, Ricksten SE, Rundqvist B, et al. Differential Effects of Levosimendan and Dobutamine on Glomerular Filtration Rate in Patients with Heart Failure and Renal Impairment: A Randomized Double-blind Controlled Trial. J Am Heart Assoc 2018;7(16):e008455.

92. Wang Q, Yokoo H, Takashina M, et al. Anti-inflammatory Profile of Levosimendan in Cecal Ligation-induced Septic Mice and in Lipopolysaccharide-stimulated Macrophages. Crit Care Med 2015;43(11):e508–20.

93. Hasslacher J, Bijuklic K, Bertocchi C, et al. Levosimendan inhibits release of reactive oxygen species in polymorphonuclear leukocytes in vitro and in patients with acute heart failure and septic shock: a prospective observational study. Crit Care 2011;15:R166.

94. Parissis JT, Adamopoulos S, Anto-niades C, et al. Effects of levosimendan on circulating proinflammatory cytokines and soluble apoptosis mediators in patients with decompensated advanced heart failure. Am J Cardiol 2004;93:1309–12.

95. Landoni G, Lomivorotov VV, Alvaro G, et al. Levosimendan for hemodynamic support after cardiac surgery. N Engl J Med 2017;376(21):2021–31.

96. Cholley B, Caruba T, Grosjean S, et al. Effect of Levosimendan on low cardiac output syndrome in patients with low ejection fraction undergoing coronary artery bypass grafting with cardiopulmonary bypass: The LICORN Randomized Clinical Trial. JAMA 2017;318(6):548–56.

97. Mehta RH, Leimberger JD, van Diepen S, et al. Levosimendan in patients with left ventricular dysfunction undergoing cardiac surgery. N Engl J Med 2017;376(21):2032–42.

98. Gordon AC, Perkins GD, Singer M, et al. Levosimendan for the Prevention of Acute Organ Dysfunction in Sepsis. N Engl J Med 2016;375(17):1638–48.

99. Luo C, Yuan D, Yao W, et al. Dexmedetomidine protects against apoptosis induced by hypoxia/reoxygenation through the inhibition of gap junctions in NRK-52E cells. Life Sci 2015;122:72–7.

100. Ji F, Li Z, Young JN, et al. Post-Bypass Dexmedetomidine Use and Postoperative Acute Kidney Injury in Patients Undergoing Cardiac Surgery with Cardiopulmonary Bypass. PLoS One 2013;8(10):e77446.

101. Cho JS, Shim JK, Soh S, et al. Perioperative Dexmedetomidine Reduces the Incidence and Severity of Acute Kidney Injury following Valvular Heart Surgery. Kidney Int 2016;89(3):693–700.

102. Peng K, Li D, Applegate RL II, et al. Effect of Dexmedetomidine on Cardiac Surgery-Associated Acute Kidney Injury: A Meta-Analysis with Trial Sequential Analysis of Randomized Controlled Trials. J Cardiothorac Vasc Anesth 2020;34(3):603–13.

103. Liu Y, Sheng B, Wang S, et al. Dexmedetomidine Prevents Acute Kidney Injury after Adult Cardiac Surgery: A Meta-analysis of Randomized Controlled Trials. BMC Anesthesiol 2018;18(1):7.

104. Turan A, Duncan A, Leung S, et al. Dexmedetomidine for Reduction of Atrial Fibrillation and Delirium after Cardiac Surgery (DECADE): A Randomised Placebo-Controlled Trial. Lancet 2020;396:177–85.
105. Menting TP, Wever KE, Ozdemir-van Brunschot DMD, et al. Ischaemic Preconditioning for the Reduction of Renal Ischaemia Reperfusion Injury. Cochrane Database Syst Rev 2017;3(3):CD010777.
106. Rozental O, Thalappillil R, White RS, et al. To Swan or Not to Swan: Indications, Alternatives, and Future Directions. J Cardiothorac Vasc Anesth 2021;35(2):600–15.
107. Hoogenberg K, Smit AJ, Girbes AR. Effects of low-dose dopamine on renal and systemic hemodynamics during incremental norepinephrine infusion in healthy volunteers. Crit Care Med 1998;26:260–5.
108. Khanna A, English SW, Wang XS, et al. Angiotensin II for the Treatment of Vasodilatory Shock. N Engl J Med 2017;377:419–30.
109. Tumlin JA, Murugan R, Deane AM, et al. Outcomes in Patients with Vasodilatory Shock and Renal Replacement Therapy Treated with Intravenous Angiotensin II. Crit Care Med 2018;46:949–57.
110. Van den Berghe G, Wouters P, Weekers F, et al. Intensive Insulin Therapy in Critically Ill Patients. N Engl J Med 2001;345(19):1359–67.
111. Finfer S, Chittock DR, Su SYS, et al. Intensive versus Conventional Glucose Control in Critically Ill Patients. N Engl J Med 2009;360(13):1283–97.
112. Shiao CC, Huang TM, Spapen HD, et al. Optimal Timing of Renal Replacement Therapy Initiation in Acute Kidney Injury: The Elephant Felt by the Blindmen? Crit Care 2017;21:146.
113. Ostermann M, Joannidis M, Pani A, et al. Patient Selection and Timing of Continuous Renal Replacement Therapy. Blood Purif 2016;42:224–37.
114. Chawla LS, Bellomo R, Bihorac A, et al. Acute Kidney Disease and Renal Recovery: Consensus Report of the Acute Disease Quality Initiative (ADQI) 16 Workgroup. Nat Rev Nephrol 2017;13(4):241–57.
115. Rachoin JS, Weisberg LS. Renal Replacement Therapy in the ICU. Crit Care Med 2019;47:715–21.
116. King JD, Kern MH, Jaar BG. Extracorporeal Removal of Poisons and Toxins. CJASN 2019;14:1408–15.
117. Cronin B, O'Brien EO. Intraoperative Renal Replacement Therapy: Practical Information for Anesthesiologists. J Cardiothorac Vasc Anesth 2022;36:2656–68.
118. Gemmell L, Docking R, Black E. Renal Replacement Therapy in Critical Care. BJA Education 2017;17(3):88–93.
119. Edrees F, Li T, Vijayan A. Prolonged Intermittent Renal Replacement Therapy. Adv Chronic Kidney Dis 2016;23(3):195–202.
120. Kellum J, Bellomo R, Ronco C. Continuous renal replacement therapy. 2nd edition. New York: Oxford University press; 2016. p. 21–35, 47-57, 63-67, 93-105.
121. Frank H, Seligman A, Fine J. Treatment of Uraemia After Acute Renal Failure by Peritoneal Irrigation. JAMA 1946;130(11):703–5.
122. Mehrotra R, Devuyst O, Davies S, et al. The Current State of Peritoneal Dialysis. J Am Soc Nephrol 2016;27:3238–52.
123. Cullis B, Al-Hwiesh A, Kilonzo K, et al. ISPD Guidelines for Peritoneal Dialysis in Acute Kidney Injury: 2020 Update (Adults). Perit Dial Int 2021;41(1):15–31.
124. Pannu N, Gibney RTN. Renal Replacement Therapy in the Intensive Care Unit. Ther Clin Risk Manag 2005;1(2):141–50.
125. Al-Hwiesh A, Abdul-Rahman I, Finkelstein F, et al. Acute Kidney Injury in Critically Ill Patients: A Prospective Randomized Study of Tidal Peritoneal Dialysis

Versus Continuous Renal Replacement Therapy. Ther Apher Dial 2018;22(4): 371–9.

126. Manns B, Doig CJ, Lee H, et al. Cost of Acute Renal Failure Requiring Dialysis in the Intensive Care Unit: Clinical and Resource Implications of Renal Recovery. Crit Care Med 2003;31:449–55.

127. Nash DM, Przech S, Wald R, et al. Systematic Review and Meta-analysis of Renal Replacement Therapy Modalities for Acute Kidney Injury in the Intensive Care Unit. J Crit Care 2017;41:138–44.

128. Chen H, Yu RG, Yin NN, et al. Combination of Extracorporeal Membrane Oxygenation and Continuous Renal Replacement Therapy in Critically Ill Patients: A Systematic Review. Crit Care 2014;18:675.

129. Paine CH, Pichler RH. Intraoperative Renal Replacement Therapy for Liver Transplantation: Is There Really a Benefit? Liver Transpl 2020;26(8):971–2.

130. Tek E, Sekerci S, Arslan G. Intraoperative Hemodialysis During Emergency Intracranial Surgery. Anesth Analg 1996;83:658–9.

131. Cooper JR, Kurtz SB, Sawyer MD, et al. Intraoperative Hemodialysis During Emergent Laparotomy. Anesthesiology 2000;93:1356–7.

132. Huang HB, Xu Y, Zhou H, et al. Intraoperative Continuous Renal Replacement Therapy During Liver Transplantation: A Meta-Analysis. Liver Transplant 2020; 26:1010–8.

133. Adelmann D, Olmos A, Liu LL, et al. Intraoperative Management of Liver Transplant Patients Without the Use of Renal Replacement Therapy. Transplantation 2018;102(5):e229–35.

134. Jeong R, Wald R, Bagshaw SM. Timing of Renal-Replacement Therapy in Intensive Care Unit-related Acute Kidney Injury. Curr Opin Crit Care 2021;27(6): 573–81.

135. Kellum JA, Bellomo R, Mehta R, et al. Blood Purification in Non-Renal Critical Illness. Blood Purif 2003;21(1):6–13.

136. Cruz DN, Perazella MA, Bellomo R, et al. Extracorporeal Blood Purification Therapies for Prevention of Radiocontrast-induced Nephropathy. Am J Kidney Dis 2006;48:361–71.

137. Atan R, Crosbie D, Bellomo R. Techniques of Extracorporeal Cytokine Removal: A Systematic Review of the Literature. Blood Purif 2012;33:88–100.

138. Wald R, Adhikari NK, Smith OM, et al. Canadian Critical Care Trials Group: Comparison of Standard and Accelerated Initiation of Renal Replacement Therapy in Acute Kidney Injury. Kidney Int 2015;88:897–904.

139. Yuan SM. Acute Kidney Injury after Cardiac Surgery: Risk Factors and Novel Biomarkers. Braz J Cardiovasc Surg 2019;34(3):352–60.

140. Evans L, Rhodes A, Alhazzani W, et al. Surviving Sepsis Campaign: International Guidelines for Management of Sepsis and Septic Shock 2021. Intensive Care Med 2021;47:1181–247.

Point-of-Care Ultrasound
A Moving Picture Is Worth a Thousand Tests

Suhas Devangam, MD[a], Matthew Sigakis, MD[a],
Louisa J. Palmer, MBBS[b], Lee Goeddel, MD, MPH[c], Babar Fiza, MD[d],*

KEYWORDS

- POCUS • FoCUS • Cardiac ultrasound • Lung ultrasound • Abdominal ultrasound
- Vascular ultrasound • Airway ultrasound • Ocular ultrasound

KEY POINTS

- Clinical applications of point-of-care ultrasound (POCUS) continue to increase in the practice of anesthesiology and critical care.
- Various pathologies common in the perioperative period can be identified rapidly by POCUS.
- Specific applications of POCUS may reduce the reliance on traditional invasive monitoring techniques.

 Video content accompanies this article at http://www.anesthesiology. theclinics.com.

INTRODUCTION

Point-of-care ultrasound (POCUS) has rapidly evolved into a crucial diagnostic adjunct in managing acutely ill patients. In the past decade, we have witnessed a remarkable growth in the clinical applications of point-of-care (POC) ultrasonography in anesthesiology. The incorporation of bedside ultrasonography skills as part of the standard Accreditation Council for Gradual Medical Education program requirements for anesthesiology and the recent introduction of the Diagnostic POCUS Certificate Program by the American Society of Anesthesiology speak to the growing recognition of the importance of this technology in the perioperative setting.

[a] Department of Anesthesiology, Division of Critical Care, University of Michigan Medical School, 1500 East Medical Center Drive, Ann Arbor, MI 48109-5048, USA; [b] Department of Anesthesiology, Division of Critical Care, Brigham and Women's Hospital, 75 Francis Street, Boston MA 02115, USA; [c] Department of Anesthesiology and Critical Care Medicine, Johns Hopkins University School of Medicine, Bloomberg 6320, 1800 Orleans Street, Baltimore, MD, USA 21287; [d] Department of Anesthesiology, Division of Critical Care Medicine, Emory School of Medicine, 1364 Clifton Road Northeast, Atlanta, GA 30322, USA
* Corresponding author. Department of Anesthesiology, Emory Critical Care Center, Emory School of Medicine, 1364 Clifton Road Northeast, Atlanta, GA 30322.
E-mail address: bfiza@emory.edu

Anesthesiology Clin 41 (2023) 231–248
https://doi.org/10.1016/j.anclin.2022.10.005
1932-2275/23/© 2022 Elsevier Inc. All rights reserved.
anesthesiology.theclinics.com

Bedside ultrasonography is an ideal tool for clinicians working in acute care settings. It enables the clinician to reach diagnoses rapidly and assess real-time intervention responses. In addition, in the intensive care unit (ICU) and perioperative environment, POCUS may decrease the utilization of conventional diagnostic modalities. This review describes the various pathologies that can be effectively and rapidly identified with the POC cardiac, lung, abdominal, vascular airway, and ocular ultrasonography, which reduce reliance on traditional diagnostic modalities.

DISCUSSION
Cardiac Ultrasound

Focused cardiac ultrasound (FoCUS) describes the use of ultrasound in a focused capacity to add anatomic, functional, and physiologic information about the heart to patient care. When evaluating hemodynamically unstable patients in the critical care and perioperative settings, FoCUS examination findings will often influence clinical management.[1,2] Below, we discuss specific applications of the FoCUS examination that may reduce traditional invasive monitoring techniques and, therefore, patient risk.

Diagnosing pulmonary embolism

Although the gold standard for diagnosing pulmonary embolism (PE) is computed tomography pulmonary angiography (CTPA), it may not always be feasible in patients with renal failure, pregnancy, or significant hemodynamic instability. Several qualitative and quantitative sonographic findings exist that support right ventricular (RV) dysfunction and the presence of PE (**Table 1**).[3] Of these, the findings most specific for acute PE are the 60/60 sign and McConnell's sign (Video 1), whereas right heart mobile thrombus is effectively diagnostic.[4] However, these findings generally have low sensitivity.[3]

An examination without RV dysfunction excludes PE with high sensitivity in hemodynamically unstable patients with suspected PE.[3] However, RV dysfunction may or may not be present in hemodynamically stable patients with suspected PE. In this case, a deep venous thromboembolism examination should be performed. A positive deep venous thrombosis (DVT) examination for proximal thrombus in combination with the presence of RV dilation yields a specificity of 100% for a diagnosis of PE.[5] Taken together, sonographic evidence of DVT or a convincing alternative diagnosis on thoracic ultrasound may reduce the need for CTPA.[6]

Table 1	
Qualitative and quantitative sonographic findings of Right Ventricular Dysfunction	
Quantitative	**Qualitative**
• RV to LV end-diastolic diameter ratio >1.0 in apical 4-chamber view	• Enlarged right ventricular outflow tract on parasternal long axis view
• IVC diameter >2 cm with <50% inspiratory collapsibility on subcostal view	• "D sign" (flattened interventricular septum on short axis view)
• "60/60 sign"—pulmonary ejection acceleration time <60 ms with peak systolic tricuspid valve gradient < 60 mm Hg	• McConnell's sign (depressed contractility of the RV free wall compared with the RV apex)
• TAPSE < 16 mm	• Thrombus in transit
• TAPSV < 9.5 cm/s	

Abbreviations: IVC, inferior vena cava; LV, left ventricle; RV, right ventricle; TAPSE, tricuspid annular plane systolic excursion; TAPSV, tricuspid annular peak systolic velocity.

Calculating cardiac output and ejection fraction

Cardiac output (CO) measurements via echocardiography provide a noninvasive alternative to traditional CO measurement tools. The CO is calculated by considering the left ventricular outflow tract (LVOT) as a cylinder, with the cross-sectional area of the aortic valve annulus as the base of the cylinder and the velocity time integral of flow across the LVOT as the height of the cylinder. The volume of the cylinder represents the stroke volume (SV). The aortic valve cross-sectional area is measured in parasternal long axis (PLAX) view, zoomed in to reduce measurement error ($\pi*(D/2)^2$) (**Fig. 1**A). Next, the apical five-chamber or apical three-chamber view is obtained to perform a pulse wave Doppler measurement of the velocity time integral of flow across the LVOT (**Fig. 1**B). The product of LVOT cross-sectional area (CSA) and velocity time integral (VTI) yields the SV, which then can be multiplied by heart rate to arrive at CO. Moderate-to-severe aortic regurgitation or subaortic obstruction precludes the accuracy of this method. Arrhythmias may result in beat-to-beat VTI variability; thus, the average of at least five VTIs is used for calculating CO.[7]

LVOT VTI variability can inform clinicians about volume status and response to volume administration or inotropic medication titration. In mechanically ventilated with no spontaneous respiratory effort, VTI variability measured during the respiratory cycle of more than 12% predicts fluid responsiveness.[8] A 12% increase in LVOT VTI during passive straight leg raise test is highly predictive of fluid responsiveness.[9] LVOT VTI can be used to track the patient's response to interventions, such as fluid challenges, vasopressor therapy, inotropic support, or relief of obstructive shock mechanisms. An increase of greater than 15% in the VTI indicates response to the intervention.[10]

Qualitative assessment of ejection fraction using FoCUS correlates well with more formal quantitative methods for calculating LVEF. E-point septal separation (EPSS) is calculated using M-mode at mitral valve anterior leaflet tip in the PLAX view (**Fig. 2**). The distance between the intraventricular septum and peak E-wave during diastole is measured to arrive at EPSS. An EPSS greater than 10 mm suggests reduced ejection fraction.[11] Other qualitative measures for assessing left ventricular (LV) function include the inward movement of the LV walls to a central point and myocardial thickening with greater than 30% endocardial thickening expected from diastole to systole.[12]

Evaluating mechanical circulatory support devices

POC echocardiography can assist in the evaluation of mechanical circulatory support devices such as ventricular assist devices or extracorporeal membrane oxygenation (ECMO) cannulas. Ultrasound imaging of the inferior vena cava (IVC) for venously placed devices or the LVOT/aorta for arterially placed devices can be used for assessing successful placement, inadvertent dislodgement, and migration of device cannulas (**Fig. 3**).[13] FoCUS can also be used for weaning of mechanical circulatory support devices using real-time monitoring of cardiac function during device turndown.

The PLAX view is used to evaluate Impella's position (types 2.5, CP [Abiomed Inc., Danvers, MA], 5.0, LD [Abiomed Inc., Danvers, MA], and 5.5), which appears as "train tracks" on 2-dimensional (2D) ultrasound (**Fig. 4**). An Impella should be positioned 3.5 cm below the aortic valve, except for the Impella 5.5 which should be positioned 5 cm below the aortic valve annulus.[14] Appropriate positioning minimizes hemolysis, suction alarms, and the chance of further migration into the ventricle.[13] The outflow area is hyperechoic in appearance relative to the adjacent cannula and should be above the aortic valve.[14] The catheter should be angled toward the apex and away from the ventricular walls and clear of the mitral valve apparatus.[14] Along with FoCUS, proper positioning of the Impella includes a verified placement signal and motor current waveforms.[15]

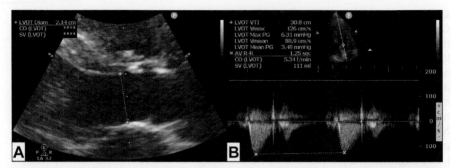

Fig. 1. (*A*) LVOT diameter measured at aortic valve annulus during end-systole using parasternal long axis view zoomed in on aortic valve annulus. LVOT area calculated (LVOT area, $\pi*(D/2)^2$). (*B*) Pulse wave Doppler on LVOT jet in apical 3-chamber (A3C) view. LVOT ejection jet is traced, with resulting area under the curve equivalent to LVOT VTI. CO is then calculated using CO, LVOT area $\times$ LVOT VTI $\times$ HR.

Focused cardiac ultrasound in undifferentiated shock

Several algorithms have been developed to rapidly assess patients with undifferentiated shock.[16,17] The most widely recognized approach is the Rapid Ultrasound in Shock (RUSH) protocol, which includes the cardiac, IVC, FAST/abdominal, aorta, and lung ultrasound examinations.[18] These components are further broken down

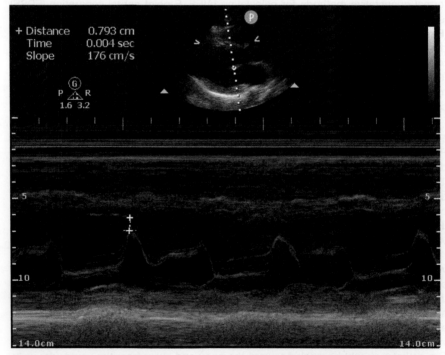

Fig. 2. Using M-mode in the PLAX view over the anterior mitral valve leaflet, measuring the minimal distance from the anterior mitral valve leaflet to the interventricular septum yields the EPSS.

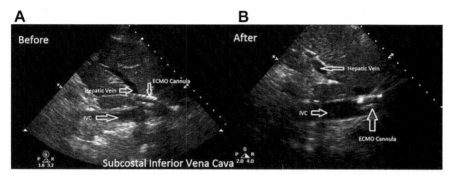

Fig. 3. Images taken from the subcostal inferior vena cava view. (*A*) Image taken during low flows on the ECMO circuit. The ECMO cannula is visualized as a hyperechoic structure located in the hepatic vein. (*B*) Resolution of low flows on ECMO circuit after catheter repositioning. The ECMO cannula is now located correctly in the lumen of the inferior vena cava. (Image reproduced in compliance with Open Access Creative Common's License.)[13]

conceptually into *pump*, *tank*, and *pipes*. *Pump* refers to cardiac function. *Tank* refers to intravascular volume status, and *pipes* refer to large vessel pathology. A meta-analysis on the application of the RUSH examination recommends that the protocol should be used to confirm suspected causes of shock rather than to definitively exclude specific etiologies.[18–20]

Pump evaluation involves assessment of pericardial effusion, global LV function, and RV:LV ratio. The presence of a pericardial effusion with collapse of the right-sided chambers during diastole is consistent with tamponade. A plethoric IVC without normal respiratory changes is also present in tamponade. Global systolic LV function is assessed in all the basic cardiac windows using qualitative or semiquantitative methods discussed previously. A hyperdynamic heart with strong ventricular contractility has greater than 80% changes in LV chamber size from diastole to systole. This can be indicative of early sepsis or hypovolemia, but also could represent underfilling from an obstructed RV outflow. An RV:LV ratio greater than 1 on apical four-chamber view suggests obstructive shock such as PE or RV infarction. The deflection of the interventricular septum from right to left or a free-floating intracardiac thrombus can also indicate this type of shock.[21]

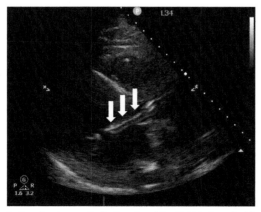

Fig. 4. Impella CP device "train tracks" visualized in PLAX view (*white arrows*). Distance from annulus to tip of train tracks should measure 5 cm for appropriate positioning.

Tank evaluation begins with assessment of the IVC size and respiratory variation to support the assessment of intravascular volume status. M-mode is used in the subcostal IVC view, 2 cm superior to the confluence of hepatic veins. In spontaneously breathing patients, an IVC diameter less than 2.1 cm with complete inspiratory collapse is associated with a CVP less than 5 mm Hg, whereas an IVC diameter greater than 2.1 cm with no inspiratory collapse is associated with a CVP of 15 mm Hg.[22] To accurately assess the IVC in the mechanically ventilated patient, the patient should be sedated to the point where the patient is not taking spontaneous breaths during measurement with the ventilator adjusted to 10 mL/kg of tidal volume. If the IVC diameter changes more than 18% during the respiratory cycle, this suggests volume responsiveness.[21]

Pipes evaluation is done by first assessing the thoracic and abdominal aorta for aneurysm or dissection. The aorta is visualized proximal to distal starting with the parasternal four-chamber view to assess the LVOT, the suprasternal view to visualizing the aortic arch, and following the aorta from thorax to abdomen by scanning down midline. The presence of aortic root dilation or an aortic intimal flap indicates dissection. The femoral and popliteal veins are assessed for compressibility. The lack of compressibility indicates DVT and obstructive shock from PE should be suspected.[21,23]

Diagnosing persistent left superior vena cava

With an incidence of 0.3% to 0.5%, persistent left superior vena cava vein (PLSVC) is a common systemic venous anomaly.[24] PLSVC is usually asymptomatic and usually discovered during central venous catheter (CVC) insertion, transjugular intrahepatic portosystemic shunt (TIPS) insertion, pulmonary artery catheter (PAC) insertion, and pacemaker insertion.[25] Case reports describe scenarios where CVCs were placed in the left internal jugular or left subclavian which appear mal-positioned in chest x-ray, often in the left chest, concerning for arterial placement.[26,27] In these cases, transduction of the CVC should support a central venous waveform and POCUS in the PLAX demonstrates a dilated coronary sinus (**Fig. 5**).[26] A bedside "bubble study," where agitated saline is injected into the distal port of the CVC, demonstrates echocardiographic visualization of the right atrium to confirm venous anatomy.[26–28] The use of ultrasonography for diagnosis of PLSVC may reduce the need for cross-sectional imaging and invasive techniques.

Lung Ultrasound

Over the years, lung ultrasound has gained a well-established role in the care of acutely ill patients. Lung ultrasonography has superior diagnostic capabilities in detecting pulmonary pathologies compared with auscultation or chest radiography during the perioperative period.[29,30] The routine use of lung ultrasonography has been associated with reducing the number of performed chest radiographs and CT scans.[31] Below, we describe some of the pulmonary pathologies commonly encountered in the perioperative environment that can be effectively and efficiently diagnosed using lung ultrasound.

Pneumothorax

Pneumothorax can be rapidly diagnosed using ultrasound which avoids the need for chest radiography, especially in the operating room where radiography may not be readily available.[32] The presence of lung-point sign on lung ultrasound examination is 100% specific for the diagnosis of pneumothorax.[33] However, it is not seen in the cases of total lung collapse. The lung-point sign describes the interface between

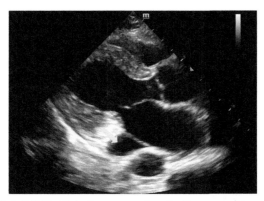

Fig. 5. Patient with left SVC, dilated coronary sinus (*yellow arrow*) present on parasternal long axis view.

the normal lung and pneumothorax. On one side of the lung point, healthy pleura is seen with normal pleural sliding—the shimmering of the hyperechoic pleura due to the sliding of visceral pleura relative to the parietal pleura—and a lack of lung sliding is noted at the site of the pneumothorax. On M-mode, the seashore sign is seen with static lines above the hyperechoic pleura, representing the stationary chest wall, and a speckled granular pattern beyond it—an artifact created by the lung sliding. In contrast, at the site of absent lung sliding, a linear pattern both above and below the pleura, the bar code sign, is seen (**Fig. 6**).[32]

Alveolar consolidation and atelectasis

Lung ultrasound has been used successfully to detect alveolar consolidation and atelectasis, including assessing the effectiveness of recruitment maneuvers in the perioperative arena.[34–36]

On ultrasonography, lung hepatization sign is noticeable when the collapsed alveoli assume tissue-like density resembling the liver (**Fig. 7**). Air bronchograms are also easily visualized on ultrasonography, and the nature of the air bronchograms can assist the clinician diagnostically compared with traditional chest radiography. In the presence of consolidation, dynamic air-bronchograms, hyperechoic opacities that move with the respiratory cycle, are visualized. These hyperechoic opacities are generated because of the higher acoustic reflectance of the aerated bronchi compared with the surrounding consolidated lung parenchyma. In contrast, in

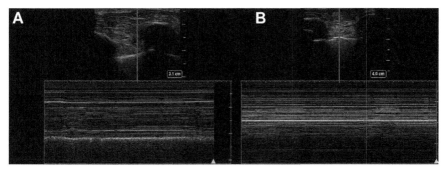

Fig. 6. Examination of the pleura on M-mode showing transition from the (*A*) seashore sign to the (*B*) barcode sign.

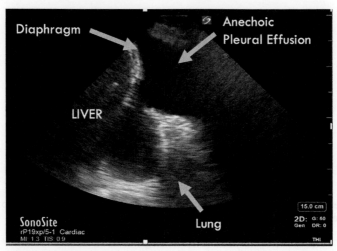

Fig. 7. This image illustrates pleural effusion and compressive atelectasis of the lung. As seen here, on ultrasonography, the collapsed lung appears similar to the liver.

resorptive atelectasis due to the result of airway obstruction, the trapped, isolated air results in the generation of static air bronchograms.[34]

Pulmonary edema

When it comes to detecting pulmonary edema, the diagnostic ability of ultrasonography is superior to that of both auscultation and chest radiography.[37,38] On ultrasonography, pulmonary edema and interstitial syndrome are visualized as B-lines. B-lines are vertical echogenic, comet-tail artifacts that move with the lung movement, arising from the pleural lines, appear as a laser beam, and spread to the edge of the screen without fading (**Fig. 8**). In contrast, A-lines are horizontal, regularly spaced hyperechogenic lines representing reverberations of the pleural line. A-lines combined with pleural sliding represent normal lung sonoanatomy (**Fig. 9**, Video 2).[39]

Pleural effusion

Auscultation and anterior-posterior chest radiography fare poorly compared with lung ultrasound for diagnosing pleural effusions.[40] In patients undergoing major surgery, detecting alveolar consolidations and pleural effusion in the PACU using ultrasound is associated with an increased risk of postoperative pulmonary complications.[41]

On ultrasonography, pleural effusions are best visualized by examining the dependent areas of the lung. They appear as homogenous anechoic structures bounded by the hemidiaphragm (see **Fig. 7**). Fibrin strands swimming in the fluid with undulations, debris, or loculations suggest complex effusion.

Endotracheal tube position confirmation

Lung ultrasound can be used effectively to identify the correct placement of a single- or double-lumen endotracheal tube (ETT) position.[42,43] Auscultation examination in the operating room environment is fraught with challenges as dorsal lung fields are difficult to reach in supine-positioned patients covered in surgical drapes, and the environment is often noisy. Ultrasound examination circumvents many of these challenges, and lung ultrasound examination is significantly more accurate compared with auscultation alone in discriminating between tracheal versus bronchial intubation.[43]

The identification of current ETT position can be achieved by evaluating for the presence or absence of lung sliding post-intubation. In the case of ETT position, lung

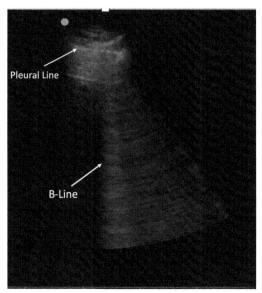

Fig. 8. B-lines or comet-tail artifacts are seen in this image. B-lines are vertical, echogenic, ray-like, reverberation artifacts that arise from the pleural line, are well-defined, spread to the edge of the screen without fading, obliterate A-lines, and move with lung sliding.

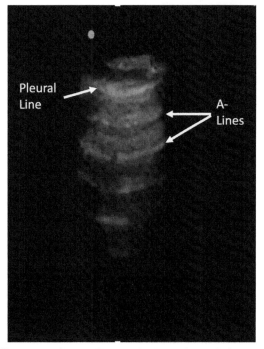

Fig. 9. This image illustrates A-lines. A-lines are horizontal, regularly spaced hyperechogenic lines representing reverberations of the pleural line.

sliding is present on both sides. However, in the case of endobronchial intubation, lung sliding will only be present on the side of the endobronchial intubation. In addition, a lack of lung sliding and lung pulse would be visualized on the contralateral side (Video 3). The lung pulse sign is seen as vibration or slight movement at the pleural line, in rhythm with the heartbeat. The lung pulse is observable when lung sliding is absent and indirectly proves an inflated but non-ventilated lung. Of note, lung pulse is a valuable sign in ruling out a pneumothorax.[44]

Diaphragmatic evaluation

Noninvasive measurements of diaphragmatic excursion and thickness on ultrasound provide for a noninvasive assessment of diaphragmatic strength. In critically ill patients, these parameters have been used to predict extubation success or failure.[45,46] Recently, similar ultrasonographic measures of diaphragmatic strength were valuable in recognizing postoperative residual curarization.[47] In addition, ultrasound can be a valuable tool in detecting diaphragmatic paralysis after neuraxial blockade procedures associated with a high risk of phrenic nerve paresis.

The anterior subcostal view is the preferred method to assess for the diaphragmatic excursion. In this method, the probe is placed in the midclavicular and anterior axillary lines in the anterior subcostal region with the transducer directed medially, cranially, and dorsally. This method allows for the visualization of the dome of the diaphragm, and the diaphragmatic movement toward or away from the transducer is observed (Video 4). The diaphragmatic excursion is measured by calculating the amplitude of the excursion on the M-mode (**Fig. 10**). The usual range of motion from the resting

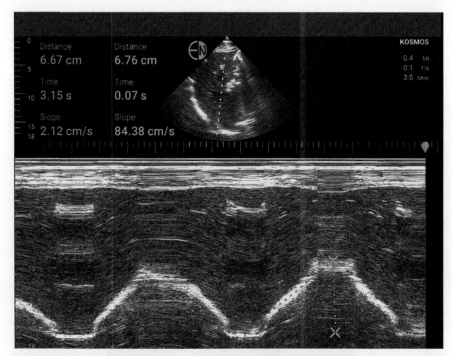

Fig. 10. Diaphragmatic motion on M-mode ultrasonography. The M-mode interrogation line is placed at the posterior one-third of the diaphragm to assess for the diaphragmatic excursion.

expiratory position to full inspiration in adults is reported to be 1.9 to 9 cm. The absence of excursion during normal breathing indicates diaphragmatic paresis or paradoxic motion on sniffing.[48]

Abdominal Ultrasound

Abdominal POCUS, applied as the FAST examination, is well established.[49] The FAST examination has greater than 90% sensitivity and specificity for detecting intraperitoneal free fluid and can detect as low as 10 mL of free fluid.[50] In the trauma setting, the routine use of POCUS has been demonstrated to decrease the time to operative intervention, need for CT scans, and hospital costs.[51]

Abdominal POCUS can also detect pneumoperitoneum with similar sensitivity, specificity, accuracy, and predictive value as an abdominal x-ray.[52] "Abdominal A-lines" or "stripe sign" may be observed, reflecting air artifact that develops at the interface of soft tissue and free air. The presence of "gut sliding," reflecting the apposition of the visceral and parietal peritoneum, allows the examiner to differentiate between pathologic abdominal free air and physiologic bowel gas. The detection of a "gut point" is pathognomonic for pneumoperitoneum, denoting a transition to loss of gut sliding and its attendant stripe sign.[53]

Gastric ultrasound has 99.8% sensitivity and 91% specificity for confirmation of intragastric tube placement and has excellent agreement with radiography.[54] Dynamic fogging in the stomach is observed when 40 cc of air or an admixture of 40 cc of saline with 10 cc of air is injected into the gastric tube.[54,55] Sonographic evaluation of the gastric antrum in the supine and right lateral decubitus position correlates well with age-adjusted predicted gastric volume, thus can be used to determine periprocedural aspiration risk.[56]

Vascular Ultrasound

Vascular ultrasound can be used in acute care settings for both procedural and diagnostic guidance. Procedural indications include assisting the placement of arterial and venous cannulas into the peripheral or central vasculature to decrease the number of failed attempts and complications.[57,58] The positioning of ECMO cannulas can also be evaluated with the use of PoCUS (see **Fig. 3**). Diagnostic usefulness of vascular ultrasound in the ICU include diagnosis of deep vein thromboses; observation of the IVC in the estimation of right atrial pressure and potential fluid responsiveness; identification of aortic aneurysms and dissections; and Doppler interrogation of the hepatic, portal, and intrarenal veins to identify venous congestion.[59,60]

Between 8% and 40% of patients develop DVTs during their ICU admission with significant associated morbidity and mortality.[61] Up to 50% of patients with proximal lower extremity DVTs may have an associated PE, making it particularly important to promptly identify these. Delays associated with ordering a formal vascular examination are reported as 13.8 hours. However, a POC DVT study, in the form of a 2D compression test, is immediately available to critical care physicians and has been shown to have comparable accuracy to a comprehensive vascular study involving color and duplex Doppler.[62,63] The protocol consists of identifying the common femoral vein (CFV) region (2 cm proximal to 2 cm distal to the intersection of the common femoral and greater saphenous veins) and popliteal vein region (distal 2 cm until its trifurcation into the peroneal, anterior, and posterior tibial veins) for a "2-point test," whereas the superficial femoral vein region (from the bifurcation of the CFV to the point at which the superficial femoral vein courses posterior through the adductor canal) is included for a "3-point test." At points separated by 2 cm increments, each area should be compressed with enough force to deform the accompanying artery. A positive test is yielded if the vein dose not completely compresses or a thrombus is visualized (**Fig. 11**). Although most DVTs are identified between the highest point of the CFV and the takeoff of the bifurcation into deep and superficial femoral veins, the 3-point test has been shown to have improved sensitivity without a significant increase in time to perform it.[64]

Airway Ultrasound

Assessment of airway anatomy is an emerging method to aid in the prediction of difficult laryngoscopy. For example, a reduced temporomandibular joint mobility (condylar translational distance < 10 mm) is correlated with a Cormack–Lehane grade 3 and 4.[65] The optimal ETT outer diameter can be estimated by measuring the subglottic transverse diameter, a technique demonstrated to be clinically superior to age-based and height-based formulas for predicting pediatric ETT size based on the tracheal leak test.[66,67] Endotracheal intubation can be confirmed by visualization of tracheal dilation during pilot balloon insufflation and the presence of bilateral lung sliding.[66]

Sonographic evaluation of the cricoid cartilage and tracheal rings is used to guide percutaneous cricothyroidotomy and percutaneous dilatational tracheostomy. The cricoid cartilage yields a thick ovoid shadow on transverse view and a "hump" appearance on longitudinal view. The tracheal rings are shaped like an "inverted U" on transverse view and a "string of beads" on longitudinal view.[67] Airway ultrasound greatly improves the accuracy of cricothyroid membrane identification compared with external palpation in patients with abnormal neck anatomy.[68] Using a dynamic sonographic technique helps to identify the cricothyroid membrane, guide the finder needle to the midline of the anterior trachea, prevent cranial misplacement, and avoid vascular structures.[69]

Ocular Ultrasound

The developing technique of ocular ultrasound has the potential to provide noninvasive monitoring and diagnostic capabilities in patients suffering from intracranial hypertension. Currently, ocular ultrasound is used to manage intubated and obtunded patients with elevated intracranial pressures due to traumatic brain injury,

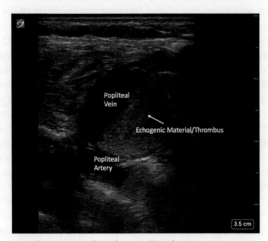

Fig. 11. A thrombus can be seen within the popliteal vein.

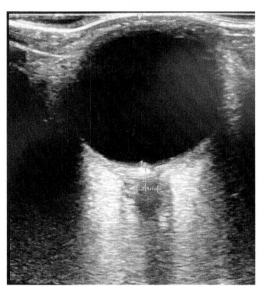

Fig. 12. Ocular ultrasound measurements of the optic sheath nerve diameter (ONSD) on ocular ultrasound. The optic nerve sheath is identified and measured approximately 3 mm posterior to the retina or lamina cribosa with the patient in the supine position.

cerebrovascular event, or acute liver failure. Clinically, one would hope that this imaging modality could prevent the need for invasive intracranial pressure monitoring or repeat CT examinations that evaluate for the progression of sequelae resulting from worsening intracranial hypertension. However, this imaging modality does not yet carry the precision or accuracy required to guide interventions to decrease intracranial hypertension or optimize cerebral perfusion pressure. Invasive intracranial devices, which have become more technologically advanced with less complications, are the gold standard. Ocular ultrasound may be a supplement to the gold standard or seem to be useful to assess intracranial hypertension when invasive monitoring is either contraindicated or unavailable.[70]

Ocular ultrasound measures the optic sheath nerve diameter (ONSD), which has been shown to increase with rising intracranial pressures. Typically, a high-frequency linear probe 5 MHz or greater is used to identify and measure the optic nerve sheath approximately 3 mm posterior to the retina or lamina cribosa with the patient in the supine position (**Fig. 12**).[71] This measurement is quickly captured and can be repeated to assess dynamic changes over time. Studies show that normal ONSD is typically less than 5.0 mm, and greater than 5.5 mm has been accurate in differentiating patients with intracranial pressure greater than 20 mm Hg on gold standard invasive monitoring.[72] More research is necessary to see how this technique can supplement critical care management when invasive monitoring is present or not present or how it may support the decision to proceed with invasive monitoring.

SUMMARY

POCUS is an impactful perioperative tool for a rapid diagnosis and management of critical illness, preventing the need for other imaging investigations and reducing the need to transport an unstable patient for further testing.

CLINICS CARE POINTS

- Point-of-care Ultrasound algorithms that combine cardiac, pulmonary, and vascular examinations can rapidly assess patients with undifferentiated shock.
- Lung ultrasonography can diagnose the exact etiologies of perioperative hypoxemia as it has superior diagnostic capabilities in detecting pulmonary pathologies compared to auscultation or chest radiography in the perioperative period.
- Gastric ultrasound for intragastric tube placement has excellent agreement with radiography, and gastric antrum evaluation can be used to determine periprocedural aspiration risk.
- Airway ultrasound improves the accuracy of cricothyroid membrane identification compared to palpation in patients with abnormal neck anatomy and can be used to safely perform percutaneous cricothyroidotomy.
- If invasive intracranial monitoring is contraindicated or unavailable, ocular ultrasound can be used to assess optic nerve sheath diameter to assess for intracranial hypertension.

FINANCIAL DISCLOSURES

None.

CONFLICTS OF INTEREST

None.

SUPPLEMENTARY DATA

Supplementary data related to this article can be found online at doi:10.1016/j.anclin. 2022.10.005.

REFERENCES

1. Kratz T, Steinfeldt T, Exner M, et al. Impact of Focused Intraoperative Transthoracic Echocardiography by Anesthesiologists on Management in Hemodynamically Unstable High-Risk Noncardiac Surgery Patients. J Cardiothorac Vasc Anesth 2017;31(2):602–9.
2. Cowie B. Focused cardiovascular ultrasound performed by anesthesiologists in the perioperative period: feasible and alters patient management. J Cardiothorac Vasc Anesth 2009;23(4):450–6.
3. Konstantinides SV, Meyer G, Becattini C, et al. 2019 ESC Guidelines for the diagnosis and management of acute pulmonary embolism developed in collaboration with the European Respiratory Society (ERS). Eur Heart J 2020;41(4):543–603.
4. Kurzyna M, Torbicki A, Pruszczyk P, et al. Disturbed right ventricular ejection pattern as a new Doppler echocardiographic sign of acute pulmonary embolism. Am J Cardiol 2002;90(5):507–11.
5. Nazerian P, Volpicelli G, Gigli C, et al. Diagnostic accuracy of focused cardiac and venous ultrasound examinations in patients with shock and suspected pulmonary embolism. Intern Emerg Med 2018;13(4):567–74.
6. Koenig S, Chandra S, Alaverdian A, et al. Ultrasound assessment of pulmonary embolism in patients receiving CT pulmonary angiography. Chest 2014;145(4): 818–23.

7. Blanco P. Rationale for using the velocity-time integral and the minute distance for assessing the stroke volume and cardiac output in point-of-care settings. Ultrasound J 2020;12(1):21.

8. Miller A, Mandeville J. Predicting and measuring fluid responsiveness with echocardiography. Echo Res Pract 2016;3(2):G1–12.

9. Levitov A, Frankel HL, Blaivas M, et al. Guidelines for the Appropriate Use of Bedside General and Cardiac Ultrasonography in the Evaluation of Critically Ill Patients-Part II: Cardiac Ultrasonography. Crit Care Med 2016;44(6):1206–27.

10. Blanco P, Aguiar FM, Blaivas M. Rapid Ultrasound in Shock (RUSH) Velocity-Time Integral: A Proposal to Expand the RUSH Protocol. J Ultrasound Med 2015;34(9):1691–700.

11. Elagha A, Fuisz A. Mitral valve E-Point to Septal Separation (EPSS) measurement by cardiac magnetic resonance Imaging as a quantitative surrogate of Left Ventricular Ejection Fraction (LVEF). J Cardiovasc Magn Reson 2012;14(Suppl 1):P154.

12. Andrus P, Dean A. Focused Cardiac Ultrasound. Glob Heart 2013;8(4):299–303.

13. Fiza B, Tang M, Maile M. Management of cardiopulmonary assist devices in critically ill patients using point-of-care transthoracic echocardiography: a case series. Crit Ultrasound J 2017;9(1):24.

14. Tran T, Mudigonda P, Mahr C, et al. Echocardiographic imaging of temporary percutaneous mechanical circulatory support devices. J Echocardiogr 2022;20(2):77–86.

15. Anderson BB, Collard CD. Images in Anesthesiology: Proper Positioning of an Impella 2.5 and CP Heart Pump. Anesthesiology 2017;127(6):1014.

16. Ha YR, Toh HC. Clinically integrated multi-organ point-of-care ultrasound for undifferentiated respiratory difficulty, chest pain, or shock: a critical analytic review. J Intensive Care 2016;4:54.

17. Volpicelli G, Lamorte A, Tullio M, et al. Point-of-care multiorgan ultrasonography for the evaluation of undifferentiated hypotension in the emergency department. Intensive Care Med 2013;39(7):1290–8.

18. Perera P, Mailhot T, Riley D, et al. The RUSH exam: Rapid Ultrasound in SHock in the evaluation of the critically Ill. Emerg Med Clin North Am 2010;28(1):29–56, vii.

19. Stickles SP, Carpenter CR, Gekle R, et al. The diagnostic accuracy of a point-of-care ultrasound protocol for shock etiology: A systematic review and meta-analysis. Cjem 2019;21(3):406–17.

20. Keikha M, Salehi-Marzijarani M, Soldoozi Nejat R, et al. Diagnostic Accuracy of Rapid Ultrasound in Shock (RUSH) Exam; A Systematic Review and Meta-analysis. Bull Emerg Trauma 2018;6(4):271–8.

21. Perera P, Mailhot T, Riley DC, et al. The RUSH Exam 2012: Rapid Ultrasound in Shock in the Evaluation of the Critically Ill Patient. Ultrasound Clin 2012;7:255–78.

22. Rudski LG, Lai WW, Afilalo J, et al. Guidelines for the echocardiographic assessment of the right heart in adults: a report from the American Society of Echocardiography endorsed by the European Association of Echocardiography, a registered branch of the European Society of Cardiology, and the Canadian Society of Echocardiography. J Am Soc Echocardiogr 2010;23(7):685–713, quiz 786-8.

23. Seif D, Perera P, Mailhot T, et al. Bedside ultrasound in resuscitation and the rapid ultrasound in shock protocol. Crit Care Res Pract 2012;2012:503254.

24. Kula S, Cevik A, Sanli C, et al. Persistent left superior vena cava: experience of a tertiary health-care center. Pediatr Int 2011;53(6):1066–9.

25. Commandeur D, Garetier M, Giacardi C, et al. Ultrasound-guided cannulation of the left subclavian vein in a case of persistent left superior vena cava. Can J Anaesth 2011;58(5):471–2.

26. Pardinas Gutierrez MA, Escobar LA, Blumer V, et al. Incidental finding of persistent left superior vena cava after 'bubble study' verification of central venous catheter. BMJ Case Rep 2017;2017. https://doi.org/10.1136/bcr-2017-220133.

27. Kumar D, Shafiq F. Successful management of septic patient with concealed left persistent superior vena cava: anaesthetic perspective. J Pak Med Assoc 2016; 66(9):1179–81.

28. Milam AJ, Tou E, Lam P, et al. Persistent left superior vena cava with partial anomalous venous return in a liver transplant patient. Anaesth Rep 2020;8(2):107–10.

29. Touw HR, Schuitemaker AE, Daams F, et al. Routine lung ultrasound to detect postoperative pulmonary complications following major abdominal surgery: a prospective observational feasibility study. Ultrasound J 2019;11(1):20.

30. Xie C, Sun K, You Y, et al. Feasibility and efficacy of lung ultrasound to investigate pulmonary complications in patients who developed postoperative Hypoxaemia- a prospective study. BMC Anesthesiol 2020;20(1):220.

31. Peris A, Tutino L, Zagli G, et al. The use of point-of-care bedside lung ultrasound significantly reduces the number of radiographs and computed tomography scans in critically ill patients. Anesth Analg 2010;111(3):687–92.

32. Fiza B, Moll V, Ferrero N. The Lung Point: Early Identification of Pneumothorax on Point of Care Ultrasound. Anesthesiology 2019;131(5):1148.

33. Lichtenstein D, Mezière G, Biderman P, et al. The "lung point": an ultrasound sign specific to pneumothorax. Intensive Care Med 2000;26(10):1434–40.

34. Hollon MM, Fiza B, Faloye A. Intraoperative Application of Lung Ultrasound to Diagnose Alveolar Consolidation. Anesthesiology 2019;131(4):894.

35. Kim BR, Lee S, Bae H, et al. Lung ultrasound score to determine the effect of fraction inspired oxygen during alveolar recruitment on absorption atelectasis in laparoscopic surgery: a randomized controlled trial. BMC Anesthesiol 2020; 20(1):173.

36. Song I-K, Kim E-H, Lee J-H, et al. Utility of Perioperative Lung Ultrasound in Pediatric Cardiac Surgery: A Randomized Controlled Trial. Anesthesiology 2018; 128(4):718–27.

37. Cox EGM, Koster G, Baron A, et al. Should the ultrasound probe replace your stethoscope? A SICS-I sub-study comparing lung ultrasound and pulmonary auscultation in the critically ill. Crit Care 2020;24(1):14.

38. Maw AM, Hassanin A, Ho PM, et al. Diagnostic Accuracy of Point-of-Care Lung Ultrasonography and Chest Radiography in Adults With Symptoms Suggestive of Acute Decompensated Heart Failure: A Systematic Review and Meta-analysis. JAMA Netw Open 2019;2(3):e190703.

39. Lichtenstein DA, Mezière GA, Lagoueyte JF, et al. A-lines and B-lines: lung ultrasound as a bedside tool for predicting pulmonary artery occlusion pressure in the critically ill. Chest 2009;136(4):1014–20.

40. Lichtenstein D, Goldstein I, Mourgeon E, et al. Comparative diagnostic performances of auscultation, chest radiography, and lung ultrasonography in acute respiratory distress syndrome. Anesthesiology 2004;100(1):9–15.

41. Zieleskiewicz L, Papinko M, Lopez A, et al. Lung Ultrasound Findings in the Postanesthesia Care Unit Are Associated With Outcome After Major Surgery: A Prospective Observational Study in a High-Risk Cohort. Anesth Analgesia 2021; 132(1):172–81.

42. Parab SY, Divatia JV, Chogle A. A prospective comparative study to evaluate the utility of lung ultrasonography to improve the accuracy of traditional clinical methods to confirm position of left sided double lumen tube in elective thoracic surgeries. Indian J Anaesth 2015;59(8):476–81.

43. Ramsingh D, Frank E, Haughton R, et al. Auscultation versus Point-of-care Ultrasound to Determine Endotracheal versus Bronchial Intubation: A Diagnostic Accuracy Study. Anesthesiology 2016;124(5):1012–20.

44. Bhoil R, Ahluwalia A, Chopra R, et al. Signs and lines in lung ultrasound. J Ultrason 2021;21(86):e225–33.

45. Zambon M, Greco M, Bocchino S, et al. Assessment of diaphragmatic dysfunction in the critically ill patient with ultrasound: a systematic review. Intensive Care Med 2017;43(1):29–38.

46. DiNino E, Gartman EJ, Sethi JM, et al. Diaphragm ultrasound as a predictor of successful extubation from mechanical ventilation. Thorax 2014;69(5):423–7.

47. Lang J, Liu Y, Zhang Y, et al. Peri-operative diaphragm ultrasound as a new method of recognizing post-operative residual curarization. BMC Anesthesiol 2021;21(1):287.

48. Sarwal A, Walker FO, Cartwright MS. Neuromuscular ultrasound for evaluation of the diaphragm. Muscle Nerve 2013;47(3):319–29.

49. Körner M, Krötz MM, Degenhart C, et al. Current Role of Emergency US in Patients with Major Trauma. Radiographics 2008;28(1):225–42.

50. Paajanen H, Lahti P, Nordback I. Sensitivity of transabdominal ultrasonography in detection of intraperitoneal fluid in humans. Eur Radiol 1999;9(7):1423–5.

51. Melniker LA, Leibner E, McKenney MG, et al. Randomized controlled clinical trial of point-of-care, limited ultrasonography for trauma in the emergency department: the first sonography outcomes assessment program trial. Ann Emerg Med 2006;48(3):227–35.

52. Braccini G, Lamacchia M, Boraschi P, et al. Ultrasound versus plain film in the detection of pneumoperitoneum. Abdom Imaging 1996;21(5):404–12.

53. Taylor MA, Merritt CH, Riddle PJ Jr, et al. Diagnosis at gut point: rapid identification of pneumoperitoneum via point-of-care ultrasound. Ultrasound J 2020; 12(1):52.

54. Mumoli N, Vitale J, Pagnamenta A, et al. Bedside Abdominal Ultrasound in Evaluating Nasogastric Tube Placement: A Multicenter, Prospective, Cohort Study. Chest 2021;159(6):2366–72.

55. Kim HM, So BH, Jeong WJ, et al. The effectiveness of ultrasonography in verifying the placement of a nasogastric tube in patients with low consciousness at an emergency center. Scand J Trauma Resusc Emerg Med 2012;20:38.

56. Perlas A, Davis L, Khan M, et al. Gastric sonography in the fasted surgical patient: a prospective descriptive study. Anesth Analg 2011;113(1):93–7.

57. Brass P, Hellmich M, Kolodziej L, et al. Ultrasound guidance versus anatomical landmarks for subclavian or femoral vein catheterization. Cochrane Database Syst Rev 2015;1(1):Cd011447.

58. Leung J, Duffy M, Finckh A. Real-time ultrasonographically-guided internal jugular vein catheterization in the emergency department increases success rates and reduces complications: a randomized, prospective study. Ann Emerg Med 2006;48(5):540–7.

59. Beaubien-Souligny W, Rola P, Haycock K, et al. Quantifying systemic congestion with Point-Of-Care ultrasound: development of the venous excess ultrasound grading system. Ultrasound J 2020;12(1):16.

60. Moreno FL, Hagan AD, Holmen JR, et al. Evaluation of size and dynamics of the inferior vena cava as an index of right-sided cardiac function. Am J Cardiol 1984; 53(4):579–85.
61. Malato A, Dentali F, Siragusa S, et al. The impact of deep vein thrombosis in critically ill patients: a meta-analysis of major clinical outcomes. Blood Transfus 2015;13(4):559–68.
62. Kory PD, Pellecchia CM, Shiloh AL, et al. Accuracy of ultrasonography performed by critical care physicians for the diagnosis of DVT. Chest 2011;139(3):538–42.
63. Roberts L, Rozen T, Murphy D, et al. A preliminary study of intensivist-performed DVT ultrasound screening in trauma ICU patients (APSIT Study). Ann Intensive Care 2020;10(1):122.
64. Zuker-Herman R, Ayalon Dangur I, Berant R, et al. Comparison between two-point and three-point compression ultrasound for the diagnosis of deep vein thrombosis. J Thromb Thrombolysis 2018;45(1):99–105.
65. Yao W, Zhou Y, Wang B, et al. Can Mandibular Condylar Mobility Sonography Measurements Predict Difficult Laryngoscopy? Anesth Analg 2017;124(3):800–6.
66. You-Ten KE, Siddiqui N, Teoh WH, et al. Point-of-care ultrasound (POCUS) of the upper airway. Can J Anaesth 2018;65(4):473–84 Échographie au point d'intervention (PoCUS) des voies respiratoires supérieures.
67. Osman A, Sum KM. Role of upper airway ultrasound in airway management. J Intensive Care 2016;4:52.
68. Siddiqui N, Yu E, Boulis S, et al. Ultrasound Is Superior to Palpation in Identifying the Cricothyroid Membrane in Subjects with Poorly Defined Neck Landmarks: A Randomized Clinical Trial. Anesthesiology 2018;129(6):1132–9.
69. Rajajee V, Fletcher JJ, Rochlen LR, et al. Real-time ultrasound-guided percutaneous dilatational tracheostomy: a feasibility study. Crit Care 2011;15(1):R67.
70. Robba C, Santori G, Czosnyka M, et al. Optic nerve sheath diameter measured sonographically as non-invasive estimator of intracranial pressure: a systematic review and meta-analysis. Intensive Care Med 2018;44(8):1284–94.
71. del Saz-Saucedo P, Redondo-González O, Mateu-Mateu Á, et al. Sonographic assessment of the optic nerve sheath diameter in the diagnosis of idiopathic intracranial hypertension. J Neurol Sci 2016;361:122–7.
72. Jeon JP, Lee SU, Kim SE, et al. Correlation of optic nerve sheath diameter with directly measured intracranial pressure in Korean adults using bedside ultrasonography. PLoS One 2017;12(9):e0183170.

Coagulopathy and Emergent Reversal of Anticoagulation

William John Wallisch, MD[a],*, Brent Kidd, MD[a], Liang Shen, MD, MPH[b],
Rachel Hammer, DO[c], Jordan Siscel, MD[a]

KEYWORDS

- Coagulopathy • Anticoagulation • Emergent reversal

KEY POINTS

- Many of the patients presenting for urgent or emergent procedures have underlying coagulopathies due to anticoagulant medications.
- Evidence-based correction of coagulopathy remains an important topic for all anesthesiologists.
- Advances over the last decade in both anticoagulant therapies and available reversal strategies require a frequent re-examination of recent literature.
- This article provides a succinct evidence-based review of current anticoagulants and their reversals.

INTRODUCTION AND CONVENTIONAL COAGULATION ASSAYS

Coagulopathy is a common finding in critically ill patients, potentially leading to life-threatening hemorrhage. The causes of coagulopathy are myriad, and frequently originate from patients' underlying pathologies. Current understanding of fibrin clot formation is based on the traditional concept of the "coagulation cascade"—a sequence of protein reactions leading to fibrin formation, as well as the more recent, nuanced view of a complex interplay of factors with built-in feedback loops.[1] Clinical laboratory tests attempt to mimic in vivo processes in an in vitro setting, and therefore cannot completely capture the complexities of true physiologic hemostasis. However, tests can still be helpful in the identification of certain coagulopathies and aid treatment.

The authors declare no relevant material or financial interests that relate to the research described in this article.
[a] Department of Anesthesiology, University of Kansas Medical Center, 3901 Rainbow Boulevard, Mail Stop 1034, Kansas City, KS 66160, USA; [b] Department of Anesthesiology, Weill Cornell Medical College, 525 East 68th Street, M324, New York, NY 10065, USA; [c] Department of Anesthesiology, Emory University, 1364 Clifton Road Northeast, Atlanta, GA 30322, USA
* Corresponding author.
E-mail address: wwallisch@kumc.edu

Anesthesiology Clin 41 (2023) 249–261
https://doi.org/10.1016/j.anclin.2022.10.006
1932-2275/23/© 2022 Elsevier Inc. All rights reserved.
anesthesiology.theclinics.com

Coagulation Cascade

When discussing in vitro coagulation in the laboratory setting, it is helpful to review the intrinsic, extrinsic, and common pathways of coagulation, which are based on the "waterfall" or "coagulation cascade" concept.[2] The intrinsic pathway is activated by blood contact with a glass test tube. The negative charge of the glass initiates the contact pathway, converting factor XII to factor XIIa, which catalyzes factor XI's conversion to factor XIa, which in turn cleaves factor IX to factor IXa. Factor XIIa also converts prekallikrein (bound to high molecular weight kininogen) to kallikrein to generate more factor XIIa in a positive feedback loop. Factor IXa then binds to its cofactor factor VIII, and this complex will activate factor X to Xa, which is the beginning of the common pathway. Factor Xa then joins its cofactor factor V to convert prothrombin (factor II) to thrombin (factor IIa). Thrombin finally converts fibrinogen (factor I) to fibrin to initiate clot formation. In summary, the intrinsic pathway involves factors XII, XI, IX, VIII, prekallikrein, and high molecular weight kininogen, whereas the common pathway uses factors X, V, II, and I.

In contrast, the extrinsic pathway requires the addition of tissue factor, phospholipid, and calcium to plasma that has been anticoagulated with citrate. Factor VII is activated to factor VIIa, which binds to tissue factor, and the resulting complex will convert factor X to factor Xa—proceeding down the rest of the common pathway.

Prothrombin Time and Activated Partial Thromboplastin Time

The most common laboratory tests used to evaluate coagulopathic patients are the prothrombin time (PT), also expressed as the international normalized ratio (INR), activated partial thromboplastin time (aPTT), and fibrinogen assays. PT and INR evaluate the extrinsic and common pathways, whereas aPTT reflects the function of the intrinsic and common pathways. Fibrinogen assays reveal abnormalities in fibrinogen function or level, depending on the specific assay used.

The PT is run by adding patient plasma, anticoagulated with sodium citrate, to a reagent containing thromboplastin and calcium chloride. The calcium initiates coagulation, and the clot formation is measured using increased impedance or turbidity, or decreased optical clarity, and expressed in seconds. PT is frequently used to monitor warfarin anticoagulation. The INR was developed to normalize differences in laboratory reference ranges for the PT and increase the ease of inter-laboratory comparisons. The aPTT is commonly used to monitor the heparin anticoagulation effect. It is performed by activating coagulation by contact with a negatively charged surface, such as kaolin, silica, or celite, along with the addition of phospholipid and calcium chloride. The time to clot formation is measured in seconds. Both the PT and aPTT can be used as screening tests for coagulopathy resulting from factor dysfunction in their respective pathways, but neither is specific as to the factor or factors affected.[1]

Tests of Fibrinogen Function

The common tests of fibrinogen function include the thrombin clotting time (TCT) and clottable fibrinogen assay (Clauss assay). Both tests add thrombin to patient plasma to directly catalyze the conversion of fibrinogen to fibrin. The TCT measures clot formation in seconds, whereas the Clauss assay calculates the amount of functional fibrinogen.

Activated Clotting Time

The activated coagulation time, also termed activated clotting time (ACT), is commonly used during surgical procedures that require the administration of heparin. It measures the intrinsic and common pathways of coagulation by activating whole blood in a test tube containing celite or kaolin, and measuring the time to clot formation in seconds. The ACT has some drawbacks, including variability of measurements depending on the device and patient characteristics, and lack of correlation with plasma heparin levels.[3] More recently, the anti-Xa assay has been increasingly used as the measurement of heparin activity. This test is a chromogenic procedure, containing exogenous factor Xa and a chromogenic substrate for that factor. The patient's own antithrombin is used, or exogenous antithrombin is added to the sample. Any heparin in the mixture will complex with antithrombin and then will inhibit factor Xa. Residual factor Xa cleaves the chromogenic substrate, releasing a yellow-colored chromophore that can be read optically. Thus, the amount of chromophore released is inversely proportional to the amount of heparin present in the sample. The anti-Xa assay can be used with unfractionated heparin (UFH), low-molecular-weight heparin (LMWH), and fondaparinux.[2]

Platelet Function Testing

Platelet function has proven somewhat difficult to measure in a rapid, useable fashion. Traditional measurements such as bleeding time are neither sensitive nor specific to evaluate for platelet abnormalities. The platelet function analyzer (PFA-100 or PFA-200) is an automated analyzer found in many labs that attempts to create high shear conditions that are expected to cause hemostasis. Platelet function is determined by measuring the amount of time needed to occlude an aperture. A prospective study found that the PFA is only marginally more useful than the bleeding time and is neither sensitive nor specific enough to preclude further platelet or von Willebrand factor (vWF) testing, and should therefore likely not be relied upon in any clinically important sense.[1]

Viscoelastic Testing

Viscoelastic tests are bedside point-of-care assays that have increased in use due to their ease of interpretation and the fact that they provide real-time measurements of clot formation and integrity. Prominent commercially available tests include thromboelastography (TEG) and rotational thromboelastometry (ROTEM).[4] These are analogous tests during which a sensory rod is placed into a cup of a small amount of citrated patient blood. The cup or rod is then rotated and the resistance to rotation is graphed over time. The graph shows the mechanics of clot formation, including time to clot initiation, clot propagation speed, and ultimate clot strength. Modifications of these tests have been made to reflect isolated fibrinogen function. These tests are frequently faster to run than conventional coagulation tests, though suffer from some drawbacks such as inability to detect platelet or vWF dysfunction.[1]

As described above, numerous tests can be used to diagnose coagulopathy, each with its own idiosyncrasies and drawbacks. No single test can elucidate all the abnormalities in the coagulation system, in part due to the origins of many of these tests as specific anticoagulant effect assays, but also due to the inherent limitations of using in vitro systems to estimate complex in vivo processes. As such, clinicians are encouraged to decide on the best course of treatment for patients based on a synthesis of history, risk factors, clinical examination, and thoughtful interpretation of coagulation test results (**Fig. 1**).

Organization of the coagulation system based on current screening assays

The intrinsic coagulation system consists of the protein factors XII, XI, IX, and VIII and prekallikrein and high-molecular-weight kininogen. The extrinsic coagulation system consists of tissue factor and factor VII. The common pathway of the coagulation system consists of factors X, V, and II and fibrinogen (I). The aPTT requires the presence

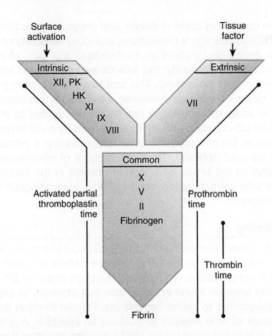

Fig. 1. Organization of the coagulation cascade based on current screening assays. (*From* Pai, M. Chapter 129: Laboratory Evaluation of Hemostatic and Thrombotic Disorders. In: R. Hoffman, E. Benz, L. Silberstein, H. Heslop, J. Weitz, J. Anastasi, M. Salama and S. Abutalib, eds. Hematology, Basic Principles and Practice, 7th ed. Philadelphia: Elsevier, 2018:1922-1931; With permission.)

of every protein except tissue factor and factor VII. The PT requires factors VII, X, V, and II, and fibrinogen. The TCT only tests the integrity of fibrinogen.

MEDICATION-INDUCED COAGULOPATHIES
Warfarin

Warfarin is a water-soluble vitamin K antagonist (VKA) that interferes with the synthesis of multiple Vitamin K-dependent clotting factors, including factors II, VII, IX, X, and Proteins C and S (**Fig. 2**). This results in clotting proteins that are only partially carboxylated, giving them reduced or absent clotting activity.[5] It typically takes 48 to 72 h after the initiation of warfarin for clotting factor levels to decrease enough to affect coagulation testing.

Warfarin activity is monitored using the PT, a test that is affected by reductions in factors II, VII, and X. This PT is converted to an INR using an equation composed of the patient's PT, the mean normal PT, and an international sensitivity index. This is done to account for any differences among various prothrombin reagents and laboratories.[5] The typical INR goal is 2.0 to 3.0 for most indications, although patients with mechanical heart valves may have higher goals ranging from 2.5 to 3.5.

Warfarin is used for a multitude of diseases requiring anticoagulation, including atrial fibrillation (AFib), mechanical heart valves, history of deep venous thrombosis or pulmonary embolism, hypercoagulable states, and left ventricular thrombus. It remains in widespread use due to its economical price, relatively stable dosing once a steady state is achieved, pharmacokinetics, and longstanding historical use proving efficacy and improved outcomes.

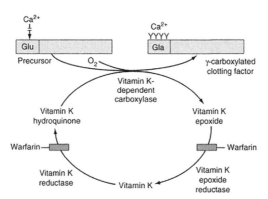

Fig. 2. Warfarin and its activity on the vitamin K-dependent coagulation factor pathway. (*From* Jaffer IH, Weitz JI. Antithrombotic Drugs. In: Hoffman R, Benz EJ, et al. Hematology: Basic Principles and Practice, 7th edition. Philadelphia: Elsevier; 2018. P. 2168-2188; With permission.)

As the population ages and medical comorbidities become more common, warfarin use has continued to be prevalent despite the advent of newer anticoagulation medications. Anesthesiologists will continue to encounter patients on warfarin requiring procedures, whether urgent or emergent. One of the advantages of warfarin is the ease with which it can be reversed. If a patient requires an urgent or emergent procedure while on warfarin, it is recommended that a patient receive 5 to 10 mg of intravenous (IV) Vitamin K infused over 30 min along with four-factor prothrombin complex concentrate (PCC) for rapid reversal of the anticoagulant effects.[6] Data show that four-factor PCC is superior to fresh frozen plasma (FFP) for rapid INR reversal and effective hemostasis in patients needing warfarin reversal for urgent surgical or invasive procedures.[7] In addition, a meta-analysis found that reversal with PCC versus FFP results in a reduction in all-cause mortality, faster and more reliable normalization of INR, and lower risk of posttransfusion volume overload.[8] In terms of choice of PCC, most societies recommend the use of four-factor PCC (KCentra) over three-factor due to the theoretically more complete reversal due to the presence of Factor VII.[9] Dosing recommendations vary by institution but are often weight-based and INR-based, which along with the time required by a Pharmacy to mix the drug, can lead to substantial delays in the administration of the medication. A recent study evaluated a fixed dose of 1000 units versus more traditional weight-based dosing and found no difference in efficacy but a faster time to administration for the fixed-dose group.[10]

Despite the clear superiority of PCC when it comes to warfarin reversal, there does exist a clinical scenario in which reversal with FFP may be preferable to PCC. If a patient is actively exsanguinating and suffering from hemorrhagic shock, FFP may prove more useful in active volume resuscitation when used with other blood components. One should keep in mind that the traditional ratio of 1:1:1 balanced blood product resuscitation may require more units of FFP to achieve normalization of the coagulation status if the patient arrived at the hospital under the effects of warfarin.

Heparin and heparinoids

Heparin was discovered in 1916 and remains one of the oldest anticoagulant medications still in use today. After being isolated from canine liver by Professor Howell at Johns Hopkins University, continued research showed human safety and efficacy.[11]

Heparin functions by activating antithrombin, an enzyme that acts as a powerful anti-coagulant by inhibiting multiple clotting factors, most notably thrombin and Factor Xa. This activation is accomplished by a specific pentasaccharide of heparin, which binds with antithrombin to form a complex. This induces a conformational change that increases antithrombin's anticoagulant activity. In addition, heparin binds thrombin and antithrombin simultaneously which causes additional thrombin inhibition. Heparin's anticoagulant effects are attenuated by its propensity for binding to vWF and Platelet Factor 4, which leads to the inactivation of the heparin molecule.[11,12]

A heparinoid's anticoagulant ability is directly affected by the length of its saccharide chain, as the length of the chain determines its ability to inhibit thrombin. Given its long saccharide chains, UFH has an equal ability to promote the inhibition of thrombin and factor Xa by antithrombin. Thus, it has an anti-factor Xa to the anti-thrombin ratio of 1:1. Low-molecular-LMWH has shorter chains, and thus cannot bridge antithrombin to thrombin as effectively. It therefore has a greater ability to inhibit factor Xa than thrombin.[12] Fondaparinux, a synthetic pentasaccharide, is too short to effectively bridge antithrombin to thrombin, and thus only accelerates inhibition of factor Xa by antithrombin.[13]

Heparinoids have different impacts on coagulation parameters. UFH results in increased aPTT, anti-Xa activity, and ACT. The coagulation parameters of patients receiving UFH must be monitored given its short half-life and need to be administered as an infusion, variable clinical response, and low bioavailability. aPTT and anti-Xa levels are the preferred monitoring strategies.[12,14] It is currently unclear which of these monitoring strategies is superior. The aPTT and anti-Xa in an individual patient are frequently discordant, and the clinical impact of this has yet to be determined.[14] In contrast, LMWH is typically not monitored. aPTT may be prolonged but is unreliable, and anti-Xa prolongation may be impacted significantly by dosing schedule and assay type used. LMWH has more consistent bioavailability than UFH and binds less avidly to other plasma proteins. As such, it has a more consistent anticoagulant effect, making monitoring less important. It also has a longer half-life and may be administered subcutaneously.[12] Similarly, fondaparinux does not require clinical monitoring. Anti-Xa levels will be elevated, but aPTT may be normal.[13] Note that none of these medications will increase the INR.

Other laboratory abnormalities that may be caused by heparinoids include thrombocytopenia, via heparin-induced thrombocytopenia (HIT). The risk of this syndrome is greatest with UFH. HIT is caused by antibodies that form the heparin-PF4 complexes. This leads to platelet activation and a procoagulant state that causes thromboses despite thrombocytopenia.[11,13]

Bleeding is a common side effect of heparin-based anticoagulation, and clinical scenarios may arise that require reversal of their effects. Reversal of heparin's anticoagulant effect is achieved with protamine, a mixture of peptides originally isolated from salmon.[12] Protamine binds heparin with high affinity, forming heparin-protamine complexes that are cleared renally. Protamine is less effective at antagonizing the anti-Xa effects of heparinoids, and thus is an incomplete reversal agent for LMWH and is not at all effective in reversing fondaparinux.[12,14] There are different dosing strategies for protamine reversal, but the time from the last UFH administration must be considered. The more time that has elapsed since the patient's last heparin dose, the less protamine will be required for reversal. For less urgent situations, reversal of UFH is not recommended, given its short half-life. Rather, waiting for monitoring parameters to return to acceptable ranges is preferred. For LMWH, reversal with 1 mg of protamine for every 1 mg of LMWH given is recommended. Additional doses of protamine may be given, up to a maximum of 50 mg.[15] Protamine itself has several side effects, which can include anaphylaxis, acute hypotension, acute severe pulmonary vasoconstriction, and bradycardia. Slow infusion is recommended to reduce this risk.[12]

In the setting of severe bleeding or intracranial hemorrhage after LMWH administration, andexanet alfa may also be used, although there is limited data to support it in this setting. Andexanet alfa, an inactive form of factor Xa, can sequester direct factor Xa inhibitors, and likely is also effective for indirect factor Xa inhibitors.[13,16] There are little data currently to guide the urgent reversal of fondaparinux. Andexanet alfa may also be effective in this case. Activated prothrombin complex concentrates (aPCC) or activated factor VII may be used, although little clinical data exist.[12,14]

Direct oral anticoagulants

VKAs have been the mainstay for oral anticoagulation in the treatment of venous thromboembolism and prevention of stroke in patients with AFib, but the arrival of direct oral anticoagulants (DOACs) has added an alternative profile that addresses many of the shortcomings of the VKAs. DOACs, as the name indicates, act by either directly inhibiting thrombin (ie, dabigatran) or factor Xa (ie, rivaraxoban, apixiban, and edoxaban). Their predictable pharmacokinetics and pharmacodynamics allow for fixed dosing and rapid onset of anticoagulant effect.[17] This also allows for less frequent laboratory monitoring and less variability of therapeutic effect from nutritional intake and drug–drug interactions.

Despite these benefits, DOACs provide a challenge when coagulation tests are needed for assessment of coagulation status or in the setting of bleeding or need for urgent reversal. Activated partial thrombin time (aPTT) and PT are prolonged by most DOACs, but the tests have an unpredictable relation to plasma concentration. TCT can be used specifically to assess the dabigatran effect but is also fairly unpredictable and unreliable.[18] The preferred test for assessing the anticoagulant activity of rivaraxoban, apixiban, and edoxaban is a chromogenic anti-Xa assay that will correlate closely with plasma drug levels, but this test is not readily available in many hospitals.[19]

All DOACs are predominantly metabolized in the kidneys. Although still approved for patients with reduced creatinine clearance, there is a concern for supratherapeutic drug levels in patients with acute kidney dysfunction and increased bleeding risk in advanced kidney disease. DOACs are contraindicated in severe hepatic impairment and pregnancy.

Studies have shown non-inferiority for DOACs compared with warfarin for the treatment of venous thromboembolism[20] and prevention of stroke in patients with AFib.[21] In addition, DOACs have been clinically used for other indications where traditionally warfarin was favored.[22] DOACs are still avoided in the anticoagulation for mechanical cardiac valves. DOACs have been shown to reduce the incidence of intracranial hemorrhage or major traumatic bleeding compared with warfarin, but the management of DOAC-induced bleeding is intricate and requires a systematic approach.[23] When feasible, one should obtain specifics from the patient such as dose, timing of last dose, and the indication for DOAC. Laboratory testing can be obtained as well. Oral activated charcoal can be considered to decrease absorption of the unabsorbed drug, if the last dose of DOAC was recent enough (~2 h). Idarucizumab (a dabigatran-specific Fab fragment) can reverse the anticoagulant effect of dabigatran, whereas Andexanet alfa is used for factor Xa inhibitors and acts as a factor Xa decoy, binding and sequestering the anticoagulant. PCCs should be considered for life-threatening bleeding or in the absence of availability of the above reversal agents.[19,24] With the increase in use of DOACs over VKAs, the lack of high-quality evidence and guidance with regards to DOAC-associated bleeding should be ameliorated as more evidence on the subject accumulates (**Table 1**).

Antiplatelet Medications

Encountering antiplatelet drugs in the operating room is quite common secondary to an ever-aging patient population and the high incidence of cardiovascular disease and subsequent interventions performed annually.[25] Although the archetype of this drug class is aspirin, other classes of drug are now available with both irreversible and reversible mechanisms of action that must be considered when managing iatrogenic coagulopathy. The indications for antiplatelet agents mean that carefully weighing risks versus benefits is a hallmark of managing this drug class.

Aspirin is a mainstay of prevention for thrombotic complications. Its mechanism of action is via inhibition of cyclooxygenase (COX) ultimately preventing thromboxane A_2 (TXA_2) creation, which inhibits platelet aggregation. This process is irreversible and can only be overcome by the generation or administration of new platelets with an average platelet lifespan of 7 to 10 days. This conveniently lends itself to the once-daily administration regimen of the drug but can be problematic in the intensive care unit (ICU) or operating room. It is worth noting that a certain percentage of patients on aspirin therapy may have a suboptimal response either from patient factors (noncompliance) or drug–drug interactions (nonsteroidal anti-inflammatory drug). True failure of aspirin in isolation to inhibit COX is thought to be extremely rare or nonexistent.

P2Y12 inhibitors such as Clopidogrel, Prasugrel, and Ticagrelor are often administered in combination with aspirin as a part of "dual-antiplatelet therapy (DAPT)." This DAPT remains the mainstay of treatment for post-acute coronary syndrome patients who have received coronary stents. These medications act through inhibition of the adenosine diphosphate (ADP) receptor via the platelet's $P2Y_{12}$ receptor.[26] This is done irreversibly in the case of Clopidogrel and Prasugrel, but reversibly by Ticagrelor and Cangrelor. Of note, Clopidogrel and Prasugrel are both prodrugs requiring conversion to their active forms in the liver. So-called nonresponders exist for both Clopidogrel and Prasugrel, with nonresponse to Clopidogrel being much more common.[27]

Glycoprotein IIB/IIIA inhibitors such as Eptifibatide and Tirofiban are given via an IV route and prevent platelet aggregation through blockade of the platelet IIB/IIA surface receptor. They both have the benefit of extremely short times to efficacy and relatively short half-lives. They may be used during acute coronary syndrome (ACS); however, DAPT and an IV anticoagulant such as heparin remain the standard of care.

Routine laboratory values often obtained on patients in the ICU or operating room will not provide useful information regarding the degree of platelet inhibition in patients using the above antiplatelet medications. Several clinically available testing mechanisms are available to guide the management of the patient on antiplatelets such as the VerifyNow PRUTest Assay, TEG PlateletMapping System, and Multiple Electrode Platelet Aggregometry.[28] The interpretation and validity of these individual tests is beyond the scope of this article but the results of these tests can be used to aid in the appropriate timing of procedural interventions, response to therapy, and degree of platelet inhibition.

Management of patients who need emergent reversal is a balance of risk versus benefit based on the severity of hemorrhage as well as the indication for antiplatelet therapy. There are no evidence-based guidelines on the treatment of life-threatening bleeding in the setting of antiplatelet medications. The first step for any clinician facing this situation should be the discontinuation of any antiplatelet medications.[29] Thankfully some of the medications in this class are reversible and/or have relatively short half-lives such as Cangrelor, Eptifibatide, and Tirofiban. Once the

Table 1
Reversal of direct thrombin inhibitors and factor Xa inhibitors

	Direct Thrombin Inhibitors (Dabigatran)	Factor Xa Inhibitor (Rivaroxaban and Apixaban Edoxaban)
Laboratory tests	PT, aPTT, and dTT	PT, aPTT, anti-factor-Xa activity
Specific reversal agent	Idarucizumab	Andexanet alfa
Prothrombic complex concentrates (PCC)	Activated PCC preferred *Four- or three-factor PCC if unavailable*	Four-factor PCC preferred *Three-factor PCC if unavailable*
Other options	Antifibrinolytics, activated charcoal, and hemodialysis	Antifibrinolytics, activated charcoal, and hemodialysis

antiplatelet agents have been stopped, adjunct therapies such as platelet transfusion and administration of Desmopressin (DDAVP) can be considered. A study using an in vitro model showed that it required ~2 to 3 aphaeresis platelet units to normalize platelet function in patients on DAPT.[30] DDAVP serves to increase the endothelial release of vWF and factor VIII. Although not yet clinically available, Bentracimab is currently in phase III clinical trials. This monoclonal antibody serves as a reversal agent for Ticagrelor as it binds reversibly to platelets via the P2Y$_{12}$ receptor. The ability of ticagrelor to move to a receptor on a new platelet means that it is not as susceptible to reversal with platelet transfusion as Clopidogrel and Prasugrel, which bind irreversibly. If approved, this drug would add a substantial tool to the armament of providers looking to emergently reverse patients on Ticagrelor.[31]

Anticoagulation for Mechanical Circulatory Devices

Mechanical circulatory support (MCS) devices have seen an increase in use over recent years with more centers beginning to perform and manage these complex devices. MCS includes left ventricular assist devices (LVADs), varying forms of extracorporeal membrane oxygenation (ECMO), and percutaneous ventricular assist devices such as Impella. These devices are associated with both high risk of bleeding and clotting related complications.[32] The exposure of whole blood to the foreign surfaces of the devices and tubing adds to the coagulation dysfunction experienced by a critically ill patient. This is compounded by the frequent use of anticoagulants such as heparin, bivalirudin, or argatroban to maintain these devices for an extended period. MCS is known to induce an acquired Von Willibrand Syndrome through the shear stress placed on vWF leading to inappropriate cleavage by ADAMTS13.[33] All these factors together induce a situation with a tenuous balance between bleeding and thrombosis that must be delicately managed. Limited evidence exists for how to appropriately manage this balance across various MCS devices and is a substantial topic that is beyond the scope of this article.

OTHER CAUSES OF COAGULOPATHY
Vitamin K deficiency

As noted in the warfarin section, Vitamin K is a crucial factor in the formation of Vitamin K-dependent clotting factors (Factors II, VII, IX, X, and Proteins C and S). It is not uncommon to encounter patients with a relative factor deficiency secondary to decreased Vitamin K absorption or intake. Patients who may be at risk for Vitamin K deficiency include those who have been on broad-spectrum antibiotics (due to the death of gut microbes involved in Vitamin K uptake), patients with poor nutritional intake, and patients with poor gut absorption (inflammatory bowel disease, cystic fibrosis). A careful history and physical can typically uncover the reason for Vitamin K deficiency. If a patient with an elevated INR due to Vitamin K deficiency requires an urgent or emergent procedure, treatment would be similar to the reversal of warfarin. Parenteral Vitamin K should be given, and although there are no guidelines for dosing, a small study showed adequate reversal with 10 mg of IV Vitamin K.[34] Depending on the urgency of the procedure, the patient may require FFP or PCC for immediate replacement of clotting factors.

Uremic bleeding

The etiology of bleeding in uremic patients is likely multifactorial but is mostly related to platelet function, both in regard to platelet–platelet interactions and platelet–vessel interactions.[35] Uremic coagulopathy is an indication for emergent dialysis if time allows. If a procedure is considered urgent or emergent and dialysis is not feasible, DDAVP may be given intravenously, subcutaneously, or intranasally. DDAVP acts by releasing vWF into the plasma that promotes platelet thrombus formation. DDAVP's activity is short-lived, however, and it loses efficacy after repeat dosing as the stores of vWF are depleted. If longer-acting hemostasis is required, some advocate for the use of conjugated estrogens, which have been shown to be safe and effective at managing uremic bleeding. Other potential therapies include tranexamic acid (TXA) or activated Factor VII.[35]

Trauma-induced coagulopathy

Trauma-induced coagulopathy (TIC) encompasses multiple coagulation issues that arise in trauma patients suffering from hemorrhagic shock. Approximately 25% to 30% of hemorrhaging trauma patients experience some form of TIC. This coagulopathy may involve issues with clot formation, thrombolysis, or vascular hemostasis. TIC has multiple causes, including inflammation caused by tissue injury and the shock state itself, activation and eventual depletion of Protein C, coagulation factor depletion, fibrinolysis, and altered platelet mechanics.[36] Therapies for TIC include appropriately balanced blood product resuscitation guided by viscoelastic coagulation studies and surgical or interventional procedures aimed at stemming active blood loss. In addition, TXA was shown to significantly reduce mortality in patients experiencing severe traumatic hemorrhage, and TXA remains a mainstay of trauma management.[37]

SUMMARY

As the population ages and becomes more medically complex, the number of patients requiring emergent reversal of their anticoagulation before an urgent or emergent procedure will continue to increase. In addition, more classes of medications will continue to be introduced. Anesthesiologists must have the ability to quickly and safely care for these patients, as an untreated or undertreated coagulopathy can lead to a multitude of postsurgical complications.

CLINICS CARE POINTS

- Prothrombin time and international normalized ratio measure the extrinsic and common pathways. Activated partial thromboplastin time reflects the intrinsic and common pathways.

- Warfarin is most effectively reversed by a combination of intravenous vitamin K and four-factor prothrombin complex concentrate (PCC). FFP is a viable option to replace PCC if volume expansion is required as well, such as in a massive trauma.
- Heparin is reversed with protamine, with dosing tailored to the amount of heparin given and the current activated clotting time
- Factor Xa inhibitors (direct oral anticoagulants) are reversed with andexanet alfa (apixaban and rivaroxaban) and four-factor PCC.
- Although there are no guidelines for the treatment of bleeding associated with antiplatelet medications, the use of Desmopressin and platelet transfusions may be useful.

REFERENCES

1. Pai M. Chapter 129: laboratory evaluation of hemostatic and thrombotic disorders. In: Hoffman R, Benz E, Silberstein L, et al, editors. Hematology, basic principles and practice. 7th ed. Philadelphia: Elsevier; 2018. p. 1922–31.
2. Winter WE, Flax SD, Harris NS. Coagulation testing in the core laboratory. Lab Med 2017;48(4):295–313.
3. Shore-Lesserson L, Enriquez L, Weitzel N. Chapter 19: coagulation monitoring. In: Kaplan J, editor. Kaplan's cardiac anesthesia. 7th ed. Philadelphia: Elsevier; 2017. p. 698–727.
4. Shen L, Tabaie S, Ivascu N. Viscoelastic testing inside and beyond the operating room. J Thorac Dis 2017;9(Suppl 4):S299–308.
5. Jaffer IH, Weitz JI. Antithrombotic drugs. In: Hoffman R, Benz EJ, Silberstein LE, et al, editors. Hematology: basic principles and practice. 7th edition. Philadelphia: Elsevier; 2018. p. 2168–88.
6. Milling TJ, Pollack CV. A review of guidelines on anticoagulation reversal across different clinical scenarios—Is there a general consensus? Am J Emerg Med 2020;38(9):1890–903.
7. Goldstein JN, Refaai MA, Milling TJ Jr, et al. Four-factor prothrombin complex concentrate versus plasma for rapid vitamin K antagonist reversal in patients needing urgent surgical or invasive interventions: a phase 3b, open-label, non-inferiority, randomized trial. Lancet 2015;385:2077–87.
8. Chai-Adisaksopha C, Hillis C, Siegal DM, et al. Prothrombin complex concentrates versus fresh frozen plasma for warfarin reversal: a systematic review and meta-analysis. Thromb Haemost 2016;116(5):879–90.
9. Frontera JA, Lewin JJ, Rabinstein AA, et al. Guideline for reversal of antithrombotics in intracranial hemorrhage: a statement for healthcare professionals from the neurocritical care society and society of critical care medicine. Neurocrit Care 2015;24:6–46.
10. Abdoellakhan RA, Khorsand N, ter Avest E, et al. Fixed versus variable dosing of prothrombin complex concentrate for bleeding complications of vitamin K antagonists—the PROPER3 randomized clinical trial. Ann Emerg Med 2022;79(1):20–30.
11. Royston D. Chapter 45: anticoagulant and antiplatelet therapy. In: Hemminds HC, Egan TD, editors. Pharmacology and physiology for anesthesia: foundations and clinical application. 2nd edition. Philadelphia: Elsevier; 2019. p. 870–94.
12. Weitz JI. Chapter 95: Hemostasis, thrombosis, fibrinolysis, and cardiovascular disease. In: Libby P, Bonow RO, Mann DL, et al, editors. Braunwald's heart disease: a textbook of cardiovascular medicine. 12th edition. Philadelphia: Elsevier; 2022. p. 1766–90.

13. Siegal DM, Curnutte JT, Connolly SJ, et al. Andexanet alfa for the reversal of factor Xa inhibitor activity. N Engl J Med 2015;373(25):2413–24.

14. Zehnder J, Price E, Jin J. Controversies in heparin monitoring. Am J Hematol 2012;87:S137–40.

15. Simon E, Streitz M, Sessions D, et al. Anticoagulation reversal. Emerg Med Clin North America 2018;36(3):585–601.

16. Connolly SJ, Crowther M, Eikelboom JW, et al. Full study report of andexanet alfa for bleeding associated with factor Xa inhibitors. N Engl J Med 2019;380(14):1326–35.

17. Wahab A, Patnaik R, Gurjar M. Use of direct oral anticoagulants in ICU patients. Part I—applied pharmacology. Anaesthesiol Intensive Ther 2021;53(5):429–39.

18. Chen A, Stecker E, Warden BA. Direct Oral Anticoagulant Use: A Practical Guide to Common Clinical Challenges. J Am Heart Assoc 2020;9:e017559.

19. Tomaselli GF, Mahaffey KW, Cuker A, et al. 2017 ACC expert consensus decision pathway on management of bleeding in patients on oral anticoagulants: a report of the american college of cardiology task force on expert consensus decision pathways. J Am Coll Cardiol 2017;70:3042–67.

20. Stevens SM, Woller SC, Baumann Kreuziger L, et al. Antithrombotic therapy for VTE disease: second update of the CHEST guideline and expert panel report. Chest 2021;160(6):e545–608.

21. Lopez-Lopez JA, Sterne JAC, Thom HHZ, et al. Oral anticoagulants for prevention of stroke in atrial fibrillation: systematic review, network meta-analysis, and cost effectiveness analysis. BMJ 2017;359:j5058.

22. Wahab A, Patnaik R, Gurjar M. Use of direct oral anticoagulants in ICU patients. Part II- Clinical evidence. Anaesthesiol Intensive Ther 2021;53(5):440–9.

23. Larsen TB, Rasmussen LH, Skjoth F, et al. Efficacy and safety of dabigatran etexilate and warfarin in "real-world" patients with atrial fibrillation: a prospective nationwide cohort study. J Am Coll Cardiol 2013;61(22):2264–73.

24. Siegal DM, Garcia DA, Crowther MA. How I treat target-specific oral anticoagulant-associated bleeding. Blood 2014;123(8):1152–8.

25. Pengo V, Pegoraro C, Cucchini U, et al. Worldwide management of oral anticoagulant therapy: the ISAM study. J Thromb Thrombolysis 2006;21(1):73–7.

26. Ding Z, Kim S, Dorsam RT, et al. Inactivation of the human P2Y12 receptor by thiol reagents requires interaction with both extracellular cysteine residues, Cys17 and Cys270. Blood 2003;101(10):3908–14.

27. Michelson AD, Bhatt DL. How I use laboratory monitoring of antiplatelet therapy. Blood 2017;130(6):713–21.

28. Mahla E, Tantry US, Schoerghuber M, et al. Platelet function testing in patients on antiplatelet therapy before cardiac surgery. Anesthesiology 2020;133(6):1263–76.

29. Yee J, Kaide CG. Emergency reversal of anticoagulation. West J Emerg Med 2019;20(5):770–83.

30. Bhal V, Herr MJ, Dixon M, et al. Platelet function recovery following exposure to triple anti-platelet inhibitors using an in vitro transfusion model. Thromb Res 2015;136(6):1216–23.

31. Kathma SJ, Wheeler JJ, Bhatt DL, et al. Population pharmacokinetic-pharmacodynamic modeling of PB2452, a monoclonal antibody fragment being developed as a ticagrelor reversal agent, in healthy volunteers. CPT Pharmacometrics Syst Pharmacol 2022;11(1):68–81.

32. Granja T, Hohenstein K, Schussel P, et al. Multi-modal characterization of the coagulopathy associated with extracorporeal membrane oxygenation. Crit Care Med 2020 May;48(5):e400–8.
33. Heilmann C, Geisen U, Beyersdorf F, et al. Acquired von Willebrand syndrome in patients with extracorporeal life support (ECLS). Intensive Care Med 2012; 38(1):62–8.
34. Harrington DJ, Booth L, Dando N, et al. Vitamin K deficiency in cancer patients referred to a hospital palliative care team with bleeding and the impact of vitamin K replacement on laboratory indicators of vitamin K status. Int J Lab Hematol 2013;35(4):457–9.
35. Galbusera M, Remuzzi G, Boccardo P. Treatment of bleeding in dialysis patients. Semin Dial 2009;22(3):279–86.
36. Kornblith LZ, Moore HB, Cohen MJ. Trauma-induced coagulopathy: The past, present, and future. J Thromb Haemost 2019;17(6):852–62.
37. Shakur H, Roberts I, Bautista R, et al. Effects of tranexamic acid on death, vascular occlusive events, and blood transfusion in trauma patients with significant hemorrhage (CRASH-2): a randomized, placebo-controlled trial. Lancet 2010;376(9734):23–32.

Impact of Intensive Care Unit Nutrition on the Microbiome and Patient Outcomes

Mara A. Serbanescu, MD[a],*, Monica Da Silva, MD[b],
Ahmed Zaky, MD, MSc, MPH, MBA[b]

KEYWORDS

- Microbiome • Nutrition • Sepsis • Soluble fiber • Short-chain fatty acids

KEY POINTS

- When possible, nutrition should be initiated early and enterally, but regardless of route, overfeeding and inadequate protein should be avoided.
- The microbiome is increasingly recognized as a contributor to outcomes in critically ill and postsurgical patients.
- Nutritional supplementation with pre-, pro-, and synbiotics has demonstrated therapeutic potential, though better characterization of individual microbial signatures is needed to identify patients that most stand to benefit from these therapies.

INTRODUCTION

The intestinal ecosystem represents a complex interface where our own intestinal and immune cells work in concert with trillions of microorganisms to provide key homeostatic and regulatory functions. The composition of these commensals and the genes they harbor (collectively referred to as the microbiome) influences not only our intestinal barrier and the absorption of necessary vitamins and nutrients but also local and systemic immune responses as well as virtually every other organ system.[1] In critical illness and other acute inflammatory states, the intestinal ecosystem is disrupted, resulting in a loss of barrier defenses and a cascade of derangements that are thought to further contribute to the progression of sepsis and multiple organ dysfunction.[2] Adequate nutrition has long been viewed as integral to the support of both intestinal defense mechanisms and the increasing metabolic demands of critical illness.[3] However, only recently are we beginning to understand and value the role of the

[a] Department of Anesthesiology, Duke University Hospital, 2301 Erwin Road, Box #3094, Durham, NC 27710, USA; [b] Department of Anesthesiology and Perioperative Medicine, University of Alabama at Birmingham, 950 Jefferson Tower, 625 19th Street South, Birmingham, AL 35249-6810, USA
* Corresponding author.
E-mail address: mara.serbanescu@duke.edu

Anesthesiology Clin 41 (2023) 263–281
https://doi.org/10.1016/j.anclin.2022.10.007
1932-2275/23/© 2022 Elsevier Inc. All rights reserved.

microbiome as an integral modulator of key processes relevant to perioperative and intensive care. Are the microbes that are present—or absent—responsible for development of infection after major intra-abdominal surgery? Are they in part responsible for the dysregulated immune responses characteristic of sepsis? By adjusting the content of enteral supplementation, can we influence our patient's microbiomes in such a way that alters clinical trajectory? The role of intensive care unit (ICU) nutrition on the microbiome is largely unexplored; however, emerging literature suggests that the microbiome may have a more significant role in critical illness than previously realized.

In this review, we first address the more familiar topic of how ICU nutritional strategies affect outcomes, summarizing the recent available evidence in this field. Next, we transition to exploring the rapidly growing field of microbiome medicine. As this area of study is new to many clinicians, we first aim to provide an introduction on composition and function of the microbiome in the context of perioperative and critical care, then move to a summary of recent clinical data implicating our microbiota as potential modulators of outcomes. Finally, we address the intersection of nutrition and the microbiome, and the growing data exploring the use of supplemental pre-, pro-, and synbiotics to influence microbial composition as a means of enhancing host responses and improving outcomes in critically ill and post-surgical patients. Our aim is to highlight the importance of medical nutritional therapy and alterations in the microbiome in critical and perioperative care (**Fig. 1**), bringing these emerging fields toward the forefront of the minds of intensivists and anesthesiologists.

Effects of Intensive Care Unit Nutritional Therapy on Patient Outcome

Malnutrition, or inadequate nutrient intake relative to an individual's metabolic demand, is associated with worse patient outcomes. This holds true for preoperative malnutrition, with adverse outcomes found following virtually all major surgeries, or that occurring in the ICU.[3,4] Preclinical studies have demonstrated impaired intestinal barrier defenses in the setting of enteral nutrient deprivation, such as reduced mucin (MUC2) secretion from goblet cells, villous atrophy, and altered cytokine production

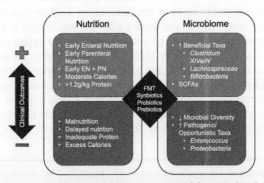

Fig. 1. Schematic of nutrition- and microbiome-associated factors that have been linked to clinical outcomes (ICU length-of-stay, duration of mechanical ventilation, or mortality) across multiple independent investigations. Factors in green boxes (up) associated with significant improvement; factors in red (below) associated with increased morbidity or mortality. Supplementation with pre-, pro-, and synbiotics, and fecal microbial transplant (FMT) lie at the intersection of nutrition and the microbiome, and represent potential emerging therapies for critically ill patients, though further studies are needed to delineate which patients most stand to benefit.

by local immunocytes.[5,6] The effects on barrier permeability seem augmented when protein malnutrition accompanies enteral nutrient deprivation.[7] However, although clinicians have long known that prevention of malnutrition is essential, recent research suggests that the provision of medical nutrition is far more nuanced than simply a question of presence or absence of therapy. Rather, content, delivery mechanism, and timing are all important factors that should be considered. There is increasing recognition that both underfeeding and overfeeding as well as providing insufficient protein may prolong ICU stay and duration of mechanical ventilation, whereas survival may be improved if therapy targets 70% of caloric needs estimated by indirect calorimetry as well as sufficient protein.[8] **Fig. 2** delineates a proposed timeline and stepwise approach for incorporating these recommendations into the ICU treatment plan.

Administration route remains important, though the superiority of enteral nutrition (EN) over parenteral nutrition (PN) has become far less definitive in recent years. Despite the negative consequences of enteral nutrient deprivation on the gut barrier, PN prescribed to meet (but not exceed) target caloric and protein needs in the setting of modern infectious control practices and improved lipid formulations may result in similar outcomes.[4] Indeed, findings from CALORIES, a pragmatic, multicenter, randomized controlled trial (RCT) of 2,400 patients admitted to mixed medical–surgical ICUs demonstrated no difference in mortality or infectious complications with initiation of early PN (EPN)versus early EN (EEN) providing equivalent caloric needs (25 kcal/kg/day to be met by 48–72 hour).[9] However, timing does matter. EEN versus delayed EN is associated with fewer infectious complications in hospitalized patients,[10] lower mortality in patients on Veno-Arterial Extracorporeal Membrane Oxygenation (VA-ECMO),[11] and reduced risk of nosocomial pneumonia in traumatic brain injury (TBI).[12]

To address the growing evidence in this field, the European Society for Clinical Nutrition and Metabolism conducted a meta-analysis and issued an updated guideline for management of medical nutritional therapy in critically ill patients.[10] The guideline advocates for a much more comprehensive approach to initiating nutrition in the ICU, at once considering the decision of route (oral vs EN vs PN) and timing of initiation,

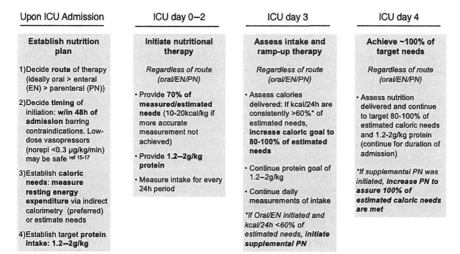

Fig. 2. Proposed step-wise approach for initiation of medical nutritional therapy for critically ill patients based on current evidence.

alongside a well-defined plan for achievement of target caloric and protein needs. Of note, irrespective of the route, a progressive ramp-up of therapy is recommended, such that less than 70% of measured energy expenditure (or estimated needs) is to be provided in the first 48 hour after admission, with escalation to 80% to 100% after day 3, all in conjunction with a targeted protein intake of 1.2-2 g/kg.[10] A recently published prospective multinational cohort study of 1172 medical ICU patients lends further support for this approach. Irrespective of timing, compared with low-caloric intake, providing 10 to 20 kcal/kg per day was associated with shorter duration of mechanical ventilation and longer survival, with the greatest benefit conveyed after day 5 of admission. Compared with low-protein intake, intake of 1.2 g/kg in the first 15 days was associated with shorter duration of mechanical ventilation.[13]

Regardless of route and timing, if oral intake is not adequate, and barring any contraindications, EN remains preferred over PN, ideally within 48 hour of admission.[10] Although the consensus cedes that the inherent heterogeneity in the critically ill population, coupled with variability in study design, execution, and evaluated outcomes challenges the ability to make generalizable statements, the guideline continues to indicate a superiority of EN over PN in severe acute pancreatitis (SAP), following gastrointestinal (GI) surgery, and in unselected critically ill patients, conveying lower infectious complications and reduced ICU stays.[10] Circulatory shock remains a contraindication to EN due to concern for bowel ischemia in the setting of increased enterocyte oxygen consumption from absorption of enteral nutrients. Nonetheless this contraindication may be debatable. The NUTRIREA-2, a pragmatic RCT comparing outcomes between EEN and EPN in 2410 mechanically ventilated patients on vasopressors admitted to primarily medical ICUs demonstrated an increased risk of nonocclusive mesenteric ischemia in the EEN group (2% vs <1% in EPN, $P = .007$).[14] However, the mean vasopressor dose in NUTRIREA-2 was 0.56 µg/kg/min norepinephrine and the mean caloric intake was 20 kcal/kg/day, and it remains possible that these findings may not hold true at reduced doses of vasopressor and lower early caloric intake.[15] To this point, data from a retrospective analysis of over 50,000 mechanically ventilated patients with shock on varying doses of vasopressor support indicate an improved survival if EEN is initiated over delayed EN in patients on lower doses of norepinephrine (<0.3 µg/kg/min), but not in patients requiring more pressor support.[16] Similarly, a recent retrospective study evaluating differences in hospital outcomes between EEN and late EN in 1700 patients receiving mechanical ventilation and vasopressor support (dose unknown) revealed no difference in mortality, and a reduction in ICU length of stay, electrolyte disturbances, and renal replacement therapy in the EEN group.[17] Taken together, these studies fall in support of EEN, even in the setting of shock.

What then, if EN fails to meet nutritional requirements? In this instance, the available literature supports supplementation with PN. Although data are limited for what defines "inadequate EN," when to initiate supplemental PN, and when to achieve target caloric needs, it seems that the best evidence exists for initiating supplemental PN when EN provides less than 60% caloric needs after 3 days following an ICU admission, with a goal of supplemental PN to achieve 100% of target caloric and protein needs (1.2 g/kg/day) between days 4 and 7. This approach showed reductions in nosocomial infections, antibiotic duration, and ICU mortality with the addition of supplemental PN versus EN alone.[4,18,19]

The Gut Microbiome in Critical and Perioperative Care

How does the effect of nutritional therapy on the microbiome contribute to the difference in outcomes observed in the clinical trials above? The short answer is simply that we do not yet know. However, before exploring what is known and unknown about the effects of perioperative nutrition on the gut microbiome, and how these interactions may shape a patient's clinical trajectory, context for this field of inquiry is necessary. Below we review the structure and function of the microbiome as it relates to critical care, why and how the microbiome of critical illness differs from health and data implicating a role for gut microbial alterations in outcomes of critically ill and postsurgical patients.

What is the gut microbiome?

The gut microbiota represents the complex group of microorganisms comprising primarily bacteria but also fungi and viruses that reside along our GI tract.[20] Advanced sequencing techniques based on recognition and amplification of the 16S ribosomal RNA gene (rRNA)—expressed by nearly all bacteria—has allowed for exponential growth in our understanding of the role of these organisms in health and disease. The addition of metagenomic sequencing has allowed for identification of the millions of genes expressed by these microbes and the functions that are encoded.[21] Within the 16s gene, there are 9 hypervariable regions (v1–v9) that differentiate between bacterial species. Primers amplify the hypervariable regions and discovered sequences can then be matched to known identifiers within a reference library, providing information on "who is there" at different taxonomic ranks (phylum, class, order, family, genus, and species), though specificity is often only possible to the genus level.[22] Researchers can then understand how much of the bacterial community in a sample is represented by each taxon (or plural taxa), measured as relative abundance, and apply analytical techniques to assess how the numbers of taxa present (diversity) differs across samples. No two individual's microbiomes are identical, and in fact, even within our GI tract, as intestinal morphology, nutrient absorption, pH, and oxygen supply varies, so too, does the microbial community.[23,24] Owing to such profound interindividual and intraindividual variability, it remains difficult to have a universal definition of a healthy human intestinal microbiome. We do, however, have some generalizable guidelines. Although hundreds of different species exist, in health, greater than 90% of these belong to either Bacteroides or Firmicutes, with less representation from Proteobacteria, Fusobacteria, and Actinobacteria.[20] At the genus-level, there seem to exist a set of 15 to 20 core genera that serve as the primary regulators of homeostatic functions affecting nearly all organ systems.[25–27] Importantly, the tens to hundreds of species within each genus exhibit different, though at times, overlapping, traits, and the representation of these species varies from person to person.

We now know that the intestinal microbiome has a role in many aspects of health that are essential in the perioperative period. The microbiome mediates host immune responses and protects against enteric pathogens via defenses such as geographic occupation, competition for nutrients, and stimulation of MUC2 by goblet cells.[28] In addition to barrier defenses, the microbiome influences immune responses both in homeostatic conditions and when acute threats are encountered, by signaling to local and distant immune cells including monocytes, macrophages, and intraepithelial lymphocytes, promoting differentiation of T-cell subsets (T_{regs}, Th_{17}), and stimulating Immunoglobulin A (IgA).[29] Importantly, different species can have widely different effects on cytokine production and immune responses.[29,30] These functions include secretion of antimicrobial peptides (Bacteroides species [spp]), and fermentation of dietary fibers into short-chain fatty acids (SCFAs) like butyrate, propionate, and acetate (Clostridium clusters IV and XIVa; Bifidobacterium; Lachnospiraceae).[23,28,31] In turn, SCFAs serve as fuel for colonocytes, and also as immunoregulatory (usually "anti-inflammatory") signaling molecules for local and systemic immune cells.[31,32] In addition, microbiota produce antioxidants, regulate insulin sensitivity, modulate neurologic processes through a bidirectional communication with the brain ("gut-brain-axis"), and transform drugs into the bioactive form.[33,34] When a disturbance in the intestinal ecosystem reduces the diversity of the microbiota and/or significantly alters the abundance of certain taxa, these downstream homeostatic processes are impaired, resulting in a state known as "microbial dysbiosis."[1,25]

There is increasing evidence that microbial dysbiosis plays an integral role in the pathobiology of sepsis,[35,36] acute respiratory distress syndrome,[37] and stress responses to surgery.[38] Preclinical models demonstrate that mass reduction in commensals directly results in increased susceptibility to sepsis from enteric pathogens,[29,39] and invasions at distal sites such as pneumonia by *Pseudomonas aeruginosa*.[40] Moreover, the isolated loss of certain specific taxa, namely SCFA-producing *Clostridiales* species (spp), has been shown to result in systemic dissemination of enteric pathogens like *Listeria monocytogenes*[41] and *Salmonella*.[42] The importance of community composition holds true for models of polymicrobial intra-abdominal sepsis, as well: Fay and colleagues[43] demonstrated that in a cecal ligation and puncture model, the variability in survival and immunophenotypes observed between mice from different vendors was attributable to differences in their fecal microbial composition. Although the precise mechanisms by which microbial dysbiosis conveys increased susceptibility to infectious insults are not certain in every model, they likely include reduced MUC2 and increased barrier permeability; unbalanced or impaired immune responses and increases in pro-inflammatory transcription factors; and increased virulence or emergence of a dominant species which easily overtakes local defense mechanisms and reaches distant sites.[29,35,44] In this context, it is evident how microbial dysbiosis could result in pathologic mechanisms that overlap with, and further worsen, the immunopathology observed in critical illness, or explain bacteremia or infection in locations unrelated to the site of surgery.

What causes microbial dysbiosis in critical illness and the perioperative period?
Multiple interventions enacted during the perioperative period alter the composition and/or function of the microbiota. Antimicrobials represent perhaps the most important and pervasive culprit, particularly when considering that most patients will receive antibiotics at some point during their hospitalization. In the United States, greater than 90% of patients undergoing major surgery receive perioperative prophylactic antimicrobials, and 50% remain on therapy beyond 24 hour.[45] Moreover, estimates show that on any given day, ~70% of ICU patients worldwide are receiving antimicrobials.[46] Extensive investigations have demonstrated that antimicrobials reduce overall gut microbial diversity, indiscriminately ablate nearly all commensals, alter metabolic activity, and lead to an increased susceptibility to invading pathogens.[47,48] Studying the effects of a 4-day course of meropenem, gentamicin, and vancomycin on the gut microbiome of healthy men, Palleja and colleagues observed a marked reduction in beneficial taxa and an overgrowth of enteric pathobionts, including *Enterococcus faecalis* and *Klebsiella pneumoniae*, with positive selection for species harboring β-lactam resistance genes. Even more concerning, for some taxa, reconstitution had not yet occurred at 180 days after administration.[49] Murine studies demonstrate that a single dose of antibiotics can cause a profound (30%–90%) loss of indigenous taxa,[50,51] as well as marked susceptibility to *Clostridium difficile* colitis.[51] Antibiotic-induced depletion of host microbiota is now such a well-established finding that it has become a mainstay of experimental design in preclinical models exploring the role of the microbiome in host response to secondary infection.[52]

However, antimicrobials are far from the sole perpetrators; in fact, many therapies routinely administered by clinicians in the operating room and ICU have been found to induce microbial dysbiosis. Our own investigations in a mouse model revealed that a 4-hour exposure to either 100% O_2, or isoflurane and 100% O_2, reduces the abundance of multiple beneficial commensals, including Clostridiales spp,[53] Ashley and colleagues[54] further demonstrated that 24 to 72 hour exposures to 100% O_2 result in alterations in gut and lung microbiota that contribute to hyperoxia-induced lung inflammation; interestingly, varying antimicrobial regimens administered before exposure enacted different effects on parameters of lung injury. In addition to reducing abundance of beneficial commensals, certain therapies additionally promote the expansion of pathogenic species. Proton-pump inhibitors taken for 4 weeks resulted in increases in taxa belonging to the *Enterococcaceae* and *Streptococcaceae* families in otherwise healthy patients and may predispose to infectious complications.[55] In preclinical models, exposure to opioids for 24 hour enhanced growth of *E faecalis* and virulence of *P aeruginosa*, effects that have been associated with an increased development of sepsis and pneumonia.[56,57]

How are these findings translated to the patients we encounter as intensivists and anesthesiologists?

Longitudinal 16S sequencing of fecal and rectal samples from critically ill patients demonstrate profound reduction in community diversity and compositional changes, even within 48 hour of ICU admission.[58,59] Moreover, certain taxonomic alterations have been replicated across multiple groups. Specifically, patients exhibit a profound loss of health-promoting commensals recognized for their roles in SCFA production and maintenance of barrier integrity, including *Faecalibacterium*,[58,60,61] *Ruminococcus, Roseburia, and Blautia*.[60,62] Functionally, the loss of SCFA producers is supported by independent reports documenting reduced fecal butyrate, propionate, and acetate in ICU patients with sepsis.[63,64] In addition to the loss of beneficial commensals, critically ill patients exhibit a significant expansion of opportunists and pathogens, which at times represent more than half of the total number of species present.[61,65] The most frequently reported findings include expansion in the phylum Proteobacteria, and dominance of the *Enterococcus* genus, but increases in *Staphylococcus*, and *Enterobacteriaceae* like *Escherichia coli* and *Shigella* are also well documented.[58,65–67] Changes in the microbiome are not unique to critically ill patients, and reduced diversity and similar alterations in community structure have also been observed after acute trauma and burns and numerous surgeries.[68–71]

These observational human studies have provided "proof" that microbial dysbiosis is rampant in the perioperative period, however the extent that iatrogenic factors versus changes in host physiology each contribute to these observations remains unknown. Although the isolated effects of antimicrobials, oxygen, and therapeutics have been demonstrated independently, we also know that the reduced intestinal perfusion in shock and sepsis increases mucosal inflammation and impairs barrier integrity, and likely also alters the microbial landscape.[37] Most findings indicating microbial dysbiosis in patients with critical illness or acute injury are based on data from samples collected at 48 to 72 hour after ICU admission, when the provision of supportive care (oxygen, lack of enteral nutrition, antimicrobials) was well underway, and both timing and site of collection can significantly influence findings.[72] This by no means undermines the relevance of these discoveries. Irrespective of the cause of dysbiosis, observational studies have additionally been able to detect conserved patterns in taxonomic alterations even within subgroups of patients. For example, expansion of *Enterococcus* in critically ill patients was independently associated with severe dysbiosis and may serve as a potential surrogate biomarker[73]; Agudelo-Ochoa and colleagues. identified 24 taxa that were differentially expressed in patients with sepsis compared with non-sepsis, including the distinctive expansion of *Bilophilia*, *Fusobacterium*, and *Parabacteroides* in sepsis, which have all been linked to pro-inflammatory pathologies in other disease states.[67]

Does microbial dysbiosis influence clinical outcomes in critically ill and postoperative patients?
Although alterations to the gut microbiome are prevalent in the postoperative period, it is understandably challenging to derive cause and effect from clinical microbiome studies. Nonetheless, several recent investigations provide compelling evidence implicating the gut microbiome in the development of infectious complications and sepsis. In a large-scale study by Prescott and colleagues, investigators examined records of nearly 11,000 patients, exploring whether three hospitalization types—non-infection-related hospitalization, infection-related hospitalization, and hospitalization with *C. difficile* infection (CDI)—were associated with increasing risk of sepsis after hospital discharge. Indeed, they found that dysbiosis was an independent predictor for the development of severe sepsis, with adjusted probabilities of 4% in the non-infectious hospitalization group, 7% for infection-related hospitalization, and almost 11% for CDI.[74] Although purely an associative study, it supports the idea that disruption of the microbial ecosystem impairs host defense mechanisms and heightens susceptibility to infection. As for the source of infection, while not explored by Prescott and colleagues, studies using high-throughput sequencing techniques indicate that enteric bacterial translocation is likely a major contributor. A landmark study of patients undergoing hematopoietic stem cell transplantation (HCT) revealed that perioperative intestinal domination ($\geq$ 30% community membership) by *Enterococcus* was associated with a 9-fold increased risk of developing vancomycin-resistant *Enterococcus* (VRE), and domination by Proteobacteria was associated with a 5-fold increased risk of gram-negative rod bacteremia.[75] Through the development and application of a novel platform (StrainSifter) that provides higher bacterial strain resolution than 16S rRNA sequencing, Tamburini and colleagues[76] demonstrated that in HCT recipients with bloodstream infections ($n = 30$), half of the pathogens (with strain level resolution) were present in the patient's stool in the weeks preceding bacteremia. Moreover, in a prospective cohort study of ~300 medical ICU patients, Freedberg and colleagues found that the presence of specific pathogens in rectal swabs (*E coli*, *Pseudomonas* spp, *Klebsiella* spp, *C difficile*, and VRE) was associated with subsequent infection by the same organism. Importantly, irrespective of VRE detection on admission, *Enterococcus* domination ($\geq$30% 16S reads) was independently associated with the increased risk of death or all-cause infection.[59] Another study separately demonstrated that in patients with sepsis, expansion of *Enterococcus* spp over the course of ICU stay was an independent predictor of death.[67]

Changes in the microbiome may also affect postoperative outcomes like anastomotic insufficiency and peritonitis after intra-abdominal surgery. In a small study of patients undergoing intestinal resection, those with post-op anastomotic disruptions or enteric infections were found to have much lower diversity in bowel specimens taken intraoperatively compared with patients that did not develop post-op complications.[77] In a longitudinal sampling of 32 patients undergoing pancreatic surgery, the incidence of post-op complications (primarily pancreatic fistula formation) was associated to the presence of distinct taxonomic alterations in fecal samples (increased *Enterobacteriaceae*, *Akkermansia*, and *Anaeroplasma* and less representation from *Lachnospiraceae* and *Prevotella* and Bacteroides).[78] Conversely, van Praagh and colleagues[79] observed an association between anastomotic disruption and *expansion* of *Lachno-spiraceae* and *Bacteroidaceae* families as well as reduced community diversity in tissue samples from patients undergoing colorectal surgery. Although results from the latter two studies seem to be at odds with each other, this information may not be contradictory, but rather a result of combinatorial factors including variable spatial resolution of taxa within and along the intestinal tract, differing mechanisms leading to disruption, and varied sampling and sequencing techniques, but underscore the difficulty in the interpretation and clinical application of microbiome studies. Nonetheless, studies like these represent the first of many exciting findings bringing us one step closer to an understanding of how the perioperative microbial landscape may influence responses to surgery and inflammation.

Intersection of Nutrition and the Microbiome

Research into the effects of nutrition on the gut microbiome in critical illness is very much in its infancy. There are only a few clinical studies exploring the effects of different ICU nutritional therapy practices on the composition of the microbiome, let alone the clinical outcomes that are associated with nutrition-induced alterations in the microbiota. However, preclinical studies have provided insight into how dietary content, as well as enteral nutrient deprivation, affect the gut microbiota. In addition to reviewing these findings, below we also summarize the recent literature from human interventional trials exploring nutrition supplementation with prebiotics, probiotics, and synbiotics to modify the gut microbiome and improve outcomes in critically ill and postsurgical patients.

Diet and enteral nutrient deprivation

Diet is one of the greatest environmental determinants of microbial composition and gene expression. Nutrients (namely indigestible carbohydrates) interact directly with gut microbes to enhance or inhibit their growth.[33] The presence of absence of certain vitamins can modify the intestinal microenvironment which, in turn, influences community structure.[80] For example, vitamin D enhances expression of epithelial tight junction proteins and decreases the abundance of *Bifidobacterium* and increases *Prevotella*.[81] In mice, diets rich in fat or deficient in fiber compromise the integrity of the gut epithelium and contribute to the production of potentially harmful metabolites.[82]

Not surprisingly, the lack of EN too affects the microbiota. In addition to increased barrier permeability and altering local cytokines (reduced Interleukin-10 (IL-10), increased tumor necrosis factor (TNF) and Interferonγ[5]), EN deprivation alongside PN fosters expansion of proteobacteria and reductions in firmicutes phyla.[83,84] Of note, provision of hypocaloric EN (20% of estimated needs) both reversed some of these changes in microbiota composition and preserved MUC2 and barrier integrity.[83] In a separate study, addition of IV butyrate to parenteral formulations also ameliorated some of the changes observed in enteral nutrient deprivation, altering both intestinal microbial composition and increasing expression of ileal mucosal tight junction proteins and antimicrobial peptides.[85]

Soluble fibers and prebiotics. There is emerging evidence that soluble fiber—either contained within enteral formulations or added as a supplement—may have a potential therapeutic role in the ICU.[86] Soluble fibers are among the most widely recognized prebiotics, a term that describes any nonviable substrate that promotes growth of beneficial commensals. Prebiotics vary in structure, which dictates the taxa and microbial-mediated metabolites they enrich.[23] When fiber (usually plant polysaccharides), is used in this context, the aim is often to enhance growth of SCFA-producing bacteria.[87] Recently, Fu and colleagues[88] demonstrated that the amount of fiber in the enteral formula of 129 critically ill patients administered from time of admission to 72 hour, influenced both fecal SCFA levels and gut microbial composition. Patients who received greater quantities of fiber had higher SCFA levels and increased abundance of SCFA-producers, as well as significantly less *Enterococcus* than other groups, without changes in GI symptoms. Although other clinical outcomes were not evaluated, the protective effect of fiber is implied by the significant reduction in *Enterococcus* spp, expansion of which has been independently associated with mortality, as detailed previously.[59,67] Nonetheless, data from RCTs evaluating the effects of fiber supplementation on infectious complications and lengths of stay in critically ill patients[89] and patients undergoing GI surgery[90] have failed to show consistent improvement in outcomes.

Probiotics and synbiotics

In contrast to prebiotics, "probiotics" are live microorganisms that confer health benefits when ingested; "synbiotics" represent a mixture of probiotics with prebiotics.[91] Importantly, the microbes within these formulations can have varying effects on immunocytes: certain *Lactobacillus* spp (*L lactis, L acidophilus, L casei,* and *L rhamnosus*) and *Bifidobacteria* (*B infantis, B longum,* and *B brevis*) favor regulatory T-cell (T_{reg}) differentiation and promote anti-inflammatory responses; *L plantarum* also increases Th_{17}, whereas *L acidophilus, L rhamnosus, B brevis,* and *E faecalis* inhibit Th_{17} differentiation.[92] Despite inherent variability in formulation, animal and interventional human studies have demonstrated benefits with probiotic administration, particularly in the treatment of GI diseases.[93] For example, supplementation with clostridium butyricum-induced IL-10 production from intestinal macrophages via toll-like receptor 2 (TLR2), preventing development of acute experimental colitis.[94,95] However, a separate study found that in the setting of enteral nutrient deprivation, reduced intestinal macrophage IL-10 is independent of the gut microbiota, but rather, due to the lack of direct stimulation by dietary amino acids.[96] Together these findings suggest that for IL-10 production and perhaps other microbial-mediated responses, augmentation through pre-/synbiotics may only be possible in the presence of EN, and the deleterious effects of complete enteral deprivation cannot be rescued by microbiota alone.

In the largest meta-analyses evaluating administration of pre-/synbiotics in nearly 3000 critically ill patients, a clear benefit was found in infectious complications, reduction in rates of ventilator-associated pneumonia (VAP), and in duration of antibiotics usage.[97] Interestingly, the recent multicenter PROSPECT trial evaluating the effects of *L rhamnosus GG* versus placebo in 2560 patients found no difference in rates of VAP (primary outcome), nor secondary outcomes, though an increased presence of *L rhamnosus* was observed in cultured sites in the therapy group (1.1% vs 0.1%, $P < .001$).[98] However, it is unclear to what extent certain methodologic considerations contributed to these findings, namely that the primary indication for admission was pneumonia in 60% of patients, and the quantity of *L rhamnosus* administered was much greater than that used by other investigations. Nonetheless, pro-/synbiotics represent a promising therapeutic avenue for critically ill patients,[99] though explorations targeted to specific subgroups of patients is necessary to better inform clinical practice.

In the postsurgical population, there is increasing evidence to suggest benefit from pro-/synbiotics, although generalizability is challenged by small sample size and variable therapy formulations and treatment lengths. Nonetheless, a meta-analysis evaluating the effects of perioperative pro-/synbiotics on infectious complications after elective intra-abdominal surgery demonstrated a significant reduction in those receiving therapy.[100] Other notable prospective placebo-controlled RCTs exploring pro-/synbiotic use in surgical populations also merit individual mention. In patients with colorectal cancer, consumption of a synbiotic preparation (L acidophilus, L casei, L rhamnosus, B lactis + 6g fructooligosaccharide; $n = 36$ vs $n = 37$ placebo) for 7 days before surgery resulted in reductions in IL-6 and CRP (post-therapy/pre-operatively) and fewer postoperative infectious complications (2.8% vs 18.9%, $P = 0.02$).[101] Similarly, in patients undergoing resection of periampullary neoplasms, administration of a synbiotic formulation (L acidophilus, L casei, L rhamnosus, B bifidum + 0.1 g fructooligosaccharide; $n = 23$ vs $n = 23$ placebo) 4 days before surgery, until post-op day 10, resulted in reduced infectious complications in the therapy group (26.1% vs. 69.6%, $P = .001$), as well as reduced incidence of delayed gastric emptying and length of stay.[102] Of note, the reduction in infectious complications included reduced incidence of surgical site infections, pneumonia, and urinary tract infections in the synbiotic group, whereas peripancreatic fistula formation was equivalent.

Nonetheless, although available evidence suggests promising results, there is no universally accepted strategy for provision of perioperative synbiotics, and virtually all studies have varying protocols in terms of timing of initiation (from several days pre- to even weeks post-op), supplement composition, and dose of therapy. Moreover, complications—though rare—can occur. Perhaps the most well-known example remains the PROPATRIA trial which demonstrated increased incidence of bowel ischemia with administration of a synbiotic formulation for 28d in patients with SAP.[103] Various aspects of this study (from design to execution) have since been questioned, and recent meta-analyses demonstrate either improved outcomes[104] or equivocal findings[105] with the use of pro- and synbiotics in SAP. Nonetheless, reports of bacteremia and sepsis from probiotic administration exist. S boulardii, a probiotic yeast used in the treatment of diarrhea, has been associated with fungemia in critically ill patients and is now avoided.[106] Moreover, in addition to PROSPECT, sepsis from Lactobacillus spp in patients receiving pro-/synbiotics been described.[107] These complications highlight that probiotics likely affect patients in differing ways, perhaps beneficial for some, while fostering selective expansion of some species in others, which may be particularly dangerous in the setting of impaired gut permeability in critical illness. Invasive sampling along the GI tract reveals that in response to probiotic administration, humans demonstrate significant person-, region-, and strain-specific colonization patterns in both microbial composition and microbial-encoded functions, which have little association with correlate analysis done on stool samples.[24] To this point, Suez and colleagues[108] demonstrated that following antibiotic administration in 21 healthy humans, probiotic administration resulted in delayed and irregular reconstitution of community structure and transcriptome responses throughout the GI tract, whereas autologous fecal microbial transplant (FMT) induced a rapid and near-complete recovery of both structure and function within days. From this respect, FMT represents perhaps the most promising therapeutic option, though also currently the least well-studied in the critically ill and postsurgical population. FMT is now a primary treatment strategy for refractory and relapsed CDI, and a recent retrospective study of 111 patients with severe CDI revealed a significant survival benefit in those who received early FMT.[109] Clinical benefit has also been demonstrated in inflammatory bowel disease, irritable bowel syndrome, and intestinal cancer[110] and may have a potential therapeutic role in ICU-associated dysbiosis.[111]

SUMMARY AND FUTURE DIRECTIONS

Our understanding of the role of the microbiome in critical illness is rapidly evolving, however, there is still much to learn. The impact of ICU nutritional therapy on the microbiome, in particular, represents a major gap in knowledge. Are the outcomes differences observed in EEN over PN and delayed EN in fact partially due to nutritional effects on the gut microbiome? We do not yet know, and exploration of this relationship should be incorporated in future trials on nutritional interventions. Biologic plausibility and recent literature support the idea that the composition of our gut microbiota figures prominently in immune responses and even the clinical course of critically ill patients. Nonetheless, we need a better understanding of the microbial signatures that are beneficial versus harmful in specific subgroups. In the perioperative space, future studies should focus on incorporating microbiome analysis in personalized perioperative risk assessment and care. Nonetheless, the inherent difficulties with execution of high-quality large-scale studies suggest that progress will be gradual: personnel is required for sample collection; rigorous bioanalytical and statistical analysis should only be performed by those with specialized training; and sample collection site, handling, and processing can all influence results. However, a diligent characterization effort could yield a future, in which the microbiome is considered equally alongside other organ systems and routinely integrated in clinical care.

For now, the current literature supports thoughtful practice decisions. A nutritional plan should be in place for every patient, integrating decisions about caloric and protein needs with route and timing. Awareness of the microbiome should be integrated into patient assessment and care: mindful provision of antimicrobials, supplemental oxygen, and other therapeutics that disrupt the microbial ecosystem; EEN when possible; and enhanced awareness that patients recently treated with antimicrobials are at greater risk of infection. In coming years, modulation of the microbiome in targeted critically ill and perioperative patients will likely be a realizable and compelling therapeutic option.

CLINICS CARE POINTS

- The impact of intensive care unit (ICU) nutritional therapy on the microbiome and how this interaction contributes to clinical outcomes represents a major gap in knowledge.
- A plan for nutrition should be made on ICU admission, factoring timing, and route alongside composition. Outcomes may be improved with early (<48 hour) initiation of nutrition (enteral, if possible), avoidance of over- and underfeeding and provision of adequate protein (1.2 g/kg)
- Initiation of nutrition for patients with shock remains debatable, though data suggest this practice may be safe—and preferred over delayed enteral nutrition —when pressor support is low
- Emerging data suggest that alterations in the microbiota—and certain microbial signatures in particular—may increase susceptibility to sepsis from enteric pathogens and may increase the incidence of complications after some intra-abdominal procedures.
- Clinicians should be thoughtful in provision of antimicrobials, supplemental oxygen, opioids, and proton pump inhibitors (PPIs) as these interventions may disrupt the microbial community and impair host defenses.
- Soluble fiber and pro-/synbiotics may improve outcomes in critical illness and after intra-abdominal procedures. However, significant heterogeneity in formulation and therapy

duration, and the inherent intraindividual and interindividual variability in patients' microbiomes challenges our current ability to apply findings to large populations of patients.

- The microbiome has significant potential as a therapeutic target, however, additional rigorously designed and executed studies are needed to identify the patient subgroups that most stand to benefit.

DISCLOSURE

None of the authors have any financial interests to disclose.

REFERENCES

1. Gilbert JA, Blaser MJ, Gregory Caporaso J, et al. Current understanding of the human microbiome. Nat Med 2018;24(4):392–400.
2. Mittal R, Coopersmith CM. Redefining the gut as the motor of critical illness. Trends Mol Med 2014;20(4):214–23.
3. Sharma K, Mogensen KM, Robinson MK. Pathophysiology of critical illness and role of nutrition. Nutr Clin Pract 2019;34(1):12–22.
4. Van Zanten ARH, De Waele E, Wischmeyer PE. Nutrition therapy and critical illness: practical guidance for the icu, post-icu, and long-term convalescence phases. Crit Care 2019;23(1). https://doi.org/10.1186/s13054-019-2657-5.
5. Ralls MW, Demehri FR, Feng Y, et al. Enteral nutrient deprivation in patients leads to a loss of intestinal epithelial barrier function. Surg (United States). 2015;157(4):732–42.
6. Buchman AL, Moukarzel AA, Bhuta S, et al. Parenteral nutrition is associated with intestinal morphologic and functional changes in humans. J Parenter Enter Nutr 1995;19(6):453–60.
7. Van Der Hulst RRWJ, Von Meyenfeldt MF, Van Kreel BK, et al. Gut permeability, intestinal morphology, and nutritional depletion. Nutrition 1998;14(1):1–6.
8. Zusman O, Theilla M, Cohen J, et al. Resting energy expenditure, calorie and protein consumption in critically ill patients: a retrospective cohort study. Crit Care 2016;20(1). https://doi.org/10.1186/S13054-016-1538-4.
9. Harvey SE, Parrott F, Harrison DA, et al. Trial of the route of early nutritional support in critically Ill adults. N Engl J Med 2014;371(18):1673–84.
10. Singer P, Blaser AR, Berger MM, et al. ESPEN guideline on clinical nutrition in the intensive care unit. Clin Nutr 2019;38(1):48–79.
11. Ohbe H, Jo T, Yamana H, et al. Early enteral nutrition for cardiogenic or obstructive shock requiring venoarterial extracorporeal membrane oxygenation: a nationwide inpatient database study. Intensive Care Med 2018;44(8):1258–65.
12. Ohbe H, Jo T, Matsui H, et al. Early enteral nutrition in patients with severe traumatic brain injury: a propensity score-matched analysis using a nationwide inpatient database in Japan. Am J Clin Nutr 2020;111(2):378–84. https://doi.org/10.1093/ajcn/nqz290.
13. Matejovic M, Huet O, Dams K, et al. Medical nutrition therapy and clinical outcomes in critically ill adults: a European multinational, prospective observational cohort study (EuroPN). Crit Care 2022;26(1):1–14.
14. Reignier J, Boisramé-Helms J, Brisard L, et al. Enteral versus parenteral early nutrition in ventilated adults with shock: a randomised, controlled, multicentre, open-label, parallel-group study (NUTRIREA-2). Lancet 2018;391(10116): 133–43.

15. Barash M, Patel JJ. Gut luminal and clinical benefits of early enteral nutrition in shock. Curr Surg Rep 2019;7(10). https://doi.org/10.1007/s40137-019-0243-z.

16. Ohbe H, Jo T, Matsui H, et al. Differences in effect of early enteral nutrition on mortality among ventilated adults with shock requiring low-, medium-, and high-dose noradrenaline: a propensity-matched analysis. Clin Nutr 2020;39(2):460–7.

17. Dorken Gallastegi A, Gebran A, Gaitanidis A, et al. Early versus late enteral nutrition in critically ill patients receiving vasopressor support. J Parenter Enteral Nutr 2022;46(1):130–40.

18. Heidegger CP, Berger MM, Graf S, et al. Optimisation of energy provision with supplemental parenteral nutrition in critically ill patients: a randomised controlled clinical trial. Lancet 2013;381(9864):385–93.

19. Alsharif DJ, Alsharif FJ, Aljuraiban GS, et al. Effect of supplemental parenteral nutrition versus enteral nutrition alone on clinical outcomes in critically ill adult patients: a systematic review and meta-analysis of randomized controlled trials. Nutrients 2020;12(10):2968.

20. Lynch SV, Pedersen O. The human intestinal microbiome in health and disease. N Engl J Med 2016;375(24):2369–79.

21. Langille MGI, Zaneveld J, Caporaso JG, et al. Predictive functional profiling of microbial communities using 16S rRNA marker gene sequences. Nat Biotechnol 2013;31(9):814–21.

22. Nguyen NP, Warnow T, Pop M, et al. A perspective on 16S rRNA operational taxonomic unit clustering using sequence similarity. NPJ Biofilms Microbiomes 2016;2. https://doi.org/10.1038/npjbiofilms.2016.4.

23. Donaldson GP, Lee SM, Mazmanian SK. Gut biogeography of the bacterial microbiota. Nat Rev Microbiol 2015;14(1):20–32.

24. Zmora N, Zilberman-Schapira G, Suez J, et al. Personalized gut mucosal colonization resistance to empiric probiotics is associated with unique host and microbiome features. Cell 2018;174(6):1388–405.e21.

25. Huttenhower C, Gevers D, Knight R, et al. Structure, function and diversity of the healthy human microbiome. Nature 2012;486(7402):207–14.

26. Li K, Bihan M, Methé BA. Analyses of the stability and core taxonomic memberships of the human microbiome. PLoS One 2013;8(5). https://doi.org/10.1371/journal.pone.0063139.

27. Krych L, Hansen CHF, Hansen AK, et al. Quantitatively different, yet qualitatively alike: a meta-analysis of the mouse core gut microbiome with a view towards the human gut microbiome. PLoS One 2013;8(5):e62578.

28. Buffie CG, Pamer EG. Microbiota-mediated colonization resistance against intestinal pathogens. Nat Rev Immunol 2013;13(11):790–801.

29. Caballero S, Pamer EG. Microbiota-mediated inflammation and antimicrobial defense in the intestine. Annu Rev Immunol 2015;33:227–56.

30. Schirmer M, Smeekens SP, Vlamakis H, et al. Linking the human gut microbiome to inflammatory cytokine production capacity. Cell 2016;167:1125–36.

31. Ivanov II, Honda K. Intestinal commensal microbes as immune modulators. Cell Host Microbe 2012;12(4):496–508.

32. Lopetuso LR, Scaldaferri F, Petito V, et al. Commensal clostridia: leading players in the maintenance of gut homeostasis. Gut Pathog 2013;5(1):23.

33. Valdes AM, Walter J, Segal E, et al. Role of the gut microbiota in nutrition and health. BMJ 2018;361:36–44.

34. Lukovic E, Moitra VK, Freedberg DE. The microbiome: implications for perioperative and critical care. Curr Opin Anaesthesiol 2019;32(3):412–20.

35. Fay KT, Ford ML, Coopersmith CM. The intestinal microenvironment in sepsis. Biochim Biophys Acta - Mol Basis Dis 2017;1863(10):2574–83.

36. Krezalek MA, Defazio J, Zaborina O, et al. The shift of an intestinal "microbiome" to a "pathobiome" governs the course and outcome of sepsis following surgical injury. Shock 2016;45(5):475.

37. Dickson RP. The microbiome and critical illness. Lancet Respir Med 2016;4(1): 59–72.

38. Alverdy JC, Hyoju SK, Weigerinck M, et al. The gut microbiome and the mechanism of surgical infection. Br J Surg 2017;104(2):e14–23.

39. Deshmukh HS, Liu Y, Menkiti OR, et al. The microbiota regulates neutrophil homeostasis and host resistance to Escherichia coli K1 sepsis in neonatal mice. Nat Med 2014;20(5):524–30.

40. Schuijt TJ, Lankelma JM, Scicluna BP, et al. The gut microbiota plays a protective role in the host defence against pneumococcal pneumonia. Gut 2016;65(4): 575–83.

41. Becattini S, Littmann ER, Carter RA, et al. Commensal microbes provide first line defense against Listeria monocytogenes infection. J Exp Med 2017;214(7): 1973–89.

42. Rivera-Chávez F, Zhang LF, Faber F, et al. Depletion of butyrate-producing clostridia from the gut microbiota drives an aerobic luminal expansion of salmonella. Cell Host Microbe 2016;19(4):443–54.

43. Fay KT, Klingensmith NJ, Chen CW, et al. The gut microbiome alters immunophenotype and survival from sepsis. FASEB J 2019;33(10):11258–69.

44. Bäumler AJ, Sperandio V. Interactions between the microbiota and pathogenic bacteria in the gut. Nature 2016;535(7610):85–93.

45. Bratzler DW, Houck PM, Richards C, et al. Use of antimicrobial prophylaxis for major surgery: baseline results from the national surgical infection prevention project. Arch Surg 2005;140(2):174–82.

46. Vincent JL, Rello J, Marshall J, et al. International study of the prevalence and outcomes of infection in intensive care units. JAMA - J Am Med Assoc 2009; 302(21):2323–9.

47. Lange K, Buerger M, Stallmach A, et al. Effects of antibiotics on gut microbiota. Dig Dis 2016;34(3):260–8.

48. Becattini S, Taur Y, Pamer EG. Antibiotic-induced changes in the intestinal microbiota and disease. Trends Mol Med 2016;22(6):458–78.

49. Palleja A, Mikkelsen KH, Forslund SK, et al. Recovery of gut microbiota of healthy adults following antibiotic exposure. Nat Microbiol 2018;3(11):1255–65.

50. Dethlefsen L, Relman DA. Incomplete recovery and individualized responses of the human distal gut microbiota to repeated antibiotic perturbation. Proc Natl Acad Sci 2011;108:4554–61.

51. Buffie CG, Jarchum I, Equinda M, et al. Profound alterations of intestinal microbiota following a single dose of clindamycin results in sustained susceptibility to clostridium difficile-induced colitis. Infect Immun 2012;80(1):62.

52. Kennedy EA, King KY, Baldridge MT. Mouse microbiota models: comparing germ-free mice and antibiotics treatment as tools for modifying gut bacteria. Front Physiol 2018;9(OCT):1534.

53. Serbanescu MA, Mathena RP, Xu J, et al. General anesthesia alters the diversity and composition of the intestinal microbiota in mice. Anesth Analg 2018;1. https://doi.org/10.1213/ane.0000000000003938.

54. Ashley SL, Sjoding MW, Popova AP, et al. Lung and gut microbiota are altered by hyperoxia and contribute to oxygen-induced lung injury in mice. Sci Transl Med 2020;12(556). https://doi.org/10.1126/SCITRANSLMED.AAU9959.

55. Freedberg DE, Toussaint NC, Chen SP, et al. Proton pump inhibitors alter specific taxa in the human gastrointestinal microbiome: a crossover trial. Gastroenterology 2015;149(4):883–5.e9.

56. Wang F, Meng J, Zhang L, et al. Morphine induces changes in the gut microbiome and metabolome in a morphine dependence model. Sci Rep 2018; 8(1):1–15.

57. Banerjee S, Sindberg G, Wang F, et al. Opioid-induced gut microbial disruption and bile dysregulation leads to gut barrier compromise and sustained systemic inflammation. Mucosal Immunol Author Manuscr Mucosal Immunol 2016;99(6): 1418–28.

58. McDonald D, Ackermann G, Khailova L, et al. Extreme dysbiosis of the microbiome in critical illness. mSphere 2016;1(4):199–215.

59. Freedberg DE, Zhou MJ, Cohen ME, et al. Pathogen colonization of the gastrointestinal microbiome at intensive care unit admission and risk for subsequent death or infection. Intensive Care Med 2018;44(8):1203–11.

60. Livanos AE, Snider EJ, Whittier S, et al. Rapid gastrointestinal loss of Clostridial Clusters IV and XIVa in the ICU associates with an expansion of gut pathogens. PLoS One 2018;13(8):e0200322.

61. Lankelma JM, van Vught LA, Belzer C, et al. Critically ill patients demonstrate large interpersonal variation in intestinal microbiota dysregulation: a pilot study. Intensive Care Med 2017;43(1):59–68.

62. Jacobs MC, Lankelma JM, Wolff NS, et al. Effect of antibiotic gut microbiota disruption on LPS-induced acute lung inflammation. PLoS One 2020;15(11): e0241748.

63. Yamada T, Shimizu K, Ogura H, et al. Rapid and sustained long-term decrease of fecal short-chain fatty acids in critically ill patients with systemic inflammatory response syndrome. J Parenter Enter Nutr 2015;39(5):569–77.

64. Valdés-Duque BE, Giraldo-Giraldo NA, Jaillier-Ramírez AM, et al. Stool short-chain fatty acids in critically ill patients with sepsis. J Am Coll Nutr 2020;39(8): 706–12.

65. Ravi A, Halstead FD, Bamford A, et al. Loss of microbial diversity and pathogen domination of the gut microbiota in critically ill patients. Microb Genomics 2019; 5(9). https://doi.org/10.1099/MGEN.0.000293.

66. Zaborin A, Smith D, Garfield K, et al. Membership and behavior of ultra-low-diversity pathogen communities present in the gut of humans during prolonged critical illness. MBio 2014;5(5).

67. Agudelo-Ochoa GM, Valdés-Duque BE, Giraldo-Giraldo NA, et al. Gut microbiota profiles in critically ill patients, potential biomarkers and risk variables for sepsis. Gut Microbes 2020;12(1). https://doi.org/10.1080/19490976.2019. 1707610.

68. Earley ZM, Akhtar S, Green SJ, et al. Burn injury alters the intestinal microbiome and increases gut permeability and bacterial translocation. PLoS One 2015; 10(7). https://doi.org/10.1371/journal.pone.0129996.

69. Howard BM, Kornblith LZ, Christie SA, et al. Characterizing the gut microbiome in trauma: significant changes in microbial diversity occur early after severe injury. Trauma Surg Acute Care Open 2017;2(1). https://doi.org/10.1136/tsaco-2017-000108.

70. Cong J, Zhu H, Liu D, et al. A pilot study: changes of gut microbiota in post-surgery colorectal cancer patients. Front Microbiol 2018;9(NOV). https://doi.org/10.3389/fmicb.2018.02777.

71. Tourelle KM, Boutin S, Weigand MA, et al. Sepsis and the human microbiome. Just another kind of organ failure? a review. J Clin Med 2021;10(21):4831.

72. Fair K, Dunlap DG, Fitch A, et al. Rectal swabs from critically ill patients provide discordant representations of the gut microbiome compared to stool samples. mSphere 2019;4(4).

73. Fontaine C, Armand-Lefèvre L, Magnan M, et al. Relationship between the composition of the intestinal microbiota and the tracheal and intestinal colonization by opportunistic pathogens in intensive care patients. PLoS One 2020;15(8 August). https://doi.org/10.1371/journal.pone.0237260.

74. Prescott HC, Dickson RP, Rogers MAM, et al. Hospitalization type and subsequent severe sepsis. Am J Respir Crit Care Med 2015;192(5):581–8.

75. Taur Y, Xavier JB, Lipuma L, et al. Intestinal domination and the risk of bacteremia in patients undergoing allogeneic hematopoietic stem cell transplantation. Clin Infect Dis 2012;55(7):905–14.

76. Tamburini FB, Andermann TM, Tkachenko E, et al. Precision identification of diverse bloodstream pathogens in the gut microbiome. Nat Med 2018;24(12):1809–14.

77. Ralls MW, Miyasaka E, Teitelbaum DH. Intestinal microbial diversity and perioperative complications. J Parenter Enter Nutr 2014;38(3):392–9.

78. Schmitt FCF, Brenner T, Uhle F, et al. Gut microbiome patterns correlate with higher postoperative complication rates after pancreatic surgery. BMC Microbiol 2019;19(1):42.

79. Van Praagh JB, De Goffau MC, Bakker IS, et al. Mucus microbiome of anastomotic tissue during surgery has predictive value for colorectal anastomotic leakage. Ann Surg 2019;269(5):911–6.

80. Zmora N, Suez J, Elinav E. You are what you eat: diet, health and the gut microbiota. Nat Rev Gastroenterol Hepatol 2019;16(1):35–56.

81. Luthold RV, Fernandes GR, Franco-de-Moraes AC, et al. Gut microbiota interactions with the immunomodulatory role of vitamin D in normal individuals. Metabolism 2017;69:76–86.

82. Rinninella E, Raoul P, Cintoni M, et al. What is the healthy gut microbiota composition? A changing ecosystem across age, environment, diet, and diseases. Microorganisms 2019;7(1):14.

83. Wan X, Bi J, Gao X, et al. Partial enteral nutrition preserves elements of gut barrier function, including innate immunity, intestinal alkaline phosphatase (IAP) level, and intestinal microbiota in mice. Nutrients 2015;7:6294–312.

84. Lucchinetti E, Lou PH, Lemal P, et al. Gut microbiome and circulating bacterial DNA ("blood microbiome") in a mouse model of total parenteral nutrition: Evidence of two distinct separate microbiotic compartments. Clin Nutr ESPEN 2022;49:278–88.

85. Jirsova Z, Heczkova M, Dankova H, et al. The effect of butyrate-supplemented parenteral nutrition on intestinal defence mechanisms and the parenteral nutrition-induced shift in the gut microbiota in the rat model. Biomed Res Int 2019;2019. https://doi.org/10.1155/2019/7084734.

86. Venegas-Borsellino C, Kwon M. Impact of soluble fiber in the microbiome and outcomes in critically ill patients. Curr Nutr Rep 2019;8(4):347–55.

87. Holscher HD. Dietary fiber and prebiotics and the gastrointestinal microbiota Dietary fiber and prebiotics and the gastrointestinal microbiota. Gut Microbes 2017;8(2):172–84.

88. Fu Y, Moscoso DI, Porter J, et al. Relationship between dietary fiber intake and short-chain fatty acid–producing bacteria during critical illness: a prospective cohort study. J Parenter Enter Nutr 2020;44(3):463–71.

89. Liu T, Wang C, Wang Y, et al. Effect of dietary fiber on gut barrier function, gut microbiota, short-chain fatty acids, inflammation, and clinical outcomes in critically ill patients: a systematic review and meta-analysis. J Parenter Enter Nutr 2022. https://doi.org/10.1002/JPEN.2319.

90. Eleftheriadis K, Davies R. Do patients fed enterally post–gastrointestinal surgery experience more complications when fed a fiber-enriched feed compared with a standard feed? A systematic review. Nutr Clin Pract 2021. https://doi.org/10.1002/NCP.10805.

91. Davison JM, Wischmeyer PE. Probiotic and synbiotic therapy in the critically ill: state of the art. Nutrition 2019;59:29–36.

92. Zeng W, Shen J, Bo T, et al. Cutting edge: probiotics and fecal microbiota transplantation in immunomodulation. J Immunol Res 2019;2019. https://doi.org/10.1155/2019/1603758.

93. McFarland LV. Use of probiotics to correct dysbiosis of normal microbiota following disease or disruptive events: a systematic review. BMJ Open 2014;4. https://doi.org/10.1136/bmjopen-2014-005047.

94. Hayashi A, Sato T, Kamada N, et al. A single strain of clostridium butyricum induces intestinal IL-10-producing macrophages to suppress acute experimental colitis in mice. Cell Host Microbe 2013;13(6):711–22.

95. Kanai T, Mikami Y, Atsushi Hayashi ●. A breakthrough in probiotics: clostridium butyricum regulates gut homeostasis and anti-inflammatory response in inflammatory bowel disease. J Gastroenterol 2015;50. https://doi.org/10.1007/s00535-015-1084-x.

96. Ochi T, Feng Y, Kitamoto S, et al. Diet-dependent, microbiota-independent regulation of IL-10-producing lamina propria macrophages in the small intestine. Sci Rep 2016;6(1):1–12.

97. Manzanares W, Lemieux M, Langlois PL, et al. Probiotic and synbiotic therapy in critical illness: a systematic review and meta-analysis. Crit Care 2016;20(1). https://doi.org/10.1186/s13054-016-1434-y.

98. Johnstone J, Meade M, Lauzier F, et al. Effect of probiotics on incident ventilator-associated pneumonia in critically ill patients: a randomized clinical trial. JAMA 2021;326(11):1024–33.

99. Bassetti M, Bandera A, Gori A. Therapeutic Potential of the Gut Microbiota in the Management of Sepsis. Crit Care 2020;24(105). https://doi.org/10.1186/s13054-020-2780-3.

100. Chowdhury AH, Adiamah A, Kushairi A, et al. Perioperative probiotics or synbiotics in adults undergoing elective abdominal surgery: A systematic review and meta-analysis of randomized controlled trials. Ann Surg 2020;271(6):1036–47.

101. Polakowski CB, Kato M, Preti VB, et al. Impact of the preoperative use of synbiotics in colorectal cancer patients: a prospective, randomized, double-blind, placebo-controlled study. Nutrition 2019;58:40–6.

102. Martins Sommacal H, Pierri Bersch V, Pascoal Vitola S, et al. Perioperative synbiotics decrease postoperative complications in periampullary neoplasms: a randomized, double-blind clinical trial. Nutr Cancer 2015;67(3):457–62.

103. Besselink MG, van Santvoort HC, Buskens E, et al. Probiotic prophylaxis in predicted severe acute pancreatitis: a randomised, double-blind, placebo-controlled trial. Lancet (London, England) 2008;371(9613):651–9.

104. Yu C, Zhang Y, Yang Q, et al. An updated systematic review with meta-analysis: efficacy of prebiotic, probiotic, and synbiotic treatment of patients with severe acute pancreatitis. Pancreas 2021;50(2):160–6.

105. Gou S, Yang Z, Liu T, et al. Use of probiotics in the treatment of severe acute pancreatitis: a systematic review and meta-analysis of randomized controlled trials. Crit Care 2014;18(2):1–10.

106. Lolis N, Veldekis D, Moraitou H, et al. Saccharomyces boulardii fungaemia in an intensive care unit patient treated with caspofungin. Crit Care 2008;12(2):414.

107. Sherid M, Samo S, Sulaiman S, et al. Liver abscess and bacteremia caused by lactobacillus: role of probiotics? Case report and review of the literature. BMC Gastroenterol 2016;16(1). https://doi.org/10.1186/s12876-016-0552-y.

108. Suez J, Zmora N, Zilberman-Schapira G, et al. Post-antibiotic gut mucosal microbiome reconstitution is impaired by probiotics and improved by autologous FMT. Cell 2018;174(6):1406–23.e16.

109. Hocquart M, Lagier JC, Cassir N, et al. Early fecal microbiota transplantation improves survival in severe clostridium difficile infections. Clin Infect Dis 2018; 66(5):645–50.

110. Choi HH, Cho YS. Fecal microbiota transplantation: current applications, effectiveness, and future perspectives. Clin Endosc 2016;49(3):257–65.

111. Alagna L, Haak BW, Gori A. Fecal microbiota transplantation in the ICU: perspectives on future implementations. Intensive Care Med 2019;45(7):998–1001.

Massive Trauma and Resuscitation Strategies

Carter M. Galbraith, MD[a], Brant M. Wagener, MD, PhD[b,c],
Athanasios Chalkias, MD, MSc, PhD, FESC, FAcadTM, FCP, FESAIC[d,e],
Shahla Siddiqui, MD, MSc, FCCM[f],*, David J. Douin, MD[g],*

KEYWORDS

- Trauma • Resuscitation • Coagulopathy • Whole blood • Component therapy
- Viscoelastic technique

KEY POINTS

- Care of the trauma patient should focus on early detection, cessation of surgical bleeding, and appropriate resuscitation.
- Whole blood and component therapy transfusion are viable techniques to support end-organ function.
- Viscoelastic techniques are useful tools to prevent and/or treat coagulopathy.
- Although there are advantages and disadvantages to both whole blood and component therapy, there is no clear consensus on the use of each therapy, societal costs, and patient benefit with either technique.

CASE PRESENTATION AND INTRODUCTION
Case Presentation

A 36-year-old man is brought into Emergency Department (ED) via helicopter after a motor vehicle accident. He was an unrestrained driver whose car was struck by a truck and was extricated from the scene within 20 minutes of first-responder arrival. Due to a Glasgow Coma Score (GCS) of 3, he was intubated with inline stabilization of the neck and a C-collar was placed. During intubation, blood was seen in the posterior oropharynx. Large bore intravenous access was obtained and 2 L of normal saline

[a] Division of Critical Care Medicine, Department of Anesthesiology and Perioperative Medicine, University of Alabama at Birmingham, 619 19th Street South, JT 845, Birmingham, AL 35249, USA; [b] Division of Critical Care Medicine, University of Alabama at Birmingham, 901 19th Street South, PBMR 302, Birmingham, AL 35294, USA; [c] Division of Molecular and Translational Biomedicine, Department of Anesthesiology and Perioperative Medicine, University of Alabama at Birmingham, 901 19th Street South, PBMR 302, Birmingham, AL 35294, USA; [d] Department of Anesthesiology, University of Thessaly, Biopolis, Larisa 41500, Greece; [e] Outcomes Research Consortium, Cleveland, OH 44195, USA; [f] Department of Anesthesia, Critical Care and Pain Medicine, Beth Israel Deaconess Medical Center, Harvard Medical School, 330 Brookline Avenue, Boston, MA 02215, USA; [g] Department of Anesthesiology, University of Colorado School of Medicine, 12401 East 17th Avenue, 7th Floor, Aurora, CO 80045, USA
* Corresponding authors.
E-mail addresses: ssiddiq4@bidmc.harvard.edu (S.S.); david.douin@cuanschutz.edu (D.J.D.)

Anesthesiology Clin 41 (2023) 283–301
https://doi.org/10.1016/j.anclin.2022.10.008
1932-2275/23/© 2022 Elsevier Inc. All rights reserved.
anesthesiology.theclinics.com

was delivered *en route*. The patient was hypotensive during transport and a phenyl-ephrine infusion was initiated.

In the ED, the patient remained unresponsive with equal, but sluggishly, reactive pupils. His vital signs were blood pressure (BP) 70/46, heart rate (HR) 125 (normal rhythm), and SpO_2 of 90% on 100% Fio_2 and initial laboratories revealed a hemoglobin (Hgb) of 6.5 g/dL and a hematocrit (Hct) of 19. A chest radiograph revealed a widened mediastinum and left hemopneumothorax and bedside ultrasound exhibited the "bar code sign" and a "lung point" on the left chest. A left-sided chest tube was placed with 500 mL fresh blood evacuated in 10 minutes. Massive transfusion protocol (MTP) was initiated, and the patient received 4 units of packed red blood cells (pRBC) and 3 units of fresh frozen plasma (FFP).

With transfusion ongoing, the patient was rushed to the operating room (OR) for a thoracotomy to determine the source of bleeding where arterial and central access was obtained. One-lung ventilation was achieved with a right-sided bronchial blocker to isolate the left lung for surgery exposure. Although the surgery team was attempting to achieve control of ongoing patient bleeding, a thromboelastorgraphy (TEG) revealed a prolonged R-time, decreased α-angle, and decreased maximum amplitude (MA). Six additional units of pRBC, 6 units of FFP, and 1 unit of platelets were transfused.

After surgical control of bleeding, a follow-up arterial blood gas (ABG) revealed a pH of 7.15, $Paco_2$ of 30, and Pao_2 of 68 on 100% Fio_2 one lung ventilation. TEG revealed improved R-time, α-angle, and MA but significant fibrinolysis with an increased LY30. Tranexamic acid (TXA) 1 g IV and 2 pools of cryoprecipitate were infused.

After surgery, the patient was transported to the intensive care unit (ICU) and continued on invasive mechanical ventilation. His TEG and coagulation status (per laboratory analysis) were near normal; however, he received active warming to treat a core temperature of 35°C. The patient was extubated 3 days after ICU admission and discharged to a rehabilitation facility 2 weeks later.

Introduction

In the case presentation, a young man suffered significant trauma in a motor vehicle accident. His injuries were severe and required emergent surgery, massive transfusion of blood products, advanced airway management, and treatment of coagulopathy among many other clinical decisions. Trauma management remains heterogeneous due to variable causes, patient variables, including age, sex, comorbidities, and so forth, and a host of other factors. This can necessitate a variety of imaging modalities to evaluate damage, laboratories to evaluate patient status, and strategies for surgical repair and patient resuscitation. The most common types of trauma and their respective management necessities are listed in **Table 1**. In the following sections, we provide a comprehensive review of evaluation, surgical objectives, and resuscitation strategies for the critically injured patient. Additionally, we discuss the use of whole blood versus component therapy for blood product resuscitation and use of coagulation monitoring techniques. We think these sections will provide anesthesiologists with the necessary information to make informed clinical decisions regarding the evaluation and resuscitation of injured patients.

INITIAL EVALUATION AND DAMAGE CONTROL RESUSCITATION
Initial Assessment

Assessment of injuries (primary survey)
The initial assessment of traumatically injured patients encompasses a structured approach (primary survey) to identify life-threatening conditions by adhering to the

Table 1
Trauma type, clinical considerations, and management options

Type of Trauma	Considerations and Possibilities	Management Options
Chest	Possible pneumothorax/hemothorax, rib fractures, aortic or cardiac injury	CXR, US, Chest CT, CT angiogram, possible surgery
Abdomen	Spleen, liver, kidney, and intestinal/omental injury; also, aortic injury, hemoperitoneum, or perforation can occur	FAST, CT/A, surgery or careful observation with serial laboratory checks
Long bones	Long bones, pelvic or facial fractures, fat emboli are possible	Consider early stabilization and monitor blood loss
Retroperitoneum	Large vessels can bleed into a large potential space	CT scan early, frequent laboratory evaluation, possible IR intervention
Neuro/spine	Fractures, contusions, bleeding, and increased intracranial pressure. Ligamentous spine injuries with potential for neurogenic shock	Stabilization, CT scan, observation, surgery
Soft tissue	Possible rhabdomyolysis	Frequent laboratory checks, monitor renal function closely
Blunt	Internal organ injury, falls, and crush injury	Hemodynamic collapse (possibly delayed), close observation
Penetrating	Gunshot injuries or knife trauma, multiple organ systems at risk	Early intervention more likely
Blast injuries	Widespread soft tissue destruction, increased chances of neurologic and myocardial injuries	Widespread damage can have delayed presentations; often polytrauma that is severe

Listed are common types of injury and the appropriate clinical considerations and management options.

Abbreviations: CT, computed tomography; CXR, chest radiograph; FAST, focused assessment with sonography for trauma; US, ultrasound.

ABCDE sequence: airway maintenance with restriction of cervical spine motion, breathing and ventilation, circulation with hemorrhage control, disability and assessment of neurologic status, and exposure/environmental control.[1] The primary survey is based on the patient's injuries and associated mechanisms, is always performed with simultaneous resuscitation of vital functions, and should be repeated frequently and whenever a patient's status changes.

Trauma airway management (difficult airway algorithm)

On initial evaluation, the airway is rapidly assessed to ascertain patency, including signs of airway obstruction by the ability of the patient to communicate verbally.[2] However, particular attention and repeated assessment are necessary to recognize progressive airway loss and ensure early intervention. Although the jaw-thrust maneuver and nasopharyngeal or oropharyngeal airways can be helpful temporarily, a definitive airway should be established in patients with nonpurposeful motor responses, altered level of consciousness (GCS of ≤8), or if there is any doubt about the patient's ability to maintain airway integrity. A cervical collar must be used to restrict cervical spine motion, yet when airway management is necessary, the cervical collar is opened and a team member should manually protect the cervical spine from excessive mobility. When endotracheal intubation is contraindicated or cannot be accomplished, the threshold to perform a surgical airway must be low.

Despite the recent definition of "difficult airway" by the American Society of Anesthesiologists (ASA), reflecting the traditional perceptions on airway evaluation and management,[3,4] increasing evidence suggest that physiologic derangements are associated with increased peri-intubation complications, and patients should be also evaluated for a physiologically difficult airway with the aim of preventing cardiovascular decompensation and other complications.[5] Physiologic derangements can be due to traumatic injuries, preexisting disease, the effects of anesthetic agents, and positive pressure ventilation. In these patients, improving peri-intubation oxygenation and hemodynamic stability is essential, especially before the first intubation attempt.[6,7]

Intravenous access

Establishing intravenous access during the primary survey is a prerequisite for the replacement of intravascular volume. In most patients, 2 large-bore peripheral venous catheters are necessary for obtaining blood samples and administering fluids, blood products, and other agents. When peripheral sites cannot be accessed, central venous/intraosseous access or venous cut down may be used.[1] In addition to venous samples, ABGs provide important information concerning the adequacy of ventilation, oxygenation, and acid–base status.

Imaging/ultrasound

Radiography can reveal potentially life-threatening injuries that require treatment or further investigation and can provide information to guide resuscitation, especially in patients with blunt trauma. Imaging can be performed in the resuscitation area to avoid delays, even in pregnant patients when necessary but should not interrupt the resuscitation process.

The implementation of point of care ultrasound has significantly affected management of trauma patients. Focused assessment with sonography for trauma (FAST) or extended FAST (eFAST) are rapid bedside ultrasound screening techniques for quick detection of intra-abdominal or intrathoracic injuries.[8,9] The presence of pathologic fluid on FAST indicates the need for surgical intervention in hemodynamically unstable patients. Nevertheless, the quality of images depends on clinician skill and experience and can be compromised in obese patients, in those with intraluminal bowel gas, and those with renal and pancreatic injuries.[10,11]

CT is important for the timely diagnosis of traumatic injuries and to determine the most suitable treatment. Currently, however, there is no agreement on an optimal CT trauma protocol. Although the Advanced Trauma Life Support (ATLS) guidelines recommend CT only if indicated, not by default, and on a selective basis, that is, for specific body regions,[1] the European Society of Emergency Radiology (ESER) guidelines distinguish patients in categories and differentiate the approaches.[12] Nevertheless, in patients without a definitive diagnosis or in patients with severe multitrauma, the ESER guidelines recommend a whole-body CT after initial resuscitation.[13,14]

Hemodynamic goals

Cardiovascular reserves vary with age and/or comorbidities. Although most hypotensive patients present with tachycardia, others, especially the elderly, may not exhibit this sign because of limited cardiac response to catecholamine stimulation, adrenal insufficiency, and hypoglycemia.[15,16] Therefore, an individualized approach should be used to correct inadequate perfusion and increase tissue oxygenation. Maintaining venous return and cardiac output is crucial for recovery from shock, and vasopressor administration should be based on the patient's hemodynamic status. Considering the multiple causes of posttraumatic shock, a physiology-guided strategy to maintain a balance between circulatory volume and vascular tone seems prudent.[17,18]

Assessment of blood consumption score

The need for MTP can be assessed during the primary survey with the use of the assessment of blood consumption (ABC) score.[19] The ABC is a well-validated score that minimizes delays in MTP initiation and focuses on 4 immediately available variables: penetrating mechanism, positive FAST, arrival systolic blood pressure (SBP) of 90 mm Hg or lesser, and arrival heart rate of 120 or greater. The ABC score is recommended by the American College of Surgeons Trauma Quality Improvement Program Massive Transfusion in Trauma Guidelines as a required trigger for MTP activation.[19]

Baseline laboratories

Laboratory tests that may be useful include Hgb or complete blood count, ABG, central venous oxygen saturation, lactate, glucose, serum electrolytes, creatine phosphokinase, coagulation profile including prothrombin time/activated partial thromboplastin time (PTT), fibrinogen, urine examination for blood, beta human chorionic gonadotropin to rule out pregnancy, viscoelastic hemostatic assays, and toxicology screening.[20,21]

Massive Transfusion Protocol

Patients with severe injuries may develop refractory hemorrhage due to dilution of clotting factors, hypothermia, and acidosis. Citrate in blood products may also lead to hypocalcemia-induced coagulopathy. This subset of patients will require aggressive early hemostatic resuscitation and MTP. The latter includes administration of pRBC, FFP, and platelets in a balanced ratio.[22]

Indications and initiation/timing

"Massive transfusion" refers to transfusion of greater than 10 units of pRBC within the first 24 hours of admission.[2,23] "Ultramassive transfusion" has been defined as the administration of 20 U or greater of pRBC in 24 hours.[24] Identification of patients who may benefit from MTP can be challenging and several scores have been developed to assist in decision-making. Currently, the American College of Surgeons Trauma Quality Improvement Program Massive Transfusion in Trauma Guidelines recommend that triggers for the activation of MTP should include an ABC score of 2 or greater, blood transfusion in the trauma bay, persistent hemodynamic instability, or active bleeding requiring intervention.[25] Because both Hgb and BP take time to decrease after the onset of bleeding, initiation of an MTP will be ultimately based on clinical judgment, especially in patients with worsening hypotension and/or vasopressor requirement. Appropriate ratios and types of blood products are described in "Determination of Coagulopathy" section.

Tenets of damage control resuscitation

Damage control resuscitation (DCR) aims for early hemorrhage control, minimizing operative time, and delaying definitive repair until the patient's physiologic status has normalized. The principles of DCR include rapid recognition of trauma-induced coagulopathy (TIC) and shock; permissive hypotension; rapid surgical control of bleeding; prevention and treatment of hypothermia, acidosis, and hypocalcemia; avoidance of hemodilution by minimizing use of crystalloids; and transfusion of pRBC, FFP, and platelets with early use of coagulation factor concentrates.[23] Transfusion strategies are discussed in "Determination of coagulopathy" section.

Rapid anatomic control
Competence in massive hemorrhage control is an essential skill for all staff involved in providing trauma care. Massive hemorrhage may be compressible or noncompressible. DCR includes 3 distinct phases: (1) a surgery limited to control of the lesions and control hemostasis, (2) temporary closure to limit the risk of abdominal compartment syndrome, and (3) preprogrammed reoperation within 24 to 48 hours. Damage control surgery should be applied only to the most seriously traumatized patients along with ongoing resuscitation. When correctly applied, damage control surgery can significantly improve patient survival rates.

Permissive hypotension and minimization of crystalloids
Permissive hypotension is the restriction of crystalloids and vasopressors to maintain a lower blood pressure (SBP 80–90 mm Hg) until bleeding is controlled to prevent dislodgement of clots by high pressure of circulating volume and improve outcomes. Nevertheless, permissive hypotension may worsen outcomes due to tissue hypoperfusion and is a temporary measure that must be used until bleeding is controlled. In patients with severe traumatic brain injury (TBI), a mean arterial pressure greater than 80 mm Hg is recommended to maintain cerebral perfusion pressure.[17]

An increasing amount of evidence suggests that excessive administration of crystalloids increases the risk of dilutional coagulopathy, acute lung injury/acute respiratory distress syndrome, hypothermia, infections, intra-abdominal hypertension/abdominal compartment syndrome, multiple organ failure, and death.[26,27] Indeed, the latest ATLS guidelines include less stringent suggestions for crystalloid administration, recommending fluid resuscitation with up to 1 L of warm saline in patients with class I or II hemorrhage, whereas early resuscitation with blood/blood products only is advised in patients with evidence of class II or greater hemorrhage.[2] This is further supported by an analysis of 10-year trends in crystalloid resuscitation reporting that the decrease in high-volume crystalloid resuscitation parallels reduced mortality.[28]

Reversal of Anticoagulants

Prothrombin complex concentrates (PCCs), primarily 4-factor-PCCs, are recommended for reversal of vitamin K antagonist (VKA), whereas several guidelines support the use of FFP for VKA reversal in life-threatening hemorrhage only if PCCs are unavailable.[17] Of note, most guidelines also recommend coadministration of vitamin K. Due to their thrombogenic profile, activated PCCs and recombinant activated coagulation factor VII (rFVIIa) are not indicated for VKA reversal, even in emergency bleeding situations.[29,30]

In patients under direct-acting oral anticoagulants (DOACs), most guidelines consider the administration (off-label) of a PCC or 3-/4F-PCC administration in cases of serious or life-threatening bleeding when specific reversal agents are not available.[31] Although some guidelines recommend the administration of rFVIIa for DOAC reversal, the associated risk of thrombosis limits its use in patients when other hemostatic measures have been ineffective.[32] The use of FFP is not recommended for reversal because the volume of FFP required for the inhibition of thrombin or Factor Xa would result in significant delays and can cause adverse effects, such as fluid overload.[33] Furthermore, most guidelines recommend the use of idarucizumab and andexanet alfa in patients with severe or life-threatening bleeding events, or before emergency surgery.[34,35] However, andexanet alfa is not indicated for edoxaban reversal, and PCC is still recommended for this purpose.[36,37]

Acute Traumatic Coagulopathy

The recognition of acute traumatic coagulopathy (ATC) is extremely important for early diagnosis and management. In many patients, coagulopathy is present even before the onset of resuscitation and correlates with severity of trauma. Despite the lack of a universally accepted definition, ATC is indicated by prolongation of the prothrombin time. Several mechanisms have been proposed to explain the development of TIC. Hyperfibrinolysis and coagulopathy seen in ATC are mainly due to the effects of shock and direct injury on the endothelium.[38] Endothelial thrombomodulin and tissue plasminogen activator are upregulated in response to tissue hypoperfusion, which together with thrombin, generated by tissue trauma, accelerate protein C activation and hyperfibrinolysis.[39,40] These, together with glycocalyx degradation and platelet and fibrinogen dysfunction eventually result in massive hemorrhage and increased mortality.[40–43]

CHOICE OF BLOOD PRODUCT
Whole Blood Resuscitation

History
Fresh whole blood transfusion was first widely adopted by the military during World War I. It remained the mainstay of treatment during the war until blood banks developed an improved fractionation process in the 1970s.[44] With the advancement of blood bank capabilities, there was a shift to component therapy as the preferred method of transfusion based on components' longer shelf life.[45] This change in transfusion strategy occurred without evidence to compare the efficacy and risks of whole blood compared with component therapy in active hemorrhage and trauma patients.[46] Apart from war, component therapy also took hold in the civilian population, with specialties now able to give specific components to correct patient pathologic condition. The Red Cross began streamlining component production and storage, thus focusing more on functional blood components, which accelerated the abandonment of whole blood in the civilian population.[47] During the US wars in Iraq and Afghanistan, whole blood again made a resurgence as a treatment on the battlefield and prehospital resuscitation. With exhausted supplies of components, the military turned to "walking blood banks" and whole blood to help treat massive trauma during wartime. Reviews of more than 8000 units of whole blood administered during that period demonstrated equivalent, if not improved, outcomes in the treatment of massive hemorrhage.[47] With increasing evidence demonstrating that balanced resuscitation (1:1:1) via component therapy is associated with better patient outcomes in the trauma population, there is a renewed interest in using whole blood alone for hemorrhagic resuscitation.[45,48]

Whole blood storage
Whole blood has taken many shapes and is delivered successfully, both warm and cold. The American Association of Blood Banks endorses the use of low titer Type O Whole Blood as a universal donor. However, a variety of whole blood is studied, from fresh warm blood used in military settings to cold-stored blood O$^-$ or O$^+$ of various titers used in civilian data.[44,45] Whole blood is collected in citrate-phosphate-dextrose-adenine solution and stored between 1°C and 6°C for 14 to 21 days.[45] A single unit of whole blood contains 500 cc and has a Hct of 38% to 50%, platelet count of 100,000 to 400,000, 100% coagulation factors, and 1000 mg of fibrinogen.[45] The use of whole blood reduces the volume of additives needed

and reduces the overall volume transfused. Type O whole blood has universal red cell compatibility but does not protect against donor plasma anti-A or anti-B antibodies.[47] Therefore, varying degrees of whole blood with low anti-A and anti-B IgM titers have been used with many institutions defining *low titer* as less than 1:256. Subsequent studies on whole blood with different titer levels did not show any significant transfusion-related reactions or increased levels of hemolysis at 24 hours.[45,47] Strandenes and colleagues used rotational thromboelastometry (ROTEM) to demonstrate that cold storage of whole blood had preserved platelet-dependent coagulation function at 2 weeks and fibrinogen-dependent coagulation function at 3.5 weeks.[49] Most centers reserve group O Rhesus (Rh)-negative whole blood for women of childbearing age and use group O Rh-positive with low titers for all men and women aged older than 50 years.[47] Given concerns for donor plasma ABO incompatibility and Rh alloimmunization, most centers restrict whole blood transfusions to 2 to 4 units, with more recent data indicating safety up to 6 units.[47]

Whole blood advantages
Intraoperatively, whole blood offers several advantages during massive resuscitation. It provides all components through a warmed rapid transfuser using the same intravenous access and improves the speed of delivery by immediate arrival to the OR without a need for product thawing. Whole blood presents a simplified product that allows clinicians to give a single unit rather than focus on balancing pRBC, FFP, and platelets while checking each unit against the patient blood type.[44] This simplification and handling of fewer blood products should lead to a reduction in administrative error.

Whole blood limitations
Despite its benefits, several limitations limit the widespread use and acceptance of whole blood in civilian hospitals. The initiation of a whole blood program to an existing blood bank can be very expensive and, on average, adds an additional US$170,000 in annual costs.[45] Although the military has streamlined the process, many civilian facilities face logistical constraints regarding shipping, handling, and storing conditions.[45] Most centers only validate the use of whole blood for 14 days, and very few centers have adopted measures to centrifuge the unit on day 15 to salvage its components.[45] Although all blood banks were affected by the coronavirus disease-2019 pandemic, it was more challenging to find suitable donors of whole blood given the combination of extensive donation limitations and the need for the ideal candidate for O$^-$ whole blood making up less than 5% of the general population.[47] However, with research to further assess the risk of hemolytic transfusion reactions and alloimmunization to the Rh antibody, the pool of available donors may drastically increase.

Component Therapy Resuscitation

Packed red blood cells definition and storage
In contrast to whole blood therapy, component therapy allows blood to be divided into separate components via differential centrifugation and, subsequently, transfused individually. The 3 primary components are pRBC, FFP, and platelets.

pRBC are the most used blood component in the United States. One unit is typically 350 cc in volume and comprised of red blood cells (250 cc), plasma (<50 cc), white blood cells, and CPDA-1 anticoagulant.[50] One unit of pRBC is stored at 1° to 6° C and maintains a Hct of 60% to 80%.[51] Many centers in the United States leukoreduce each unit of pRBC to deplete the leukocyte content to less than 5×10^6 per unit to reduce the risk of alloimmunization and transfusion reactions.[52] One unit of pRBC will raise the Hct by 3% and the Hgb by 1 g/dL but must be compatible with the patients' plasma ABO antibodies.[50]

Fresh frozen plasma definition and storage

Used initially as a volume expander, FFP is a mainstay for hemorrhage management and preventing coagulation abnormalities. FFP is derived from a single unit of whole blood into a citrate-containing anticoagulant solution and frozen within 8 hours. FFP is stored at temperatures between $-18°C$ and $-30°C$ and remains viable for up to 1 year. FFP must be ABO compatible, with AB being the universal donor because it lacks both anti-A and anti-B antibodies. Each unit is approximately 250 cc and contains all the necessary clotting factors, including up to 700 mg of fibrinogen per unit.[53] FFP must be used within 4 hours once thawed or factors V and VIII begin to decline.[53] Providers give FFP in a balanced resuscitation for bleeding or a surgical setting with an international normalized ratio (INR) greater than 1.6 or PTT greater than 55. The initial dosing recommendations are 10 to 15 cc/kg.[53]

Platelet definition and storage

Platelet concentrates are prepared from a unit of whole blood or via apheresis. Once collected, platelets require storage at approximately 22°C, which facilitates the possible growth of bacterial contaminants. The volume of one apheresed unit of platelets is approximately 200 to 400 cc, whereas 4 to 6 units of platelets from whole blood are pooled to equal the same amount.[50] Platelets must be used within 5 days, which frequently causes system-wide shortages. Dosing is 10 to 15 cc per kg, raising the platelet count by 30,000 to 50,000. Platelets must be ABO and Rh compatible with the recipient.

Cryoprecipitate definition and storage

Cryoprecipitate, formulated to treat hemophilia A in the 1950s, is now used to replenish fibrinogen in coagulopathic patients, particularly in the trauma and obstetric setting.[54] Prepared from FFP, cryoprecipitate contains high concentrations of factor VIII, factor XIII, and fibrinogen.[54] Cryoprecipitate is prepared from a small pool of donors rather than administered as single units as each unit is approximately 10 to 15 cc.[54] Ten pooled units should replenish the fibrinogen level by 65 to 70 mg/dL. Although hospital-specific, cryoprecipitate is typically indicated with a fibrinogen level less than 150 mg/dL in the setting of acute bleeding or surgery.

Antifibrinolysis therapy

Aminocaproic acid and TXA target the fibrinolysis pathway, reducing the bleeding during trauma. There is an acute imbalance between the coagulation cascade and fibrinolytic pathway in trauma patients, often leading to an overall hyperfibrinolytic state.[55] Aminocaproic acid and TXA act to block plasminogen's lysine binding site irreversibly. Plasminogen is then unable to be activated to plasmin, thus stopping fibrinolysis.[55] Data has not indicated a detrimental prothrombic effect in the trauma population. TXA in the trauma population was studied explicitly in the CRASH-2 study and demonstrated significantly reduced bleeding rates with no increase in thromboembolic events.[55] Today, many institutions administer TXA in the trauma population within 3 hours of injury and encourage continued monitoring of the fibrinolysis pathway via TEG.

Balanced transfusion therapy

In trying to maintain a balanced resuscitation via component therapy, many questions have arisen as to the appropriate balance of components during the management of massive trauma. The Pragmatic, Randomized, Optimal Platelet and Plasma Ratios

(PROPPR) trial offers the best evidence of massive transfusion component ratio. They compared the ratios of 1:1:1 and 2:1:1 in pRBC:FFP:platelets. Although unable to find a statistically significant difference in mortality at 24 hours and 30 days, Holcomb and colleagues did demonstrate that the 1:1:1 ratio achieved faster hemostasis and fewer deaths due to exsanguination at 24 hours.[22]

Other individual component strategies

In Europe, there has been a push for individual administration of clotting factors to assist in massive hemorrhage. Although beneficial in specific coagulation disorders, there may be limited use in the trauma population because many patients in the initial hemorrhage have a global coagulopathy that is not factor specific. PCC may be the exception because it can provide a mixture of vitamin K-dependent coagulation factors (factors II, VII, IX, and X).[53] Derived from FFP, the concentrated nature of PCC results in 25 times higher clotting potential than plasma alone. Although there is good rationale for the addition of PCC to trauma resuscitation, more data are required for its inclusion in component therapy in addition to FFP.

Early Identification of Blood Type

Early identification of blood type is essential to hemostatic resuscitation but significant delays may occur in administrating recommended treatment. Initiating DCR as early as possible after severe trauma is pivotal for survival but identification of trauma patients who need MTP is a real challenge.[56] Health-care systems must notify the blood bank early to avoid delays in delivery of blood products. However, in a patient without unexpected antibodies, crossmatched erythrocytes can be available in about an hour after the blood bank receives the sample, which can be lengthier in patients with a positive antibody screen.[57] In patients with severe shock, the risk of administering noncrossmatched erythrocytes is low and outweighs the risks of waiting for crossmatched pRBC, and thus, transfusion of the former can be lifesaving.[58]

Transfusion End Points

Targets of resuscitation must be individualized in the setting of MTP. In general, end points include MAP 60 to 65 mm Hg (or higher in TBI), Hgb 7 to 9 g/dL, INR less than 1.5; fibrinogen greater than 1.5 to 2 g/L, PLTs greater than 50 K/μL, pH 7.35 to 7.45, and core temperature greater than 35°C.[1,17]

Component Therapy Disadvantages

The delivery of blood components inherently comes with the risks of hemolytic reactions, transfusion-related lung injury, bacterial contamination, virus transmission, and blood group mismatch.[59] Although extensive measures are in place to minimize these risks, there are more common intraoperative sequelae that require close monitoring during a massive transfusion. Such abnormalities include citrate toxicity, hypothermia, acid–base balance, and potassium derangements.[59] Citrate comprises all forms of anticoagulant preparations for blood component storage. Citrate's primary purpose is to prolong viability for each unit but when transfused will bind calcium in vivo leading to hypocalcemia.[59] Although physiologically unavoidable, close attention must be paid to calcium depletion during massive transfusion, particularly when transfusing more than one unit every 5 minutes. Citrate undergoes hepatic metabolism, and thus in hepatic failure or dysfunction, close attention should be paid to calcium levels. With massive transfusion, all efforts to warm blood products and fluids should be made before administration. Hypothermia from massive transfusion can lead to worsening acidosis and leave the patient susceptible to malignant arrhythmias.[59] Stored blood products are acidotic before administration due to citrate and accumulation of metabolites.[51] During massive resuscitation, a well-perfused liver will appropriately metabolize both citrate and lactate to bicarbonate, leading to a compensatory metabolic alkalosis. Furthermore, close monitoring of a patient's potassium levels is critical during transfusion as extracellular potassium will accumulate in stored blood products. The rate of product transfusion is positively correlated with the risk of hyperkalemia, so close monitoring is key during massive transfusion.

As with whole blood therapy, component therapy has several restrictions and limitations, many of which are institution-dependent. As described, each component has a slightly different storage modality, which leads to the need for more storage space and different protocols. With each unit separately transfused, there is a logistical burden placed on in-room providers to check each unit with the patient's blood type and appropriately verify the unit. pRBC and FFP are administered through a rapid infuser that likely will have a warming mechanism but the AABB recommends against the infusion of platelets and cryoprecipitate through a warmer.[59] Thus, at least 2 access points will need to be available for blood product delivery. Moreover, there can be a delay for the proper thawing of FFP and cryoprecipitate to be readily available for transfusion, which may prolong administration time.

Institutional Variation

Significant differences in mortality have been demonstrated between Level I trauma centers, which may be accounted for by transfusion practices.[60] Significant variability in the reporting of quality indicators has also been demonstrated, reflecting the lack of international consensus and benchmarks. In order to understand trends in MTPs and institutional variation, a standard and universally accepted definition of massive transfusion is imperative.[61]

DETERMINATION OF COAGULOPATHY
Point of Care Viscoelastic Tests of Coagulation

Viscoelastic test introduction
Because our understanding of TIC has improved, the need for a targeted, precise approach to trauma resuscitation has become more apparent.[62] Viscoelastic coagulation tests, such as TEG and ROTEM, provide real-time feedback to guide transfusion during massive trauma. These point of care tests offer a visual representation of coagulation through 3 distinct phases of the clot life-cycle: propagation, stabilization, and dissolution.[63] Given the challenging logistics of using conventional coagulation assays (CCAs) in a suitable timeframe, TEG and ROTEM not only provide a rapid alternative assessment of coagulation but also improve survival when compared with CCAs in severely injured patients receiving massive transfusion.[64] Both TEG and ROTEM have been increasingly incorporated into algorithms to diagnose and treat bleeding in a variety of clinical applications, including massive trauma.[63]

Viscoelastic test introduction
Assessment of clot formation/dissolution kinetics and strength for both ROTEM and TEG are measured via rotational force. Specifically, a continuously applied rotational force is transmitted to an electromechanical transduction system, which produces a real-time display of clot dynamics.[63] A similar cylindrical cup containing 340 μL of whole blood is used for each system. For TEG, the cylindrical cup rotates 4° 45′ every 5 seconds through a pin on a torsion wire. Because viscoelastic clot strength increases, more rotation is transmitted to the torsion wire and detected by the electromagnetic transducer. For ROTEM, the cylindrical cup remains fixed while a ball-

bearing suspended pin rotates 4° 75′ every 6 seconds through the application of a constant force. Because viscoelastic clot strength increases, pin rotation is impeded. The impedance is detected via a charge-coupled device image sensor system. The operating characteristics of TEG and ROTEM are summarized in **Table 2**. Notably, a TEG device is capable of analyzing 2 samples simultaneously, whereas a ROTEM device can analyze 4 samples at once. Both devices are sensitive to vibration and must be maintained on a stable surface.

Viscoelastic test process

Information regarding clot formation kinetics, strength, and dissolution are very similar between ROTEM and TEG. However, the 2 tests use different nomenclature to describe the same parameters (**Figs. 1** and **2**).[65] The time in minutes required for the tracing to reach an amplitude of 2 mm is defined as the clotting time (CT) for ROTEM and reaction rate (R) for TEG. Similarly, the time necessary for clot amplitude to increase from 2 to 20 mm is defined as clot formation time (CFT) for ROTEM and kinetics time (K) for TEG. Angle (α) is measured by creating a tangent line from the point of clot initiation (CT or R) to the slope of the developing curve. Peak amplitude of the clot, a surrogate for clot strength, is defined as the maximum clot firmness (MCF) for ROTEM and MA for TEG. TEG assesses clot lysis at 30 minutes (LY30) by measuring the percent reductions in the area under the curve that occurs 30 minutes after MA is achieved. However, ROTEM assesses clot lysis index at 30 minutes (LI30) by measuring the percent reduction in MCF when amplitude is measured 30 minutes after CT is detected.

Viscoelastic test transfusion guidelines

In massive trauma, ROTEM and TEG have become key elements of resuscitation algorithms to treat hemorrhage and mitigate TIC. Transfusion of red blood cells can therefore be augmented with targeted transfusion of additional component blood products by assessing the viscoelastic tracing produced in real-time by ROTEM and TEG.[64] Recently published algorithms are available to guide transfusion of individual components.[62] FFP should be considered when R is greater than 10 minutes (TEG) or InTEM CT is greater than 200 seconds (ROTEM). Fibrinogen (in the form of cryoprecipitate or fibrinogen concentrate) should be administered for an α-angle less than 55° or K > 3 minutes, or MA less than 20 mm (TEG); or an ExTEM α-angle less than 65°, ExTEM CFT greater than 140 seconds, or a FibTEM MCF less than 10 mm (ROTEM). Platelets should be transfused when MA less than 50 mm (TEG) or when ExTEM MCF less than 50 mm and FibTEM greater than 10 mm (ROTEM). In cases of

Table 2		
Rotational thromboelastometry and thromboelastography operating characteristics		
	ROTEM	**TEG**
Cup motion	Fixed	Rotates
Pin motion	Rotates	Fixed
Angle of rotation	4° 75′/6 s	4° 45′/5 s
Detection method	Rotation impedance	Pin transduction
Temperature regulation	Heated metal block	Heated cup
Temperature control	30°C–40°C	24°C–40°C
Cup interior	Ridged (0.6–0.9 mm)	Smooth

Summary of operational considerations for each analytical method.

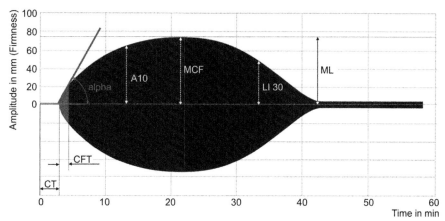

Fig. 1. Components of ROTEM. Representation of normal ROTEM evaluation of blood. Different analytical times, angles, and components are listed with abbreviations defined in the figure. Previously published materials that are unchanged from the source: "From Anderson L, Quasim I, Steven M, et al. Interoperator and intraoperator variability of whole blood coagulation assays: a comparison of thromboelastography and rotational thromboelastometry. J Cardiothorac Vasc Anesth. Dec 2014;28(6):1550-7. https://doi.org/10.1053/j.jvca.2014.05.023; with permission". A10, amplitude 1 minute after CT; alpha, alpha-angle; CT, clotting time; CFT, clot formation time; LI30, lysis index 30 minutes after CT; MCF, maximum clot firmness; ML, maximum lysis.

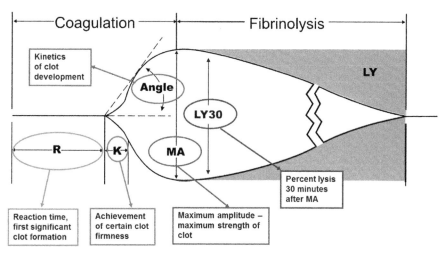

Fig. 2. Components of thromboelastography (TEG). Representation of normal TEG evaluation of blood. Different analytical times, angles, and components are listed with abbreviations defined in the figure. Previously published materials that are unchanged from the source: "From Anderson L, Quasim I, Steven M, et al. Interoperator and intraoperator variability of whole blood coagulation assays: a comparison of thromboelastography and rotational thromboelastometry. J Cardiothorac Vasc Anesth. Dec 2014;28(6):1550-7. https://doi.org/10.1053/j.jvca.2014.05.023; with permission".

hyperfibrinolysis (LY30 > 8% for TEG and ExTEM LI30 < 94% for ROTEM), TXA should be considered based on results from the landmark CRASH-2 trial.[66]

Viscoelastic tests in clinical practice

Although we encourage the use of ROTEM and TEG in clinical practice, we acknowledge they are not perfect assays. When compared head-to-head against CCAs such as PTT and INR in trauma patients, viscoelastic assessments of coagulation are sometimes inaccurate.[67] Clinicians using ROTEM or TEG—versus CCAs—may transfuse blood products excessively or when no longer indicated, increasing the risk of adverse reactions.[68] However, these pitfalls are largely outweighed by the advantages for viscoelastic assays. ROTEM and TEG-guided massive transfusion improves survival compared with CCA-guided resuscitation.[64] Therefore, the precise accuracy of viscoelastic tests may be immaterial to the bleeding patient. In fact, patients who received TEG-guided resuscitation received fewer plasma and platelet transfusions in the early phase of resuscitation.[64] TEG and ROTEM are point-of care tests that are usually available for clinical interpretation much earlier than CCAs. Ease of use, rapidity of results, speed of interpretation, and improved survival are all advantages for viscoelastic assessments compared with CCAs. We therefore strongly encourage either TEG or ROTEM guided resuscitation be used during massive transfusion in trauma patients.

WHOLE BLOOD OR COMPONENT PRODUCTS—WHICH TO CHOOSE?

Currently, heterogeneity reigns supreme regarding the transfusion of whole blood. A recent meta-analysis identified significant variations in both the storage of whole blood and the definition of what constitutes whole blood transfusion.[44] Some military settings use fresh warm blood, whereas civilian settings tend to use cold-stored O$^+$ or O$^-$ blood. Some whole blood units are leukoreduced; others are not. For research purposes, whole blood transfusion has been defined as patients exclusively receiving whole blood or those who received mixtures of whole blood with other components. Ultimately, no significant difference in 24 hour or in-hospital mortality was reported in the meta-analysis.[44]

SUMMARY

In conclusion, we have provided a comprehensive examination of trauma, hemorrhage, patient evaluation modalities, resuscitation strategies, and specific considerations for products and tests available for appropriate patient resuscitation. Initial evaluation should be focused on the best use of resources for to best care for the patient. Thereafter, any surgical intervention should be dedicated to control of bleeding and resuscitation should support end-organ function with the prevention and/or treatment of acute blood loss anemia and coagulopathy. As to appropriate blood product resuscitation, it is clear that the use of whole blood is returning in the military and some larger civilian medical centers. Although whole blood removes some problems with subsequent coagulopathy, it is a resource-intensive process that is not achievable for every institution. Component therapy is a viable option for the patient who produces good clinical outcomes with appropriate transfusion ratios and use of viscoelastic techniques to guide therapy. Finally, questions remain that call for more research, including, but not limited to: short-term and long-term outcomes associated with whole blood versus component therapy and health-care utilization associated with both strategies.

CLINICS CARE POINTS

- Prompt initiation of resuscitation and addressing surgical bleeding remain the pillars of trauma resuscitation
- Point-of-care viscoelastic coagulation testing should be regularly used to guide resuscitation during massive transfusion
- Both whole blood and component therapy may be used during trauma resuscitation, pending robust clinical trials
- Point-of-Care Ultrasound (POCUS) is a valuable tool for guiding volume responsiveness

AUTHOR CONTRIBUTIONS

All authors made significant contributions to the conception and design of the study, drafting of the article, critical revision of the article for intellectual content, and approve the final article for publication.

DISCLOSURE

None of the authors has any conflicts to disclose. Funding for this article was provided by R01GM127584 to B.M. Wagener.

REFERENCES

1. James D, Pennardt AM. Trauma care principles. Treasure Island, FL: StatPearls; 2022.
2. Galvagno SM Jr, Nahmias JT, Young DA. Advanced Trauma Life Support((R)) update 2019: management and applications for adults and special populations. Anesthesiol Clin 2019;37(1):13–32.
3. Detsky ME, Jivraj N, Adhikari NK, et al. Will this patient be difficult to intubate?: The rational clinical examination systematic review. JAMA 2019;321(5):493–503.
4. Apfelbaum JL, Hagberg CA, Connis RT, et al. 2022 American Society of Anesthesiologists practice guidelines for management of the difficult airway. Anesthesiology 2022;136(1):31–81.
5. Russotto V, Myatra SN, Laffey JG, et al. Intubation practices and adverse peri-intubation events in critically ill patients from 29 countries. JAMA 2021;325(12):1164–72.
6. Karamchandani K, Wheelwright J, Yang AL, et al. Emergency airway management outside the operating room: current evidence and management strategies. Anesth Analg 2021;133(3):648–62.
7. Kornas RL, Owyang CG, Sakles JC, et al, Society for Airway Management's Special Projects C. Evaluation and management of the physiologically difficult airway: consensus recommendations from society for airway management. Anesth Analg 2021;132(2):395–405.
8. American Institute of Ultrasound in M, American College of Emergency P. AIUM practice guideline for the performance of the focused assessment with sonography for trauma (FAST) examination. J Ultrasound Med 2014;33(11):2047–56.
9. Grunherz L, Jensen KO, Neuhaus V, et al. Early computed tomography or focused assessment with sonography in abdominal trauma: what are the leading opinions? Eur J Trauma Emerg Surg 2018;44(1):3–8.

10. Tsui CL, Fung HT, Chung KL, et al. Focused abdominal sonography for trauma in the emergency department for blunt abdominal trauma. Int J Emerg Med 2008; 1(3):183–7.

11. Sato M, Yoshii H. Reevaluation of ultrasonography for solid-organ injury in blunt abdominal trauma. J Ultrasound Med 2004;23(12):1583–96.

12. Wirth S, Hebebrand J, Basilico R, et al. European Society of Emergency Radiology: guideline on radiological polytrauma imaging and service (short version). Insights Imaging 2020;11(1):135.

13. Stengel D, Mutze S, Guthoff C, et al. Association of low-dose whole-body computed tomography with missed injury diagnoses and radiation exposure in patients with blunt multiple trauma. JAMA Surg 2020;155(3):224–32.

14. Yoong S, Kothari R, Brooks A. Assessment of sensitivity of whole body CT for major trauma. Eur J Trauma Emerg Surg 2019;45(3):489–92.

15. Stein DM, Jessie EM, Crane S, et al. Hyperacute adrenal insufficiency after hemorrhagic shock exists and is associated with poor outcomes. J Trauma Acute Care Surg 2013;74(2):363–70 [discussion: 370].

16. Rushworth RL, Torpy DJ, Falhammar H. Adrenal crisis. N Engl J Med 2019;381(9): 852–61.

17. Spahn DR, Bouillon B, Cerny V, et al. The European guideline on management of major bleeding and coagulopathy following trauma: fifth edition. Crit Care 2019; 23(1):98.

18. Gelman S, Bigatello L. The physiologic basis for goal-directed hemodynamic and fluid therapy: the pivotal role of the venous circulation. Can J Anaesth 2018;65(3): 294–308. https://doi.org/10.1007/s12630-017-1045-3. Les fondements physiologiques de la therapie hemodynamique et liquidienne ciblee: le role fondamental de la circulation veineuse.

19. Nunez TC, Voskresensky IV, Dossett LA, et al. Early prediction of massive transfusion in trauma: simple as ABC (assessment of blood consumption)? J Trauma 2009;66(2):346–52.

20. Bhandarkar P, Pal R, Munivenkatappa A, et al. Distribution of laboratory parameters in trauma population. J Emerg Trauma Shock 2018;11(1):10–4.

21. Volod O, Bunch CM, Zackariya N, et al. Viscoelastic hemostatic assays: a primer on legacy and new generation devices. J Clin Med 2022;(3):11. https://doi.org/ 10.3390/jcm11030860.

22. Holcomb JB, Tilley BC, Baraniuk S, et al. Transfusion of plasma, platelets, and red blood cells in a 1:1:1 vs a 1:1:2 ratio and mortality in patients with severe trauma: the PROPPR randomized clinical trial. JAMA 2015;313(5):471–82.

23. Camazine MN, Hemmila MR, Leonard JC, et al. Massive transfusion policies at trauma centers participating in the American College of Surgeons Trauma Quality Improvement Program. J Trauma Acute Care Surg 2015;78(6 Suppl 1):S48–53.

24. Matthay ZA, Hellmann ZJ, Callcut RA, et al. Outcomes after ultramassive transfusion in the modern era: an Eastern Association for the Surgery of Trauma multicenter study. J Trauma Acute Care Surg 2021;91(1):24–33.

25. Cotton BA, Dossett LA, Haut ER, et al. Multicenter validation of a simplified score to predict massive transfusion in trauma. J Trauma 2010;69(Suppl 1):S33–9.

26. O'Mara MS, Slater H, Goldfarb IW, et al. A prospective, randomized evaluation of intra-abdominal pressures with crystalloid and colloid resuscitation in burn patients. J Trauma 2005;58(5):1011–8.

27. Duchesne JC, Kaplan LJ, Balogh ZJ, et al. Role of permissive hypotension, hypertonic resuscitation and the global increased permeability syndrome in patients with severe hemorrhage: adjuncts to damage control resuscitation to

prevent intra-abdominal hypertension. Anaesthesiol Intensive Ther 2015;47(2): 143–55.

28. Harada MY, Ko A, Barmparas G, et al. 10-Year trend in crystalloid resuscitation: reduced volume and lower mortality. Int J Surg 2017;38:78–82.

29. Kozek-Langenecker SA, Ahmed AB, Afshari A, et al. Management of severe perioperative bleeding: guidelines from the European Society of Anaesthesiology: first update 2016. Eur J Anaesthesiol 2017;34(6):332–95.

30. Association of Anaesthetists of Great B, Ireland, Thomas D, et al. Blood transfusion and the anaesthetist: management of massive haemorrhage. Anaesthesia 2010;65(11):1153–61.

31. Milling TJ, Pollack CV. A review of guidelines on anticoagulation reversal across different clinical scenarios - Is there a general consensus? Am J Emerg Med 2020;38(9):1890–903.

32. Frontera JA, Lewin JJ 3rd, Rabinstein AA, et al. Guideline for reversal of antithrombotics in intracranial hemorrhage: a statement for healthcare professioNALS from the Neurocritical Care Society and Society of Critical Care Medicine. Neurocrit Care 2016;24(1):6–46.

33. Burnett AE, Mahan CE, Vazquez SR, et al. Guidance for the practical management of the direct oral anticoagulants (DOACs) in VTE treatment. J Thromb Thrombolysis 2016;41(1):206–32.

34. Pollack CV Jr, Reilly PA, van Ryn J, et al. Idarucizumab for dabigatran reversal - full cohort analysis. N Engl J Med 2017;377(5):431–41.

35. Frontera JA, Bhatt P, Lalchan R, et al. Cost comparison of andexanet versus prothrombin complex concentrates for direct factor Xa inhibitor reversal after hemorrhage. J Thromb Thrombolysis 2020;49(1):121–31.

36. Cuker A, Burnett A, Triller D, et al. Reversal of direct oral anticoagulants: guidance from the anticoagulation forum. Am J Hematol 2019;94(6):697–709.

37. Raval AN, Cigarroa JE, Chung MK, et al. Management of patients on non-vitamin K antagonist oral anticoagulants in the acute care and periprocedural setting: a scientific statement from the American Heart Association. Circulation 2017; 135(10):e604–33.

38. Brohi K, Cohen MJ, Ganter MT, et al. Acute coagulopathy of trauma: hypoperfusion induces systemic anticoagulation and hyperfibrinolysis. J Trauma 2008; 64(5):1211–7 [discussion: 1217].

39. Cap A, Hunt BJ. The pathogenesis of traumatic coagulopathy. Anaesthesia 2015; 70(Suppl 1):96–101, e32-e34.

40. Duque P, Mora L, Levy JH, et al. Pathophysiological response to trauma-induced coagulopathy: a comprehensive review. Anesth Analg 2020;130(3):654–64.

41. Meizoso JP, Karcutskie CA, Ray JJ, et al. Persistent fibrinolysis shutdown is associated with increased mortality in severely injured trauma patients. J Am Coll Surg 2017;224(4):575–82.

42. Hagemo JS, Christiaans SC, Stanworth SJ, et al. Detection of acute traumatic coagulopathy and massive transfusion requirements by means of rotational thromboelastometry: an international prospective validation study. Crit Care 2015;19:97.

43. Gall LS, Vulliamy P, Gillespie S, et al. The S100A10 pathway mediates an occult hyperfibrinolytic subtype in trauma patients. Ann Surg 2019;269(6):1184–91.

44. Crowe E, DeSantis SM, Bonnette A, et al. Whole blood transfusion versus component therapy in trauma resuscitation: a systematic review and meta-analysis. J Am Coll Emerg Physicians Open 2020;1(4):633–41.

45. Hanna M, Knittel J, Gillihan J. The use of whole blood transfusion in trauma. Curr Anesthesiol Rep 2022;1–6. https://doi.org/10.1007/s40140-021-00514-w.

46. Avery P, Morton S, Tucker H, et al. Whole blood transfusion versus component therapy in adult trauma patients with acute major haemorrhage. Emerg Med J 2020;37(6):370–8.

47. McCoy CC, Brenner M, Duchesne J, et al. Back to the future: whole blood resuscitation of the severely injured trauma patient. Shock 2021;56(1S):9–15.

48. Black JA, Pierce VS, Kerby JD, et al. The evolution of blood transfusion in the trauma patient: whole blood has come full circle. Semin Thromb Hemost 2020; 46(2):215–20.

49. Strandenes G, Austlid I, Apelseth TO, et al. Coagulation function of stored whole blood is preserved for 14 days in austere conditions: A ROTEM feasibility study during a Norwegian antipiracy mission and comparison to equal ratio reconstituted blood. J Trauma Acute Care Surg 2015;78(6 Suppl 1):S31–8.

50. Osterman JL, Arora S. Blood product transfusions and reactions. Hematol Oncol Clin North Am 2017;31(6):1159–70.

51. Yoshida T, Prudent M, D'Alessandro A. Red blood cell storage lesion: causes and potential clinical consequences. Blood Transfus 2019;17(1):27–52.

52. Fadeyi EA, Saha AK, Naal T, et al. A comparison between leukocyte reduced low titer whole blood vs non-leukocyte reduced low titer whole blood for massive transfusion activation. Transfusion 2020;60(12):2834–40.

53. Nordmann GR, Obal D. Is fresh frozen plasma still necessary for management of acute traumatic coagulopathy? Curr Anesthesiol Rep 2020;10:297–307.

54. Nascimento B, Goodnough LT, Levy JH. Cryoprecipitate therapy. Br J Anaesth 2014;113(6):922–34.

55. Ortmann E, Besser MW, Klein AA. Antifibrinolytic agents in current anaesthetic practice. Br J Anaesth 2013;111(4):549–63.

56. Spahn DR, Bouillon B, Cerny V, et al. Management of bleeding and coagulopathy following major trauma: an updated European guideline. Crit Care 2013; 17(2):R76.

57. Tormey CA, Fisk J, Stack G. Red blood cell alloantibody frequency, specificity, and properties in a population of male military veterans. Transfusion 2008; 48(10):2069–76.

58. Yazer MH, Waters JH, Spinella PC, Aabb/Trauma HORNWP. Use of uncross-matched erythrocytes in emergency bleeding situations. Anesthesiology 2018; 128(3):650–6.

59. Sihler KC, Napolitano LM. Complications of massive transfusion. Chest 2010; 137(1):209–20.

60. Wade CE, del Junco DJ, Holcomb JB, et al. Variations between level I trauma centers in 24-hour mortality in severely injured patients requiring a massive transfusion. J Trauma 2011;71(2 Suppl 3):S389–93.

61. McQuilten ZK, Flint AW, Green L, et al. Epidemiology of massive transfusion - a common intervention in need of a definition. Transfus Med Rev 2021;35(4):73–9.

62. Baksaas-Aasen K, Van Dieren S, Balvers K, et al. Data-driven development of ROTEM and TEG algorithms for the management of trauma hemorrhage: a prospective observational multicenter study. Ann Surg 2019;270(6):1178–85.

63. Whiting D, DiNardo JA. TEG and ROTEM: technology and clinical applications. Am J Hematol 2014;89(2):228–32.

64. Gonzalez E, Moore EE, Moore HB, et al. Goal-directed hemostatic resuscitation of trauma-induced coagulopathy: a pragmatic randomized clinical trial comparing a

viscoelastic assay to conventional coagulation assays. Ann Surg 2016;263(6): 1051–9.

65. Anderson L, Quasim I, Steven M, et al. Interoperator and intraoperator variability of whole blood coagulation assays: a comparison of thromboelastography and rotational thromboelastometry. J Cardiothorac Vasc Anesth 2014;28(6):1550–7.

66. CRASH-2 Trial Collaborators. Effects of tranexamic acid on death, vascular occlusive events, and blood transfusion in trauma patients with significant haemorrhage (CRASH-2): a randomised, placebo-controlled trial. Lancet 2010; 376(9734):23–32.

67. Hunt H, Stanworth S, Curry N, et al. Thromboelastography (TEG) and rotational thromboelastometry (ROTEM) for trauma-induced coagulopathy in adult trauma patients with bleeding. Cochrane Database Syst Rev 2015;2. https://doi.org/10. 1002/14651858.CD010438.pub2.

68. Fraga GP, Bansal V, Coimbra R. Transfusion of blood products in trauma: an update. J Emerg Med 2010;39(2):253–60.

Health and Well-Being of Intensive Care Unit Physicians

How to Ensure the Longevity of a Critical Specialty

John C. Klick, MD, FCCP, FCCM[a], Madiha Syed, MD[b],
Ron Leong, MD[d], Haley Miranda, MD[c], Elizabeth K. Cotter, MD[c],*

KEYWORDS

- Burnout • COVID-19 • Moral distress • Wellness • ICU staffing • Diversity
- Inclusion

KEY POINTS

- There is a high incidence of burnout among physician intensivists.
- The stresses of our specialty leave the intensivist particularly vulnerable to burnout syndrome.
- The COVID-19 pandemic has only exacerbated the incidence and severity of burnout among physician intensivists.
- The shortage of physician intensivist could potentially lead to even higher rates of burnout syndrome in the specialty.
- Institutions need to make a concerted effort to prevent and treat burnout in the specialty of critical care medicine.
- Institutions and individuals do have options to lessen the burden of burnout syndrome in critical care medicine.

The authors have nothing to disclose.
[a] Department of Anesthesiology, University of Vermont Medical Center, University of Vermont Larner College of Medicine, 111 Colchester Avenue, Burlington, VT 05401, USA; [b] Department of Intensive Care & Resuscitation, Anesthesiology Institute, Cleveland Clinic Foundation, 9500 Euclid Avenue, Mail Code G58, Cleveland, OH 44195, USA; [c] Department of Anesthesiology, Pain and Perioperative Medicine, University of Kansas Medical Center, 3901 Rainbow Boulevard, MS 1034, Kansas City, KS 66160, USA; [d] Thomas Jefferson University Hospital, Sidney Kimmel Medial College, 111 South 11th Street, Gibbon Building, Suite 8130, Philadelphia, PA 19107, USA
* Corresponding author.
E-mail address: Ecotter2@kumc.edu

Anesthesiology Clin 41 (2023) 303–316
https://doi.org/10.1016/j.anclin.2022.10.009
1932-2275/23/© 2022 Elsevier Inc. All rights reserved.
anesthesiology.theclinics.com

INTRODUCTION

A second epidemic coexists with the coronavirus disease 2019 (COVID-19) pandemic; it has been smoldering for many years, and the extreme pressures of COVID-19 have only fueled the flames. Physicians, and specifically those providing critical care services, are suffering from anxiety and burnout at an alarming rate.[1,2] This epidemic of burnout has now reached a crisis level; it has driven droves of physicians to scale back work hours or leave health care altogether.[3] Without acknowledging the health and well-being of the critical care physician, the survival of the specialty is at risk. This review provides a brief history of the burnout epidemic, examines the impact of the COVID-19 pandemic on intensivists, explores how burnout may disproportionally affect different groups of individuals, and discusses possible solutions to preserve the specialty of critical care.

Before the onset of COVID-19, there was a yearly net loss of critical care physicians that led to uncertainty surrounding the critical care workforce. Despite increasing fellowship spots and alternate pathways for entry into critical care, this gap was anticipated to widen.[4] Contributing factors included the aging population of the United States, an increasing burden of disease, a move toward 24/7 physician coverage of the intensive care unit (ICU), and expansion of intensivists outside of the ICU.[4] Another contributing factor to the yearly net loss of critical care physicians was the trainees' direct observation of a burnt out work force.[5] In 2016 there was a call to action from the Critical Care Societies Collaborative (an organization made up of representatives from the American College of Chest Physicians, American Thoracic Society, Society of Critical Medicine, and American Association of Critical Care Nurses) to address the issue of burn out among critical care providers.[6] Contemporaneous surveys indicated that more than half of critical care practitioners were experiencing burnout.[7] In a survey of anesthesia intensivists, nearly 10% of respondents felt burnt out "all the time" and 75% reported at least "sometimes" feeling burnt out.[8]

In the wake of that call to action, the academic community has responded with numerous publications discussing the effect of burnout on health care workers. To date, most research includes surveys and assessments to identify risk factors and consequences of burnout (**Table 1**).[7,9–13] Although these risk factors may ring true for many health care professionals, critical care providers appear to be affected at an increased rate due to the unique, high-acuity environment of the ICU where physicians are repeatedly exposed to high levels of stress, conflict, and moral distress.[13] Left unchecked, burnout is associated with high personal and organizational costs. In fact, in the United States the estimated cost associated with replacing health care workers due to departure or reduced hours is about $4.6 billion annually.[3]

Table 1	
Contributing factors and consequences of burnout in physicians	
Factors Contributing to Burnout in Physicians	**Consequences of Burnout in Physicians**
• Women	• Health and well-being of physician
• Younger age	• Decreased quality of health care
• Trainees	• Medical errors
• Midcareer faculty	• Reduced patient satisfaction
• Patient work loads	• Increased cost of care
• Long hours	• Reduced effectiveness at work
• Stressful work environment	• Less commitment to job/organization
• Unsatisfactory work environment	• High turnover and associated costs
• Conflicts with colleagues	• Difficult interpersonal relationships
• Administrative tasks	• Loss of mentorship for junior faculty

These concerns, which presented a clear and present danger to the specialty in 2016, were amplified and brought to the public eye during the COVID-19 pandemic. Since that time, anesthesiologists and other non–critical care physicians had to pivot and step into unfamiliar roles, often with high stakes.[5] Intensivists and anesthesiologists alike were asked to care for more patients with fewer resources, including critical resources that are designed to keep them safe such as personal protective equipment. ICU bed capacity was rapidly increased and extended into areas such as the postanesthesia recovery unit and operating rooms.[5] Although there initially seemed to be a collective resolve to tackle the virus, repeated onslaughts have pushed critical care providers beyond their limits. Since the initial wave of COVID-19, surveys indicate that burnout is even more pervasive now than prepandemic.[14]

The current culture of medicine will be one of the more difficult areas to generate reform of because it is so deeply ingrained. Arnold-Forster and colleagues[15] point out 3 aspects of the culture of medicine that will need to be addressed: medical exceptionalism, medicalization, and individual responsibility. Medical exceptionalism is the idea that to practice medicine one must be self-sacrificing; this leads to unhealthy behaviors and unsafe work practices and leaves physicians vulnerable to exploitation by the health care system to the system's benefit. Medicalization is the notion that physicians with mental health or substance abuse problems are not fit to practice; this has the untoward effect of disincentivizing current practicing physicians from seeking help for mental health conditions. Finally, individual responsibility places the responsibility on the physician to maintain their own wellness. Although physicians should have ownership of their own well-being, this concept, in effect, provides a dispensation to employers; it allows minimal change or implementation of low-cost programs that "support" the physicians to be considered permissible solutions.[15]

Burnout Syndrome: Prevalence, Risk Factors, and Diagnosis

A combination of increased expectations, relative lack of workplace support, and longer hours has led to an increase in work-related stress. Burnout syndrome (BOS) has become a worldwide phenomenon among members of high-stress professions, such as critical care physicians. The term "burnout syndrome" was first defined in the 1970s. BOS refers to a work-related constellation of symptoms and signs that usually occur in people with no prior history of psychological or psychiatric disorders.[16] BOS is triggered by a difference between the expectations and ideals of the employee and the actual requirements of the position. Symptoms generally develop gradually and build over time. Initially, physicians may feel emotional stress and disillusionment with the job; they later develop an inability to adapt to the work environment and demonstrate negative attitudes toward their job, their coworkers, and even their patients. The 3 classic symptoms are exhaustion, depersonalization, and reduced personal accomplishment. The result is a physician who questions the value or worth of his or her work and generalized poor professional self-esteem. Feelings of frustration, anger, fearfulness, and anxiety are quite common. The physician may express an inability to feel happiness or pleasure. Physical symptoms such insomnia, muscle tension, headaches, and gastrointestinal problems may develop.[17]

Prevalence

Collectively, physicians are 36% more likely to develop BOS when compared with other high-school graduates. Among physicians, those in acute care specialties such as intensivists, report the highest rates of BOS in medicine, as high as 50%[6]; this is not only stressful for the individual but also may adversely affect the physician's ability to properly care for patients. High patient morbidity and mortality, high prevalence of moral and ethical issues, and challenging work routines all add to the psychological stress. Chronic psychological stress may lead to feelings of being overwhelmed and can result in physical conditions such as insomnia, fatigue, irritability, anxiety, and depression. These feelings and symptoms can accelerate and intensify when it is perceived that there is insufficient time or unduly limited resources to properly care for patients.[17]

The shortage of critical care physicians, along with the increased demand for overnight ICU coverage, has raised the awareness of BOS and its recognitions among physicians. Up to 50% of critical care physicians have reported symptoms of severe BOS. The situation is even worse in pediatric critical care physicians, with up to 71% of physicians reporting symptoms of severe BOS, which is double the rate of general pediatricians. Among physicians in general, critical care physicians report the highest prevalence of BOS, with emergency medicine physicians a close second.[17]

Diagnosis

BOS is most commonly diagnosed via the Maslach Burnout Inventory (MBI). The MBI is a questionnaire that asks respondents to score themselves on a Likert scale the frequency that they experience certain feelings related to their work. The MBI score grades the presence and severity of a decreased sense of personal accomplishment, emotional exhaustion, and depersonalization. Those who score beyond a cutoff value on the MBI are diagnosed with BOS. Unfortunately, there are no established cutoff values for intensivists, making comparisons among different studies difficult.[17]

Other overlapping conditions with BOS include compassion fatigue, moral distress, and even a perceived delivery of inappropriate care. Moral distress occurs when the practitioner feels constrained from taking the ethical and appropriate action; this may be due to self-doubt, conflict avoidance, or perceived imbalances of power. Cost reduction, concern for legal ramifications, and poor communication strategies may also play into moral distress. Perceived examples of inappropriate care may occur in situations such as care of noncompliant patients, perceived futility of aggressive care, perceived inadequate quality of care, or observation of a patient's wishes being ignored. Compassion fatigue is the gradual reduction in compassion over time due to mounting frustrations with the individual practitioner's situation or environment. Inappropriate administration of care has been perceived in 25% of critical care nurses and up to 32% of ICU physicians.[17]

Risk factors

Certain personal attributes are known to be associated with BOS, including being self-critical, having poor coping strategies, sleep deprivation, and overall poor work-life balance. Idealism, perfectionism, and individual overcommitment are also known to contribute to BOS, along with having an inadequate social support system. Interestingly, younger physicians show nearly twice the prevalence of BOS when compared with older physicians. These symptoms may appear as early as residency training.[17]

Organizational factors associated with BOS include an increased workload, inadequate rewards, poor sense of community, and lack of control over the work environment. For critical care physicians, the number of night shifts per month and time since the last nonworking week has clearly been associated with the incidence of BOS.[17] Having to make repeated ethical decisions is also associated with a high rate of BOS. Poor working relationships and workplace conflict are other factors at play; this represents one potentially modifiable risk factor.[17]

End-of-life care is a risk factor for BOS, and higher individual ICU mortality rates have been associated with higher BOS rates. Caring for dying patients and involvement in decisions to forego life-sustaining treatments are clear stressors.[17]

Sleep disruption is an often-unavoidable consequence of shift work. Insufficient and interrupted sleep is much more common than among those working normal daytime schedules. Interestingly, working in a university hospital setting has also been associated with a higher incidence of BOS, possibly related to the typical higher acuity found in these settings.[17] **Fig. 1** summarizes the potential risk factors for burnout.

Consequences of burnout

A survey conducted by the European Society of Intensive Care Medicine (ESICM) in 2020 revealed an incidence of depression, anxiety, and severe burnout as high as 30% to 50% among intensivists.[18] In late 2021, the American Society of Anesthesiologists (ASA) Committee on Critical Care Medicine conducted its own survey in the United States. This survey incorporated members of the ASA, the Society of Critical Care Anesthesiologists, and the Anesthesiology Section of the Society of Critical Care Medicine. Of note, 65% of the respondents practiced in academic medical centers. Results showed that 42% of respondents met criteria for generalized anxiety disorder, whereas 32% of respondents demonstrated severe symptoms of anxiety. These symptoms were particularly common in females and younger respondents. Seventy-three percent of female, compared with 58% of male respondents, reported that working as an ICU physician during the COVID-19 pandemic had increased their feelings of burnout.

Frighteningly, 75% of respondents considered institutional wellness resources to be unhelpful. Sixty-four percent of respondents felt their participation in critical care

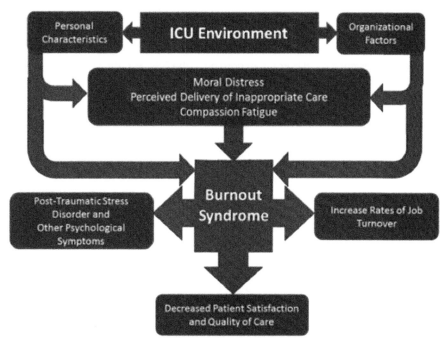

Fig. 1. Risk factors associated with burnout syndrome. Moss M, Good VS, Gozal D, Kleinpell R, Sessler CN. An Official Critical Care Societies Collaborative Statement: Burnout Syndrome in Critical Care Healthcare Professionals: A Call for Action. Crit Care Med. 2016;44(7):1414–1421.

clinical duties increased during the pandemic, whereas 28% of respondents felt their satisfaction with their professional life declined during the pandemic. Of note, this survey was conducted before the widespread availability of COVID-19 vaccination for medical providers.[1] Collectively, these data demonstrate a high incidence of generalized anxiety disorder and a high level of burnout among critical care anesthesiologists.[1]

The consequences of BOS among critical care practitioners can be catastrophic; it may result in posttraumatic stress disorder (PTSD), drug or alcohol abuse, and even suicidal thoughts. Physicians in general have been shown to have higher rates of alcohol abuse than the general population. PTSD may be the result of frequent exposure to traumatic events or the result of one catastrophically traumatic event. Participation in end-of-life issues, caring for combative patients and family members, postmortem care, caring for massive hemorrhage, and feelings of being overextended are all recognized triggers associated with PTSD.[17]

The impact of BOS on the workforce is detrimental, to say the least. The loss of practitioners results in increased health care costs, lower productivity, poor morale, an overall reduction in quality of patient care, and higher patient mortality rates. A recent study estimated the total cost of burnout among Canadian physicians to be more than $200 million. There is a strong linear relationship between burnout scores and medical errors as well.[17]

Impact of Coronavirus Disease 2019 on Intensive Care Unit Providers

The recent COVID-19 pandemic has put unprecedented stress on the world's critical care resources. Data from the ESICM show that the pandemic has had an overwhelming psychological impact on practicing intensivists. Between February and May 2020 alone, there were more than 350,000 deaths directly attributable to the severe acute respiratory syndrome coronavirus 2. The increased work hours and limited logistic support placed incredible stress on practicing intensivists. Scarcity of resources such as personal protective equipment, ICU beds, and ventilators only increased the psychological burden. According to the ESICM data, symptoms of anxiety during the pandemic exceeded 46.5%, depression was reported by 30.2% of intensivists, and severe burnout symptoms were reported by 51% of intensivists. Female gender, younger age, living in a city of more than 1 million inhabitants, and higher religiosity were all associated with higher reported rates of anxiety and severe burnout. Intensivists who reported symptoms of anxiety, depression, or severe burnout reported significantly higher rates of taking sleeping pills and smoking. Interestingly, the number of patients with COVID-19 managed did not seem to be associated with an increase in psychological distress.[18]

Improving Wellness in Critical Care

Since 2016, the pandemic has no doubt moved burnout into the mainstream as a central issue in health care, with most now acknowledging it as an issue pervasively affecting the medical community at large.[19] Efforts at burnout mitigation, however, have not significantly adapted to meet the needs of the critical care practitioner. For a specialty that demonstrated great adaptability during the pandemic in terms of shifting to meet the needs of the public, current efforts to address burnout mitigation seem inadequate. The classic "more research is needed" is often a common conclusion of health care research involving wellness committees and other efforts combating burnout. When burnout is an issue causing increasing rates of alcohol abuse, dysfunction in personal relationships, self-isolation, and depression, it should be clear that there is no time to waste.[20] Ignoring this progressive public health problem will not only be a stain on the moral compass of the health care system but also may ultimately result in its collapse.

The good news is that simple steps are easily accessible. Less than half of physicians report their workplaces offer a wellness program to reduce stress and/or burnout. More than 40% of physicians report they avoid seeking help for burnout or depression because of fears of risking disclosure to medical boards. When asked what would most help reduce burnout, a more manageable work schedule was the primary choice of all survey respondents, followed by increased compensation to avoid financial stress. In addition, greater respect from colleagues and the health care team, and improved autonomy were important solutions.[20]

In the setting of a worsening intensive care workforce shortage and rising burnout, an important question arises surrounding what the optimal patient load-to-intensivist ratio is to maintain quality of care and physician wellness.[21,22] Several studies have sought to address this question in various ICU settings with inconclusive results.[23–26] Two studies looking at ICUs in the United Kingdom and France showed hospital mortality worsened above a certain threshold of patient beds-to-intensivist ratio.[23,25] Gershengorn and colleagues[23] demonstrated a U-shaped association with hospital mortality when both lower (below 7) and higher (above 12.5) patient-to-intensivist ratios led to higher mortality. This U-shaped relationship implies there is an optimal range for patient-to-intensivist ratio whereby having a patient load too low leads to compromised care due to inexperience and a patient load too high leads to detrimental care due to overwork and ineffectiveness. On the other hand, studies in the United States, Australia, and New Zealand populations did not find an association between patient-to-intensivist ratio with hospital mortality.[24,26] Although hospital mortality did not differ, Dara and Afessa[26] did find ICU length of stay was longer when the ratio was 15 or more.

Multiple studies have investigated various critical care schedules and team models with indeterminate results. There is evidence to support limiting the number of consecutive ICU days (less than 7) worked for an intensivist, leading to shorter patient ICU length of stay without increased ICU readmissions and hospital mortality.[27] In addition, Ali and colleagues[28] demonstrated that weekend cross-coverage for intensivists to reduce the number of weekends worked led to less provider burnout and better job satisfaction without adversely affecting hospital mortality or length of stay. Two studies compared a day/night shift work model with an on-demand staffing model with a daytime intensivist who was available by phone at night and found that the shift work model had lower provider burnout without differences in patient outcomes.[29,30] However, evidence regarding 24-hour intensivist staffing has not yielded a clear consensus on patient outcomes and cost-effectiveness.[31]

Efforts have been made to extend intensivist coverage and offload the ICU work burden with other health care professionals, trainees, and telemedicine. Advanced practice providers (nurse practitioners and physician assistants) are increasingly being integrated into the ICU care team model and have been shown to provide quality care through improved continuity of care, adherence to best practice guidelines, and collaboration in the ICU.[32] Furthermore, the use of residents and fellows can improve intensivist efficiency while providing a rich critical care educational experience. It is important to stress that the education of the trainee should remain a priority, which, at times, can place increased demand on the intensivist. In addition, non–critical care boarded physicians, such as hospitalists, have been safely utilized in the ICU without worsening ICU mortality or ICU length of stay.[33,34] With appropriate competency-based training and close collaboration with consultation services, non–critical care boarded physicians provide considerable value to ICUs in community hospitals and rural settings.

There has been an emerging interest in telemedicine since its origin in 1977.[35] With the ability to provide critical care expertise remotely, telemedicine has the potential to significantly alleviate the ICU workforce burden. However, there are inherent limitations without the physical intensivist presence, and questions persist whether telemedicine is cost-effective in the setting of inconclusive patient outcomes.[36–39] There are more convincing data to support telemedicine in ICU settings with low-intensity daytime intensivist staffing and sicker patients.[40] Unfortunately, studies investigating the effect of telemedicine on intensivist's burnout, quality of life, and job satisfaction are lacking, and this remains an area of significant interest.

Never more evident than in the past two years during the COVID-19 pandemic, the unexpected imbalance in critical care needs and patient volume with available ICU resources further strains the ICU workforce and leads to health care provider burnout.[22,41,42] All these factors must be considered to determine the appropriate staffing model for a particular ICU.

Diversity, Equity, and Inclusion in Critical Care

An important part of improving wellness in health care is to create a genuine sense of belonging and being valued for our unique experiences and skills. The population in the United States has become more ethnically and racially diverse over time, and it is projected that there might be no racial majority group by 2035.[43] This growing diversity, however, is not reflected in the US health care workforce providing care for this population. The lack of diversity can significantly impact culturally mindful delivery of health care.[44]

The Association of American Medical Colleges collects data on diversity, and their report from 2019 shows that women comprise 35.8% of the physician workforce.[45] This representation has increased over time with the greatest increase seen in the less than 34-year age group. Encouragingly, at the undergraduate level, female students have achieved parity with male students.

However, black and Latino physician representation has remained at a standstill; in 2013 it was 4.2% and 4.6%, respectively, and in 2018 it increased to 5% and 5.8%. This finding represents a deficit when compared with these minorities' representation in the general population. These disparities are also seen in anesthesiology and critical care (**Table 2**).

There are significant advantages to tackling issues of inequality. Unconscious bias regarding women, for instance, can be tackled by increasing the visibility and representation of women in leadership. "You can't be what you can't see," a quote attributed to Marian Wright Edelman, holds true to this situation. Increasing representation of underrepresented minorities allows opportunities for inspiration and mentorship for those starting out in their career. A study from the United Kingdom also showed that

Table 2			
Demographic composition of anesthesiology and US physician cohort			
Demographic	Academic Anesthesiology Faculty Cohort	Anesthesiology Resident Cohort	US Physician Cohorts
Women	26%	33%	36%
Black	4.80%	4.97%	5%
Hispanic	5%	5%	5.80%
Native American	0.30%	0.13%	0.30%

Obtained with permission from Nwokolo OO et al.[60]

health care organizations with higher diversity of gender and race in their boards tended to be more innovative and had higher performance levels.[46] A diverse team can lead to fresh perspectives, innovative ideas, increased productivity, and competitive advantage.[46,47] Diverse teams can also lead to greater patient satisfaction, improved access to care for underserved populations, and a more expansive research agenda.[47] A systematic meta-analysis showed patient and provider racial concordance, improved communication, and patient satisfaction.[48]

Women and underrepresented minorities

In 2017, Lane-Fall and colleagues[43] published their work on the emerging demographic trends in Critical Care Fellow recruitment from 2004 to 2017. Their work highlighted the significant increase in female fellows from 29.5% in 2004 to 38.3% 2014 ($P < 0.001$). The number of Hispanic fellows increased from 7.7% in 2005 to 8.4% ($P = 0.015$), whereas the absolute number of black fellows increased, but it was not significant ($P = .92$). The number of American Indian/Alaskan Native/Native Hawaiian/Pacific Islander fellows decreased from 1% to 0.3% ($P < .001$) over the same time.[43] Overall, women and racial/ethnic minorities continue to be underrepresented.

Despite improving recruitment at the undergraduate and medical school levels, women continue to be underrepresented in some specialties, including critical care, and in leadership roles in all specialties. Workforce demographics surveys from the United States, United Kingdom, and Australia show that the proportion of female intensivists is 14% to 26%. The Women in Intensive Care Study, published in 2018, confirmed these data.[49] The study surveyed 84 critical care societies and received responses from 70.1% of their membership, with most information coming from higher-income countries. The study used pooled data to generate an estimate that the proportion of women was about 37% ± 11% (range 26%–50%). The study also shed light on female representation in critical care societies, as presidents or as part of the membership (**Tables 3** and **4**).

Research productivity, funding, and publications are integral to advancement in academic medicine. Women continue to be underrepresented in this area as well; less than one-third of first authors in critical care journals are women, and they count for only one-fourth of senior authors.[50] Miller and colleagues[51] examined the

Table 3
Representation of women in presidential roles of critical care medicine organizations

Society	Number (%) of Female Presidents 2000–2017
ESICM[a]	0/9 (0%)
SCCM (http://www.sccm.org/About-SCCM/Leadership/Past-Presidents)	7/17 (41)%
ANZICS (http://www.anzics.com.au/www.anzics.com.au/about-us.html)	1/9 (11%)
WFSICCM	1/5 (20%)
CICM of Australia and New Zealand[b] (http://www.cicm.org.au/About/Honours-Awards#PastPresidentsandDeans)	0/5 (0%)

Abbreviations: ANZICS, Australia and New Zealand Intensive Care Society; CICM, College of Intensive Care Medicine; SCCM, Society of Critical Care Medicine; WFSICCM, World Federation Society of Intensive and Critical Care Medicine.
[a] Personal correspondence with Prof. Andrew Rhodes, past president of ESICM.
[b] Data for CICM only from 2010, the date of inception of the college.
Obtained with permission from Venkatesh et al.[49]

Table 4			
Academic representation in major scientific meetings: proportion of female faculty			
Meeting	2015 (%)	2016 (%)	2017 (%)
ESICM	15	15	16.9
SCCM[a]	29	30	27
ISICEM	7.5	11.4	7.8
CICM of Australia and New Zealand	7.7	17.2	34

Abbreviations: CICM, College of Intensive Care Medicine; ESICM, European Society of Intensive Care Medicine; ISICEM, International Society of Intensive Care and Emergency Medicine; SCCM, Society of Critical Care Medicine.
[a] SCCM includes a proportion of nonphysician participants.
Obtained with permission from Venkatesh et al.[49]

representation of women in 2 academic anesthesiology journals (Anesthesiology and Anesthesia & Analgesia) over 4 years (2002, 2007, 2012, and 2017) and showed an increase in female first authorship, senior authorship, and editorial board membership by 10%, 9%, and 6%, respectively. Women are also less likely to be on expert panels at conferences or on the editorial boards of journals.

Some of the causes of this disparity have been attributed to women having a higher proportion of family responsibilities compared with male counterparts, women having not been in the system long enough (pipeline theory), or women not being considered natural born leaders.[52] Women frequently suffer from "imposter syndrome" and undervalue their own achievements. Women may not apply for a job if they do not fulfill 100% of the criteria.

The aging workforce

Another area that may be frequently overlooked is the aging critical care workforce. According to the American Medical Association Council, the number of practicing physicians aged greater than 65 years had increased by 374% between 1975 and 2013.[53] Most studies focus on younger trainees or competency assessment related to aging; there is a lack of literature on the impact of burnout on older physicians and successful aging.

How does burnout impact older physicians? What accommodations may be required to assist physicians as we age? How do we assess competency yet maintain dignity? An Australian study assessed the impact of burnout on older physicians (age 61 years or greater) and found less psychological distress, burnout, and suicidal ideation than younger and middle-aged colleagues. Risk for psychological distress was highest for older physicians with a preexisting mental health disorder. Activities that caused the most amount of stress for older physicians were public speaking, working long hours, litigation fears, and having too much to do at work. Older physicians had fewer financial stressors but higher personal stressors (health issues, caregiver role, deaths in the family) compared with their younger colleagues.[54]

Several studies demonstrate the impact of aging as cognitive decline, manifesting as decreased processing speed, limited ability to complete complex tasks, and increased difficulty deciphering irrelevant information among other findings.[53] However, due to a lack of direct correlation with age, variability of results, and concerns regarding age-based discrimination, most societies recommend voluntary physical examination or cognitive testing after 65 to 70 years of age. Another common problem that may affect ICU physicians at one time or another is chronic fatigue from working long hours, especially at night. Some studies suggest that night shifts may have more adverse effects on older physicians.[55] Possible solutions could be an age-based decrease in call responsibility or allowing flexibility for part time work.

Physicians with disabilities

There is also limited data on physicians with disabilities in anesthesia and critical care. Reports suggest that about 2% of currently employed physicians are disabled.[56] A recent survey identified that physicians aged greater than 54.8 years reported more disabilities. Of those with disabilities, 9.2% identified as a racial or ethnic minority, and 14.7% had served on active military duty.[57] Physicians with disabilities may be capable to perform with increased communal support and advice. Progressive technological support and increased acceptance by society may allow physicians to continue their practice and serve as a source of mentorship and inspiration.

Many challenges lie ahead of our specialty. The Great Resignation[58,59] in health care that has led to the departure of many colleagues en masse as well as the lack of diversity and inclusivity represent 2 areas of primary concern. It is of vital importance that the workplace amplifies voices and highlights leadership roles of underrepresented minorities and creates a genuine sense of belonging and respect. As we face a world where the effects of COVID-19 have forever changed the landscape, changes at the institutional level are needed. Creating diversity among work groups, ensuring gender/racial balance in committees or conference invites, actively recruiting women and people of color for leadership roles, and providing flexible work schedules for both men and women to allow optimal balance of professional versus personal life are plausible starting points. In addition, burnout mitigation efforts need to start from the top down. The systems needs to support the workforce, and the workforce should not be crushed under the weight of a broken system. The goal should be to foster a healthy workforce that engenders a sense of value for unique abilities and experiences, provides equal opportunities to attain promotion and recognition, and ultimately retains our talented workforce for a long time.

CLINICS CARE POINTS

- Exhaustion, depersonalizaion and reduced personal accomplisment are three classic symptoms of burn out syndrome.
- Depression, anxiety and feelings of burnout are highly prevalent in critical care physicians.
- Women and racial or ethnic minorities continue to be underrepresented in critical care medicine.

REFERENCES

1. Siddiqui S, Tung A, Kelly L, et al. Anxiety, worry, and job satisfaction: effects of COVID-19 care on critical care anesthesiologists. Can J Anaesth 2022;69(4):552–4.
2. Moll V, Meissen H, Pappas S, et al. The coronavirus disease 2019 pandemic impacts burnout syndrome differently among multiprofessional critical care clinicians-a longitudinal survey study. Crit Care Med 2022;50(3):440–8.
3. Sinsky CA, Brown RL, Stillman MJ, et al. COVID-related stress and work intentions in a sample of us health care workers. Mayo Clin Proc Innov Qual Outcomes 2021;5(6):1165–73.
4. Khanna AK, Majesko A, Johansson M, et al. The multidisciplinary critical care workforce: an update from SCCM. Soceity of critical care medicine. Critical connections

Web site. 2022. Available at: https://www.sccm.org/Communications/Critical-Connections/Archives/2019/The-Multidisciplinary-Critical-Care-Workforce-An. Accessed May 8, 2022.

5. Hussain RS, Kataria TC. Adequacy of workforce - are there enough critical care doctors in the US-post COVID? Curr Opin Anaesthesiol 2021;34(2):149–53.

6. Moss M, Good VS, Gozal D, et al. An official critical care societies collaborative statement: burnout syndrome in critical care healthcare professionals: a call for action. Crit Care Med 2016;44(7):1414–21.

7. Pastores SM. Burnout syndrome in ICU caregivers: time to extinguish. Chest 2016;150(1):1–2.

8. Siddiqui S, Bartels K, Schaefer MS, et al. Critical care medicine practice: a pilot survey of US anesthesia critical care medicine-trained physicians. Anesth Analg 2021;132(3):761–9.

9. Pai Cole S. Burnout prevention and resilience training for critical care trainees. Int Anesthesiol Clin 2019;57(2):118–31.

10. Lilly CM, Cucchi E, Marshall N, et al. Battling intensivist burnout: a role for workload management. Chest 2019;156(5):1001–7.

11. Sessler CN. Intensivist burnout: running on empty? Chest 2019;156(5):817–9.

12. Pastores SM, Kvetan V, Coopersmith CM, et al. Workforce, workload, and burnout among intensivists and advanced practice providers: a narrative review. Crit Care Med 2019;47(4):550–7.

13. Kleinpell R, Moss M, Good VS, et al. The critical nature of addressing burnout prevention: results from the critical care societies collaborative's national summit and survey on prevention and management of burnout in the ICU. Crit Care Med 2020;48(2):249–53.

14. Kok N, van Gurp J, Teerenstra S, et al. Coronavirus disease 2019 immediately increases burnout symptoms in ICU professionals: a longitudinal cohort study. Crit Care Med 2021;49(3):419–27.

15. Arnold-Forster A, Moses JD, Schotland SV. Obstacles to physicians' emotional health - lessons from history. N Engl J Med 2022;386(1):4–7.

16. Maslach C, Leiter M. The truth about burnout: how organizations cause personal stress and what to do about it. San Francisco, CA: Jossey-Bass; 1997.

17. Moss M, Good VS, Gozal D, et al. A critical care societies collaborative statement: burnout syndrome in critical care health-care professionals. A call for action. Am J Respir Crit Care Med 2016;194(1):106–13.

18. Azoulay E, De Waele J, Ferrer R, et al. Symptoms of burnout in intensive care unit specialists facing the COVID-19 outbreak. Ann Intensive Care 2020;10(1):110.

19. Brooks M. COVID continues to take a toll on neurologists' well-being. WebMD LLC. Medscape Medical News Web site. https://www.medscape.com/viewarticle/968874. Accessed April 2022.

20. Physician Burnout & Depression Report 2022: Stress, Anxiety, and Anger. WebMD LLC. https://www.medscape.com/slideshow/2022-lifestyle-burnout-6014664. Accessed April 2022.

21. Kelley MA, Angus D, Chalfin DB, et al. The critical care crisis in the United States: a report from the profession. Chest 2004;125(4):1514–7.

22. Kerlin MP, Silvestri JA, Klaiman T, et al. Critical Care Clinician Wellness during the COVID-19 Pandemic: A Longitudinal Analysis. Ann Am Thorac Soc 2022;19(2):329–31.

23. Gershengorn HB, Harrison DA, Garland A, et al. Association of intensive care unit patient-to-intensivist ratios with hospital mortality. JAMA Intern Med 2017;177(3):388–96.

24. Gershengorn HB, Pilcher DV, Litton E, et al. Association of patient-to-intensivist ratio with hospital mortality in Australia and New Zealand. Intensive Care Med 2022;48(2):179–89.
25. Neuraz A, Guerin C, Payet C, et al. Patient mortality is associated with staff resources and workload in the ICU: a multicenter observational study. Crit Care Med 2015;43(8):1587–94.
26. Dara SI, Afessa B. Intensivist-to-bed ratio: association with outcomes in the medical ICU. Chest 2005;128(2):567–72.
27. Gershengorn HB, Pilcher DV, Litton E, et al. Association between consecutive days worked by intensivists and outcomes for critically ill patients. Crit Care Med 2020;48(4):594–8.
28. Ali NA, Hammersley J, Hoffmann SP, et al. Continuity of care in intensive care units: a cluster-randomized trial of intensivist staffing. Am J Respir Crit Care Med 2011;184(7):803–8.
29. Gajic O, Afessa B, Hanson AC, et al. Effect of 24-hour mandatory versus on-demand critical care specialist presence on quality of care and family and provider satisfaction in the intensive care unit of a teaching hospital. Crit Care Med 2008;36(1):36–44.
30. Garland A, Roberts D, Graff L. Twenty-four-hour intensivist presence: a pilot study of effects on intensive care unit patients, families, doctors, and nurses. Am J Respir Crit Care Med 2012;185(7):738–43.
31. Nizamuddin J, Tung A. Intensivist staffing and outcome in the ICU: daytime, nighttime, 24/7? Curr Opin Anaesthesiol 2019;32(2):123–8.
32. Kleinpell RM, Ely EW, Grabenkort R. Nurse practitioners and physician assistants in the intensive care unit: an evidence-based review. Crit Care Med 2008;36(10):2888–97.
33. Wise KR, Akopov VA, Williams BR Jr, et al. Hospitalists and intensivists in the medical ICU: a prospective observational study comparing mortality and length of stay between two staffing models. J Hosp Med 2012;7(3):183–9.
34. Tenner PA, Dibrell H, Taylor RP. Improved survival with hospitalists in a pediatric intensive care unit. Crit Care Med 2003;31(3):847–52.
35. Fuhrman SA, Lilly CM. ICU telemedicine solutions. Clin Chest Med 2015;36(3):401–7.
36. Chen J, Sun D, Yang W, et al. Clinical and economic outcomes of telemedicine programs in the intensive care unit: a systematic review and meta-analysis. J Intensive Care Med 2018;33(7):383–93.
37. Thomas EJ, Lucke JF, Wueste L, et al. Association of telemedicine for remote monitoring of intensive care patients with mortality, complications, and length of stay. JAMA 2009;302(24):2671–8.
38. Collins TA, Robertson MP, Sicoutris CP, et al. Telemedicine coverage for postoperative ICU patients. J Telemed Telecare 2017;23(2):360–4.
39. Udeh C, Perez-Protto S, Canfield CM, et al. Outcomes associated with ICU telemedicine and other risk factors in a multi-hospital critical care system: a retrospective, cohort study for 30-day in-hospital mortality. Telemed J E Health 2022;28(10):1395–403.
40. Venkataraman R, Ramakrishnan N. Outcomes related to telemedicine in the intensive care unit: what we know and would like to know. Crit Care Clin 2015;31(2):225–37.
41. Opgenorth D, Stelfox HT, Gilfoyle E, et al. Perspectives on strained intensive care unit capacity: a survey of critical care professionals. PLoS One 2018;13(8):e0201524.

42. Kok N, Hoedemaekers A, van der Hoeven H, et al. Recognizing and supporting morally injured ICU professionals during the COVID-19 pandemic. Intensive Care Med 2020;46(8):1653–4.

43. Lane-Fall MB, Miano TA, Aysola J, et al. Diversity in the emerging critical care workforce: analysis of demographic trends in critical care fellows from 2004 to 2014. Crit Care Med 2017;45(5):822–7.

44. Takeshita J, Wang S, Loren AW, et al. Association of racial/ethnic and gender concordance between patients and physicians with patient experience ratings. JAMA Netw Open 2020;3(11):e2024583.

45. Diversity in medicine: facts and figures. 2019. Available at: https://www.aamc.org/data-reports/workforce/report/diversity-medicine-facts-and-figures-2019. Accessed April 6, 2022.

46. Patel R, Moonesinghe SR. A seat at the table is no longer enough: practical implementable changes to address gender imbalance in the anaesthesia workplace. Br J Anaesth 2020;124(3):e49–52.

47. Estime SR, Lee HH, Jimenez N, et al. Diversity, equity, and inclusion in anesthesiology. Int Anesthesiol Clin 2021;59(4):81–5.

48. Shen MJ, Peterson EB, Costas-Muniz R, et al. The effects of race and racial concordance on patient-physician communication: a systematic review of the literature. J Racial Ethn Health Disparities 2018;5(1):117–40.

49. Venkatesh B, Mehta S, Angus DC, et al. Women in Intensive Care study: a preliminary assessment of international data on female representation in the ICU physician workforce, leadership and academic positions. Crit Care 2018; 22(1):211.

50. Vincent JL, Juffermans NP, Burns KEA, et al. Addressing gender imbalance in intensive care. Crit Care 2021;25(1):147.

51. Miller J, Chuba E, Deiner S, et al. Trends in authorship in anesthesiology journals. Anesth Analg 2019;129(1):306–10.

52. Sreedharan R, Perez-Protto S. Women in critical care medicine. Crit Care Connections 2017. Accessed April 8, 2022.

53. Dellinger EP, Pellegrini CA, Gallagher TH. The aging physician and the medical profession: a review. JAMA Surg 2017;152(10):967–71.

54. Wijeratne C, Johnco C, Draper B, et al. Older physicians' reporting of psychological distress, alcohol use, burnout and workplace stressors. Am J Geriatr Psychiatry 2021;29(5):478–87.

55. Maltese F, Adda M, Bablon A, et al. Night shift decreases cognitive performance of ICU physicians. Intensive Care Med 2016;42(3):393–400.

56. LA D, del Carmen Forrest M. A diverse perioperative physician workforce includes those with disabilities. ASA Monitor 2019;83:20–2.

57. Nouri Z, Dill MJ, Conrad SS, et al. Estimated prevalence of US physicians with disabilities. JAMA Netw Open 2021;4(3):e211254.

58. Cook I. Who is driving the great resignation. Harv Business Rev 2021. Available at: https://hbr.org/2021/09/who-is-driving-the-great-resignation. Accessed August 8, 2022.

59. Gordon D. Amid healthcare's great resignation, burned out workers are pursuing flexibility and passion. Forbes; 2022. Available at: https://www.forbes.com/sites/debgordon/2022/05/17/amid-healthcares-great-resignation-burned-out-workers-are-pursuing-flexibility-and-passion/?sh=13248eb57fda. Accessed August 8, 2022.

60. Nwokolo OO, Coombs AAT, Eltzschig HK. Butterworth JFt. Diversity and Inclusion in Anesthesiology. Anesth Analg 2022;134(6):1166–74.

Moving?

Make sure your subscription moves with you!

To notify us of your new address, find your **Clinics Account Number** (located on your mailing label above your name), and contact customer service at:

Email: journalscustomerservice-usa@elsevier.com

800-654-2452 (subscribers in the U.S. & Canada)
314-447-8871 (subscribers outside of the U.S. & Canada)

Fax number: 314-447-8029

Elsevier Health Sciences Division
Subscription Customer Service
3251 Riverport Lane
Maryland Heights, MO 63043

*To ensure uninterrupted delivery of your subscription, please notify us at least 4 weeks in advance of move.

Printed and bound by CPI Group (UK) Ltd, Croydon, CR0 4YY

08/05/2025

01864720-0001